CHALLENGES IN
Prostate Cancer

CHALLENGES IN

Prostate Cancer

EDITED BY

Winsor Bowsher

St Joseph's Hospital
Newport
South Wales
UK

and

Adam Carter

Royal Gwent Hospital
Newport
South Wales
UK

SECOND EDITION

Blackwell
Publishing

Blackwell Publishing, Inc., 350 Main Street, Malden, Massachusetts 02148-5020, USA
Blackwell Publishing Ltd, 9600 Garsington Road, Oxford OX4 2DQ, UK
Blackwell Publishing Asia Pty Ltd, 550 Swanston Street, Carlton, Victoria 3053, Australia

First published 2000
Second edition 2006

Library of Congress Cataloging-in-Publication Data

Challenges in prostate cancer / edited by Winsor Bowsher and
   Adam Carter. – 2nd ed.
     p. ; cm.
   Includes bibliographical references and index.
   ISBN-13: 978-1-4051-0752-5
   ISBN-10: 1-4051-0752-9
   1. Prostate Cancer. I. Bowsher Winsor. II. Carter, Adam, Dr.
   [DNLM: 1. Prostatic Neoplasms. WJ 752 C48 2006]
RC280.P7C48 2006
616.99'463–dc22

2005031967

ISBN-13: 978-1-4051-0752-5
ISBN-10: 1-4051-0752-9

A catalogue record for this title is available from the British Library

Set in 10/13.5 pt Sabon by Newgen Imaging Systems (P) Ltd, Chennai, India
Printed and bound in Singapore by Fabulous Printers Pte Ltd

Commissioning Editor: Stuart Taylor
Editorial Assistant: Saskia Van der Linden
Development Editor: Rob Blundell
Production Controller: Kate Charman

For further information on Blackwell Publishing, visit our website:
http://www.blackwellpublishing.com

Dedication

The shock of Winsor Bowsher's sudden and unexpected death, from a coronary thrombosis in May 2004, was felt at all levels of the local community in and about Newport. The enormous respect and affection felt for him was evident from the huge congregation that overflowed the lovely church of St Mary in Usk at his funeral on 20th May.

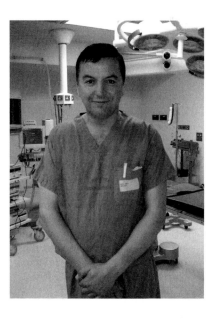

In 1993, Winsor joined the consultant staff of the Royal Gwent Hospital with a formidable reputation. Previously, he had won a string of prestigious awards, such as the ICRF Research Fellowship, two awards from the Royal College of Surgeons, and two Travelling Fellowships in 1990, that enabled him to further his training in Australia while senior registrar with Professor John Blandy at The Royal London Hospital. This took him to St Vincent's Hospital, Melbourne for 18 months, as Senior Registrar and Visiting Fellow, and it must be a measure of their high regard for him, that he was appointed Staff Consultant. It was at St Vincent's that he learned the skills of radical prostatectomy and laparoscopic nephrectomy.

Wales was not a strange country to Winsor, for his SHO and registrar posts had been at Cardiff, prior to posts at The Institute of Urology and St Bartholemew's. Therefore, when he arrived in Newport, he had an extensive clinical background, and brought to us new dimensions of urological care; in particular, his mastery of radical prostatectomy for early prostate cancer and his experience with laparoscopic nephrectomy for kidney cancer, which he set up in Newport, were firsts in Wales.

He soon became deeply committed to post-graduate training, with courses to teach laparoscopic techniques for urologists, training days for consultants, and especially courses for urological nurses to learn about endoscopic equipment and methods.

Winsor was a very bright person. His research and clinical studies led to 63 publications in peer urological journals, chapters in several books on prostate cancer, and in 1999, he was asked by Blackwell Science to compile a review volume entitled 'Challenges in Prostate Cancer' published in 2000. This volume is successor to that book and was half completed when he died; we are grateful to his colleague, Adam Carter, for completing the task.

Winsor's precise analytical mind sometimes made others feel uncomfortable, for he did not beat about the bush with trivialities and irrelevancies. This was reflected in his lecturing style: he was a stimulating communicator, making about 80 learned presentations, 41 as a consultant. He made several videos of urological techniques, and was Medical Advisor to BBC2 for a series called 'The Male Survival Guide', which won 6 BMA Gold Awards, along with Awards in Canada and from the Royal Television Society.

I was not surprised, therefore, at his appointment to the Editorial Committee of The British Journal of Urology, and as Deputy Editor of the Update Series of The European Board of Urology.

Had fate given him a chance, Winsor would have scaled the heights of achievement for his dedication, determination, and an exceptional intelligence that is given to few. He was a fine surgeon whose dexterity and attention to detail put him in the top bracket and which I admired greatly.

The true worth of a man such as Winsor Bowsher is not measured solely against the judgements of his colleagues and peers. It is really measured by the respect, affection and regard of his juniors, his staff and above all by his patients and their families. This was present in abundance.

As a colleague, I will remember Winsor as a fine urologist who contributed more in his shortened career than most achieve in a whole professional lifespan.

However, to those of us who were his friends, Winsor will be missed for the enthusiasm for everything that he did, for his wide interests in music and art, for his outdoor activities with fishing and mountaineering (he had walked up Mont Blanc two weeks before he died), for his excitement at rugby internationals with his son, but especially for his company.

Brian Peeling
Newport, December 2005

Contents

List of contributors, x

....

Part 3: Initial Treatment Policies

Part 4: Monitoring Progress and Secondary Treatment

Colour plates appear after p. 84

Preface

Prostate cancer continues to be one of surgery's most enigmatic tumours, which is why it is so fascinating. Slowly but surely the wall of mystery surrounding many aspects of the disease is being chipped away. It is timely that a new addition of Challenges in Prostate Cancer is written, building on and developing from the First Edition published in 2000.

The former edition was so successfully edited by Winsor Bowsher. It was his wish and intention to oversee a completely re-written summary of up-to-date current opinion. This was to cover challenging aspects prostate cancer using a completely new set of authors. His efforts however were cut short by his untimely death. Using his book plan I have completed the work Winsor initially started. It draws together many strands of the prostate cancer puzzle summarised in chapters written by prostate cancer experts and enthusiasts.

A collection of chapters is presented, written by independent authors, which address many of the most interesting aspects of the disease in an accessible and readable way. Topics range from the changes in prostate cancer epidemiology, biochemical investigation, operative and non-operative treatment of localised disease, salvage for failed local treatment and chemotherapy for advanced disease. I believe the result is a volume of work which Winsor would have been proud and that you will enjoy reading. I wish to thank the authors for all of their efforts and Blackwell Publishing for their continuing support.

Adam Carter
Newport, December 2005

List of Contributors

EDITORS

Winsor Bowsher (deceased), *St Joseph's Hospital, Newport, South Wales, UK*

Adam Carter, *Department of Urology, Royal Gwent Hospital, Cardiff Road, Newport, NP20 2UB, UK*

CONTRIBUTORS

Christopher Bangma, Professor of Urology and Head of Department, Department of Urology, Erasmus Medical Centre, Rotterdam, The Netherlands

Ludger Barthelmes, Specialist Registrar, Department of General Surgery, Morriston Hospital, Swansea, UK

Gail Beese, Department of Urology, Royal Gwent Hospital, Cardiff Road, Newport, UK

Michael Blute, Consultant and Professor of Urology, Department of Urology, Mayo Clinic College of Medicine, Rochester, MN, USA

Bernhard Brehmer, Consultant of Urology, Clinic of Urology, University Hospital Aachen, Germany

Barrie Cassileth, Laurance S. Rockefeller Chair in Integrative Medicine and Chief, Integrative Medicine Service, Memorial Sloan-Kettering Cancer Center, New York, USA

Richard Clements, Consultant Radiologist, Department of Radiology, Royal Gwent Hospital, Newport, UK

Stijn de Vries, Urology Resident in Training, Department of Urology, Erasmus Medical Centre, Rotterdam, The Netherlands

Gary Deng, Assistant Attending, Assistant Member, Integrative Medicine Service, Memorial Sloan-Kettering Cancer Center, New York, USA

Bob Djavan, Professor of Urology, Vice Chairman, Department of Urology, Director Prostate Disease Center and Co-Director Ludwig Boltzman Institute for Prostatic Disease, Department of Urology, University of Vienna, Austria

Michael Dobrovits, Resident of Urology, Department of Urology, University of Vienna, Austria

Christopher Edmunds, Nsf Information Co-ordinator, Welsh Assembly for Wales, Cardiff, UK

Neil Fenn, Consultant Urologist, Department of Urology, Morriston Hospital, Morriston, Swansea, UK

Christopher Gateley, Consultant General and Breast Surgeon, Royal Gwent Hospital, Newport, UK

Anuj Goyal, Research Registrar in Urology, Department of Urology, Southampton Hospitals NHS Trust, UK

David Griffiths, Senior Lecturer in Pathology, Honorary Consultant Histopathologist, Department of Pathology, University of Wales College of Medicine, University Hospital of Wales, Cardiff, UK

Simon Hayward, Assistant Professor of Urologic Surgery and Cancer Biology, Department of Urologic Surgery, Vanderbilt University Medical Center, Nashville, TN, USA

Emma Hudson, Velindre Hospital, Whitchurch, Cardiff, UK

Owen Hughes, Consultant Urological Surgeon, SpR in Urology, Department of Urology, University Hospital of Wales, Cardiff, UK

Rhidian Hurle, Specialist Registrar in Urology, University Hospital of Wales, Cardiff, UK

Kenichiro Ishii, Department of Urologic Surgery, Vanderbilt University Medical Center, Nashville, TN, USA

Gerhard Jakse, Clinic of Urology, University Clinic Aachen, Germany

Paul Jones, Specialist Registrar, Department of Urology, Royal Gwent Hospital, Newport, UK

Amir Kaisary, Lead Clinician in Urological Cancer, Consultant Urological Surgeon and Honorary Senior Lecturer, The Royal Free Hospital NHS Trust, The Royal Free and University College London Medical School, London, UK

Jamie Kearsley, Urology Fellow, Department of Surgery, St Vincent's Hospital, East Melbourne, Australia

Tim Lane, Lecturer in Urological Oncology and Specialist Registrar in Urology, Department of Medical Oncology, St Bartholomew's Hospital, London, UK

Jason Lester, Consultant Clinical Oncologist, Velindre Hospital, Cardiff, UK

Antonios Makris, Clinic of Urology, University Clinic Aachen, Germany

Michael Marberger, Department of Urology, University of Vienna, Austria

Malcolm Mason, Professor of Clinical Oncology, Department of Oncology and Palliative Medicine, Cardiff University, Velindre Hospital, Cardiff, UK

Leslie Moffat, Chairman of Scottish Urological Audit Group (SUCA), Senior Lecturer, Consultant Urologist, Aberdeen Royal Infirmary, Aberdeen, UK

Robert Myers, Consultant and Professor of Urology, Mayo Clinic College of Medicine, Rochester, MN, USA

Owen Niall, Consultant Urologist, St Vincent's Hospital, East Melbourne, Australia

R. Timothy Oliver, Sir Maxwell Joseph Professor of Medical Oncology, Department of Medical Oncology, St Bartholomew's Hospital, London, UK

Steven Oliver, Senior Lecturer in Population Studies, Department of Health Studies, University of York, UK

Stephen Schatz, Senior Resident in Urology, Mayo School of Graduate Medical Education, Mayo Clinic College of Medicine, Rochester, MN, USA

Fritz Schröder, Professor of Urology, Department of Urology, Erasmus Medical Centre, Rotterdam, The Netherlands

John Staffurth, Velindre Hospital, Cardiff, UK

Jon Strefford, Lecturer in Medical Oncology, The Orchid Cancer Appeal, Department of Medical Oncology, St Bartholomew's Hospital, London, UK

R. Houston Thompson, Senior Resident in Urology, Mayo School of Graduate Medical Education, Mayo Clinic College of Medicine, Rochester, MN, USA

Murali Varma, Consultant Histopathologist, Department of Histopathology, University Hospital of Wales, Cardiff, UK

Mark Wright, Consultant Urological Surgeon, Bristol Royal Infirmary, Bristol, UK

Part 1: Biological and Scientific Aspects

1: An Update on Biotechnology in the Assessment of Prostate Cancer

Tim Lane, Jon Strefford and Tim Oliver

INTRODUCTION

Prostate cancer represents the second most common cancer in men (after lung cancer) in both the United Kingdom and the European Union and is the most common cancer in men in the United States. With over 20 000 new cases diagnosed in the United Kingdom every year (and 134 000 in Europe as a whole), the disease has a significant impact on the health of the nation. It is a large and growing problem, with the annual cost of treating prostate cancer in England and Wales alone likely to exceed €100 million [1].

Prostate cancers however differ widely in their aggressiveness and as a result their relative prognoses vary accordingly. Efforts aimed at understanding the underlying pathogenesis of the disease process serve to highlight both new and improved biological markers of disease initiation and progression, which may be of diagnostic or prognostic significance. In recent years, there has been a proliferation of innovative techniques that have served to probe malignant prostate growth at both the genomic and proteomic levels. Such advances, the majority of which have been pioneered by workers in the biotechnology industry, have resulted in both highly unique and specific tools for investigating the changes paralleling tumourigenesis. The techniques involved have inevitably become automated and advanced by improvements in microtechnology, which has further facilitated the rapid throughput of high-quality research data.

In this opening chapter, we seek to describe a variety of innovative tools alongside the improved understanding of prostate tumour biology, which have been accrued as a result.

PROSTATE CANCER GENOMICS

In the vast majority of prostate cancers, there are no inherited defects affecting high-penetrance susceptibility genes and malignant transformation results instead from a series of acquired somatic changes affecting many genes on several chromosomes. Understanding the genetic changes involved in the development of prostate cancer is pivotal to a rational approach to both diagnosis and therapeutic intervention. It has been estimated that anywhere between 5 and 10 genes are deleted [putative tumour-suppressor genes (TSG)] before malignant transformation occurs and that a further series of gains (amplification of oncogenes) arise with the advent of metastases [2]. A number of techniques have been used to investigate these changes. While classical cytogenetics and loss of heterozygosity (LOH) studies have been the mainstay for investigators for the last few decades, these techniques have been increasingly superseded by a number of alternative strategies.

Fluorescent *In Situ* Hybridisation

Fluorescent *in situ* hybridisation (FISH) represents an established and widely used tool in the investigation of both DNA and RNA targets. Its use has become synonymous with the hybridisation of DNA probes to specific chromosomal regions and in the investigation of tumour genomes (Plate 1). It allows for a more comprehensive surveillance of chromosomal aberrations and with a higher degree of accuracy than standard GTG-banding techniques (which might otherwise be sufficient for constitutional applications). Such DNA *in situ* hybridisation has had a pivotal role in the elucidation of patterns of deletion and amplifications in tumour. It has been employed as a useful method in the detection of gene and chromosome anomalies in cell lines, touch preparations from fresh tissue, isolated nuclei from formalin-fixed paraffin-embedded tissue and routine histologic sections from paraffin blocks [3].

Given existing cytogenetic evidence indicating that the gain of chromosome 7 was associated with higher tumour grade, Jenkins *et al.* (1998) utilised FISH probes to investigate prostate specimens using a chromosome 7 centromere and five loci mapped to 7q31 [4]. In their study, they noted that gain of 7q31 was strongly associated with tumour Gleeson score. It was noted that the DNA probe for D7S522 spanned the common fragile site FRA7G at the 7q31 position and the authors postulated that the instability in this fragile site could explain both loss and gain of this region as noted by a number of authors. Bostwick *et al.* likewise investigated allelic imbalance at 7q31 and noted that its imbalance was greater in prostate cancer foci than in prostatic intraepithelial neoplasia (PIN) suggesting a role in the progression of precursor lesions to carcinoma [5].

The 8p22 region has also been implicated in prostate tumourigenesis by FISH analysis and widely examined by a number of authors. For example, Emmert-Buck found loss of 8p12-21 in 63% of PIN and 91% of cancer foci – work independently supported by Bostwick [6]. Given the number of authors highlighting regions of loss on the 8 *p-arm*, it is likely there are a number of putative tumour-suppressor genes located therein, one of which is likely to be the leucine zipper protein, FEZ1 and another the lipoprotein lipase gene (*LPL*) at the 8p22 position. In addition to losses on the 8 *p-arm*, a number of gains on the 8 *q-arm* have also been reported using FISH-based methodologies. Qian *et al.* [7] initially observed that gain of chromosome 8 was the most frequent chromosomal anomaly in metastatic foci and that the frequency was much higher in PIN and in carcinoma. Subsequent to this Jenkins *et al.* implicated the *c-myc* gene (8 *q-arm*) in 22% of meta-static foci which appeared at a higher frequency in these when compared to their primary (9%) counterparts [8]. It appears that an increase in copy number of the *c-myc* gene is associated with both systemic progression and early death of the patient. In this respect, it has been hypothesised that an over-expression of *c-myc* causes the breakdown of p27*kip*1 and a resulting activation of cyclin-dependent kinase 2 and cell proliferation. Of greater interest, however, was the demonstration that those with co-existent loss of 8p22 and gain of *c-myc* had the poorest outcomes overall [9].

Comparative Genomic Hybridisation

In contradistinction to FISH-based methodologies, comparative genomic hybridisation (CGH) represents a powerful molecular cytogenetic technique, which utilises tumour DNA to provide a genome-wide screen for sequence copy number aberrations in a single hybridisation reaction; a marked con-trast to the single locus specific probes employed in classical FISH procedures (Plate 2). With tumour and reference DNA labelled differentially (with con-trasting fluorophores), samples are mixed and co-hybridised onto normal metaphase chromosomes. By quantifying the hybridisation intensity vari-ations between test and reference DNA samples, relative gains and losses of chromosomal regions can be assessed. Arguably, its principle advantage is that all chromosome regions can be screened for gains and losses simultan-eously, giving an unparalleled data mining tool. Visakorpi and others have used this technique to examine in great detail the changes involved in pro-state cancer initiation and progression [10]. Indeed, changes at the genomic level (in terms of sequence copy number changes) appear to affect some 74% of primary prostate cancers. The fact that regions of loss are almost five times as common as regions of gain in early disease, is taken by many to suggest the importance of TSG loss in the initiation of tumourigenesis. The regions of loss identified include 6q, 8p, 9p, 13q, 16q and 18q – regions of LOH also implicated in FISH-based studies. The application of CGH has addi-tionally been employed to assess the progressive changes involved with the transition from benign disease, through high-grade prostatic intraepithelial neoplasia (HGPIN), to localised and eventually metastatic hormone resistant prostate cancer. At the most basic level it appears clear, for example, that genetic aberrations in recurrent tumours are three times higher than in primary tumours, with the number of regions noted as gained almost five times greater than their primary counterparts. Of particular importance in relation to disease progression, however, appears to be the association of 5q loss and gains in 7p, 8q and Xq, in the progression to hormone resistant disease. The candidate genes involved in these regions are keenly sought. Unfortunately however, CGH, with its relatively low resolution (the method can only detect deletions greater than 10 Mb in size) does not allow for any degree of useful specificity – a deficiency that CGH-based microarrays have been able to address directly.

Genomic Microarrays

While chromosome-based CGH (with its whole-genome screening capability) is significantly faster and less laborious than methods examining for single-target dosage changes (Southern blotting, PCR and FISH), there are technical aspects that have limited its usefulness. Principle amongst these is its resolution. Because DNA within chromosomes is tightly coiled and condensed, a 10 Mb span is required to detect a deletion and a 2 Mb length to detect gains – both in part dependent on amplicon size. While providing a starting point for positional cloning studies, the regions contain far too many genes to localise sequences of interest. Another principle limitation is the need to identify individual chromosomes – something even experienced cytogeneticists may find difficult from the inverted DAPI images available. As a result of these difficulties (and with the recent advances in microarray technology), CGH-based microarrays have been developed, which use genomic DNA sequences as targets (Plate 3). DNA targets for these microarrays can be derived from yeast artificial chromosomes (YAC, 2 Mb), bacterial artificial chromosomes (BAC, 300 Kb) and cosmids (45 Kb) all of which are several magnitudes of size smaller than chromosome targets in conventional CGH. As such, they provide for an increase in resolution of copy number over traditional CGH.

We have used commercially available (Vysis) CGH-based microarrays to explore loss of TSG in early stage prostate cancer and the variable gain in copy number of a wide variety of putative oncogenes in the progression to hormone resistant disease. Using prostate cancer cell lines, fresh frozen tissue and tumour material isolated by laser capture microscopy (LCM) from formalin-fixed paraffin-embedded tissue, we have identified a number of common regions of loss and gain in disease initiation and progression.

Using a series of 50 microdissected tumour specimens, we have identified a series of 60 regions that are consistently either amplified or deleted and known to harbour candidate genes. This minimum dataset appears to represent the beginnings of a genomic fingerprint, the significance of which has yet to be fully appreciated. It seems likely however that loss and gain of genomic material in pre-cancerous or early stage disease will identify putative TSGs in disease initiation, while the gain of additional material with progression to the androgen-resistant state will define novel targets for therapeutic intervention [11].

Multiplex FISH and Spectral Karyotyping

While relative loss and gain of genomic material can be assessed by FISH and CGH, it is clear that such approaches cannot reflect the complexity of chromosomal abnormalities in prostate cancer in their entirety. Of particular interest in this respect, is the growing realisation that chromosomal translocations may harbour influential fusion genes that have a significant impact on disease initiation and progression. This has most clearly been demonstrated in the field of haematological malignancy in which a translocation involving chromosomes 9 and 22 brings the *Abl* gene onto chromosome 22. As a result, the Philadelphia chromosome is formed and represents a derivative chromosome 22 : t (9;22). As a result, a fusion protein (termed Bcr-Abl) is formed, a product of chimeric mRNA arising as a consequence of the translocation. This Bcr-Abl product, functions as a constitutively activated tyrosine kinase, which is essential for the transforming function of the protein and plays a pivotal role in chronic myeloid leukaemia (CML). Following a high-throughput screen of chemical libraries searching for compounds with kinase inhibitory activity, a series of compounds originally optimised against the platelet derived growth factor (PDGF) receptor was shown to have equipotent activity against the *Abl* tyrosine kinase. ST1571 or Gleevec is the therapeutic agent that has resulted. Its rapid clinical success in the treatment of CML has already rendered existing treatment algorithms obsolete overnight [12].

Assessing such complex chromosomal translocations in solid tissue malignancies has traditionally been limited, both because of the restrictions imposed by traditional cytogenetics and the difficulties involved in establishing primary prostatic cultures. However, recently developed molecular cytogenetic techniques in the form of spectral karyotyping (SKY) and multiplex FISH (M-FISH) have greatly facilitated these processes. M-FISH is a combinatorial technique that allows the identification of human chromosomes by painting them with a spectrum of DNA probes labelled with a unique combination of five fluorochromes, such that individual human chromo-somes can be identified in 24 discrete pseudo-colours (Plate 4). The SKY methodology represents an essentially similar technique but in the latter case, instead of relying on a series of multiple excitation and emission filters, it relies on Fourier spectroscopy to identify individual chromosomes.

Pan *et al.* [13] were among the first to characterise chromosomal abnor-malities in prostate cancer cell lines using SKY. In doing so, a number of novel chromosomal abnormalities were identified, which had remained pre-viously unidentified by conventional cytogenetics – suitably demonstrating the increased sensitivity of the technique. Subsequent to this, Strefford *et al.* [14] reported M-FISH data on a similar group of commercially available malignant prostate cell lines and drew comparisons between those features identified in both SKY and M-FISH studies. One such chromosomal aberra-tion that was identified as common to a number of studies was a reciprocal translocation involving chromosomes 1 and 15. Given the relative rarity of such translocations (especially ones that are recurrent) they postulated a potentially significant role for it in either the initiation or progression of the disease.

This work on M-FISH has recently been extended from work on pro-state cancer lines to the analysis of primary cultures. Using a low calcium serum-free medium (PrEGM), we have established a number of malignant primary cell cultures from tissue harvested fresh from radical prostatectomy specimens. [15]. Though generally less complex in terms of karyotype than their immortalised cell counterparts, a number of novel chromosomal trans-locations have nevertheless been identified, some of which have also been previously identified in cell lines [16].

Some of the translocations identified by a variety of these authors appear common to a number of cell lines and cell cultures. In doing so, it raises the intriguing possibility that one or more breakpoint translocations may be giv-ing rise to common fusion proteins involved in the initiation or progression of the disease. As such, it is possible that novel therapeutic interventions in the form of new drug treatments could herald innovative treatments in much the same way as ST1571 has revolutionised the management of haematological malignancies.

EPIGENETIC CHANGES IN PROSTATE CANCER

While the direct loss of a gene can have a fairly obvious effect on the func-tional phenotype of a cell, changes relating to promoter hypermethylation have been shown to represent an alternative to Knudson's 'two hit' hypo-thesis where TSGs are inactivated [17,18]. In essence, it reflects changes in a promoter region (which represents a regulatory DNA sequence upstream of a gene) that involves an increased binding of methyl groups to so-called

CpG islands. The modification of this critical region, which is thought to have significant regulatory effects, causes loss of gene expression insofar as this reversible and epigenetic event inhibits the transcription of genes into mRNA. While the mechanisms involved remain stubbornly obscure, the list of aberrant methylation genes in cancer is rapidly growing. For example, frequent methylation of *DAPK* and *RAR2* has been reported in both lung and breast cancer respectively and there has been widespread speculation about its diagnostic and prognostic implications. Likewise, there has also been growing interest in a possible aberrant promoter methylation profile in prostate cancer and its relationship to clinicopathological features.

Using a *methylation-specific polymerase chain reaction* (MSP) Maruyama and co-workers [19] examined a series of 100 prostate cancer specimens (and 32 benign controls) for promoter hypermethylation in a series of 10 preselected genes. Six of these genes, *RARβ*, *RASSF1A*, *GSTP1*, *CDH13*, *APC* and *CDH1* were found to be selectively methylated. Although in this study, the proportion of samples demonstrating *GSTP1* methylation was relatively low at 36%, other authors have demonstrated its much more pervasive involvement in prostatic malignancy. For example, Jeronimo *et al.* [20] using a fluorogenic and quantitative real-time MSP analysed cytidine methylation in the *GSTP1* promoter in a series of 69 patients with prostate cancer and 31 patients with benign prostatic hyperplasia. With the relative level of methylated *GSTP1* DNA in each case being determined by the ratio of MSP-amplified *GSTP1* to *MYOD1* (a reference gene), 91% of the malignant and 53% of the HGPIN specimens displayed *GSTP1* hypermethylation. Importantly however, some of the tissues from patients with BPH also displayed *GSTP1* hypermethylation. However, the distribution of the ratios of *GSTP1 : MYOD1* differed significantly when plotted on a log scale. Using this fluorogenic quantitative approach, its sensitivity in the detection of prostate cancer was 85% and its positive predictive values was an impressive 100%. On the basis of these initial results, the authors investigated whether quantitative *GSTP1* methylation could be used to detect prostate cancer in small biopsy specimens. Using a cut-off value of 10 for the methylation ratio, the authors correctly predicted the histologic diagnosis of prostate cancer in 90% of the sextant biopsies and successfully excluded a diagnosis of malignancy in all the 10 patients whose biopsy specimens showed no evidence of malignancy.

The application of this fluorescent MSP technology to the detection of promoter hypermethylation of the *GSTP1* gene in DNA isolated from body fluids has more recently proved a potentially exciting and non-invasive tool for the detection of prostate cancer [21]. In this respect, Goessl and colleagues have isolated DNA from plasma, semen and post-prostatic massage urine in patients with prostate cancer and benign diseases alike. The authors detected *GSTP1* promoter hypermethylation in 94% of tumours, 72% of plasma, 50% of ejaculate and 36% of urine in patients with prostate cancer and in doing so, proposed MSP as a specific tool for the molecular diagnosis of prostate cancer in bodily fluids.

EXPRESSION PROFILING USING MICROARRAYS

Genetic alterations, regardless of the mechanisms that bring them about, often result in changes in mRNA expression levels which in turn have an impact on the protein expression pattern of a cell and its subsequent phenotype. The use of cDNA arrays allows the quantitative measurement of mRNA in many thousands of genes in a single biological sample. Its conceptual basis is the hybridisation of a complex probe derived from tissue RNA (Complementary DNA, cDNA) to DNA fragments that represent target genes arrayed on a glass slide. The tissue-derived probes are produced by the reverse transcription of RNA accompanied by simultaneous labelling. It is a complex probe, insofar as it contains in solution many different sequences of cDNA in various amounts, corresponding to the number of copies of the original mRNA species extracted from the tissue specimen. This labelled probe is then allowed to hybridise to the array, which may contain thousands of targets derived from PCR-amplified cDNA inserts or oligonucleotides – each representing a gene of interest (or part of a gene). The amount of labelled probe binding to arrays is directly proportional to the level of RNA in the original sample and as such provides a measure of its expression in tissues.

One of the most widely used commercial systems is manufactured by Affymetrix (Santa Clara, CA, United States). In this particular system, manufacture depends on the utilisation of hundreds of thousands of oligonucleotides synthesized directly *in situ* on glass chips by means of a photochemical reaction combined with an innovative masking technology. Each target gene under investigation is represented by a series of oligonucleotides in addition to appropriately mismatched sequences, which provide necessary internal controls. With test and reference probes labelled with different fluorescent markers (in much the same way as with CGH-based microarrays) expression is assessed directly by high-resolution scanners and sophisticated imaging software. Given that, it is now routinely possible to spot many thousands of targets of interest on less than a square centimetre of such arrays, the information provided by such systems are immense and has spawned a rapidly diversifying bioinformatics industry.

One of the most frequently employed systems of data interpretation is based around a hierarchical clustering algorithm [22] originally described by Eisen (1998). With a step-wise analysis of gene expression levels (involving the establishment of a similarity metric), all genes are incorporated into a dendrogram that connects genes (or nodes) generated by the clustering. Importantly, the length of each branch in the dendrogram reflects the degree of similarity between connected nodes or genes. Finally, software analysis allows the representation of correlated genes, which share similar expression patterns over large groups of specimens analysed, to provide a visual display of similarities between what might have originally appeared as a disparate group of specimens.

A number of research groups have applied this emerging technology to the investigation of both initiation and progression in prostate cancer. Luo *et al.* (2001) performed gene expression profiling on both benign and malignant prostate tissue in an attempt to identify fundamental differences [23]. Using cDNA microarrays consisting of 6500 genes, a series of 210 genes were identified as distinguishing benign and malignant disease. When ranked according to the ability to differentiate benign prostatic hyperplasia (BPH) from malignancy – the number one ranked gene was *hepsin*, a gene that encodes for a transmembrane serine protease, previously implicated in cell growth. Subsequent reverse transcriptase-polymerase chain reaction (RT-PCR) analysis was used to determine expression level of the *hepsin* gene in a number of benign and malignant samples. This analysis confirmed the high expression of *hepsin* in tumour specimens with low or minimal signal in benign specimens. While many of the other identified genes were not independently verified by PCR-based methods, the authors noted that a database search revealed other confirmatory evidence of differential expression of many of the genes identified by microarray.

Dhanasekaran *et al.* [24] in a seminal paper of the same year similarly applied microarray technology to the investigation of benign and malignant prostatic disease. Using a 9984 element cDNA microarray they analysed a variety of benign, hyperplastic and malignant specimens in addition to a number of cell lines with the principal aim of establishing a molecular classification of prostate cancer. Using several methods of gene selection to create a more limited set of targets for further analysis, the authors selected 200 genes (those with the largest effect sizes). From these, a number of candidate genes were identified including *HPN* (*hepsin*), *PIM1*, *LIM*, *TIMP2*, *HEVIN*, *RIG* and *THBS1* (thrombospondin 1) – amongst others. Selected genes identified by microarray were corroborated by northern analysis. *Hepsin*, for example, was 4.3-times up-regulated by microarray and 11.3-fold up-regulated by northern analysis. Subsequent *hepsin* immunohistochemistry on a total of 738 arrayed tissue samples using an affinity purified *hepsin* peptide antibody demonstrated preferential staining of malignant over benign tissue specimens. A similar approach was undertaken with *PIM1* kinase checking expression on high-throughput tissue microarrays;

PIM1 expression being observed as moderate or high in over half of the prostate cancer specimens.

The approach taken by both these sets of researchers, amply demonstrates the ability of DNA microarrays to identify new and potentially useful markers of disease for which diagnostic and prognostic utility appears likely. Their use is set to increase and with larger numbers of genes being analysed with the latest generation of DNA microarrays, further candidate genes are likely to come to the fore.

PROTEOMICS AND PROSTATE CANCER

While there are considerable number of researchers who are content to limit their work to the transcript level, most would agree that any meaningful interpretation of their data ultimately requires an extrapolation of that information to the protein level. An unquestioning acceptance of the validity of this extrapolation is clearly not sufficient. Principal amongst a number of widespread concerns relating to this assumption is the apparent discordance of mRNA expression measurements and co-existent protein levels [25]. As a result, it is crucial to verify such findings at the transcription level by assessing protein expression directly because the phenotype of a given cell is ultimately determined by the composition and activation status of its proteins. In addition, there are a host of post-translational modifications, which can only be determined by proteomic methodologies. As a result there has been growing enthusiasm for both qualitative and quantitative proteomic measurements.

One of the principal tools in the emerging field of proteomics, curiously is not new by itself, in that two-dimensional electrophoresis has been widely used as an investigative tool for more than two decades. Essentially, it involves the resolution of proteins on both their isoelectric point as well as molecular weight. Given its current level of refinement, however, two-dimensional gels rarely resolve more than 1000 proteins. As a result, it has become frequent to apply a series of affinity-based purification strategies to crude lysates to isolate a desired set of proteins before performing electophoresis. In this sense, two-dimensional electrophoresis is not too dissimilar from DNA microarrays – the difference being that instead of giving a transcript expression pattern, a protein expression pattern is achieved instead. A variety of computer software packages are currently available to align gel images and assign cluster indices and gauge relative abundance of proteins at select spots. It is, however, in the combination of two-dimensional electrophoresis and mass spectrometry that proteomics achieves its greatest resolution. Proteins are at first separated by gel electrophoresis and subsequently digested by sequence specific proteases (endo-peptidase), such that a peptide mixture can be eluted for further processing. Using matrix-assisted laser desorption and ionisation (MALDI) a mass spectrum or peptide-mass fingerprint is obtained. By fragmenting individual peptides to gain sequence information and submitting masses to a database search, individual matches can be made. If the protein is not identified (because of its novel nature or post-translational modification) it can be analysed by tandem mass spectroscopy. A sequence tag can be used for a more specific search or sometimes identified directly from the tandem mass spectroscopy. An alternative strategy involves using surface-enhanced laser desorption ionisation (SELDI) spectrometry. It is a highly sensitive, specific and high-throughput technology for the study of protein lysates. It differs from the conventional MALDI in that it does not rely on pre-clearing complex biological mixtures by high performance liquid chromatography or gas chromatography.

Proteins of interest are directly applied to a surface, utilising a defined chemical chromatographic characteristic such that it allows the construct of reproducible protein profiles. Using an essentially two-dimensional gel approach to the analysis of benign and malignant prostatic disease, Guevara *et al.* (1986) were one of the first groups to demonstrate the utility of a proteomic approach to the identification of new and informative biomarkers in prostate cancer [26]. In their study, a series of nine proteins were identified as being common to a number of malignant samples (and absent from benign tissue) and a further three were only identified in benign tissue (and significantly absent from the malignant cases identified). Present day investigators, who have continued this work, now benefit from recent advances in the biotechnology industry such that they can now begin to accurately identify the proteins identified in these early pioneering studies. For example, Alaiya *et al.* (2001), using a two-dimensional gel electrophoresis followed by gel digestion and MALDI mass spectrometry, compared tissue harvested from patients with benign prostatic disease and those with prostatic carcinoma [27]. In addition to a 40 kDa protein (identified as prostatic acid phosphatase) that decreased two-fold between benign and malignant disease, the authors reported the increased expression of heat shock protein 70 and a decreased expression of tropomyosin 1 in malignant tissue – the significance of which was uncertain.

Larger studies have now demonstrated the ability to differentiate normal, pre-malignant and malignant prostatic tissue on the basis of proteomics alone. Cazares *et al.* (2002) using SELDI spectrometry examined benign, malignant and high-grade PIN tissue obtained from radical prostatectomy specimens [28]. In turn, they determined several small molecular mass peptides and proteins which were up-regulated in prostate cancer and pre-malignant lesions. While there was no single protein alteration observed in all

PIN and prostate cancer specimens, it became readily apparent that the combination of a number of these markers had utility in distinguishing between tissue pathologies. Using a logistic regression analysis involving seven differentially expressed proteins resulted in a predictive equation that correctly distinguished pathological specimens with a sensitivity and specificity of 93.3% and 93.8% respectively.

A particularly innovative application of this proteomic fingerprinting has more recently been applied to the serum of patients with prostate cancer by Bao-Ling *et al.* [29]. The authors noted that while prostate-specific antigen (PSA) measurements had played a major part in increasing awareness and improving disease management, its lack of specificity had seriously limited its usefulness. The authors reasoned that the evaluation of a proteomic signature for prostate cancer could be established from the patient's sera using the protein profiling technologies detailed above. Using SELDI mass spectroscopy combined with an artificial learning algorithm, protein profiles of sera from 167 prostate cancer patients were examined along with age-matched normal controls. Using a nine-protein mass pattern decision tree, the authors correctly assigned 96% of the samples. A subsequent blinded series demonstrated a sensitivity of 83% and specificity of 97% with a positive predictive value of 96% for correctly identifying patients with prostate cancer.

Such proteomic-based approaches (which appear to be growing in popularity for the identification of occult disease in a number of solid tissue malignancies) rely not on individual biomarkers but alternatively on complex patterns or signatures of disease. Given the heterogeneous nature of prostatic malignancy, this approach appears to have at last offered the potential for a reliable and non-invasive test on which the selection of patients for histological sampling might reasonably be based – something which a range of individual biomarkers has so conspicuously failed to do over the last decade.

CONCLUSION

For decades it has been clear that the limitations imposed by standard scientific methodologies on data acquisition, represented the single most important barrier to the elucidation of a variety of clinically significant markers in both disease initiation and progression. Over a period of less than 5 years, however, this stance has radically changed. In contrast to previous decades, scientific and translational researchers are now faced with a deluge of information. The challenge, therefore, appears to be not how much data can be acquired, but how much can be deemed significant above the inevitable hiss of background noise. In this respect, it is likely that researchers will no longer focus on individual markers but instead examine the pattern of changes (whether at a genomic or proteomic level) associated with malignant transformation. And as is now becoming increasingly clear, the challenge of the future is one of data handling, a role that the emerging field of bioinformatics will have to grasp firmly if we stand any chance of benefiting from the rapid advances of recent years.

REFERENCES

1 Cancer Research Campaign. Scientific Year Book. 2000–2001. CRC.

2 Fearon E *et al.* A genetic model for colorectal tumorigenesis. *Cell* 1990; **61**: 759–67.

3 Schwarzacher and Heslop-Harrison. *Practical in-situ hybridisation.* Bios Scientific Publishers Ltd. (2000).

4 Jenkins R *et al.* A molecular cytogenetic analysis of 7q31 in prostate cancer. *Cancer Res* 1998; 57: 524–31.

5 Bostwick D. Independent origin of multiple foci of PIN. *Cancer* 1998; **83**: 1995–2002.

6 Emmert-Buck MR *et al.* Allelic loss on chromosomes 8p12-21 in microdissected PIN. *Cancer Res* 1995; **55**: 2959–62.

7 Qian J *et al.* Determination of gene and chromosome dosage in PIN and carcinoma. *Annal Quant Cytol Histol* 1998; **20**: 373–80.

8 Jenkins R et al. Detection of *c-myc* oncogene amplification and chromosome anomalies in metastatic prostate carcinoma by FISH. *Cancer Res* 1997; **57**: 524–31.

9 Sato L *et al.* Clinical significance of alterations of chromosome 8 in HGPIN and prostate carcinoma. *J Natl Cancer Ins* 1999; **91**: 1574–80.

10 Visakorpi T *et al.* Genetic changes in primary and recurrent prostate cancer by comparative genomic hybridisation. *Cancer Res* 1995; **55**: 342–7.

11 Lane TM *et al.* Genomic microarrays in the analysis of prostate cancer progression. *J Med Genet* 2002; **39**: S59.

12 Druker B *et al.* Perspectives on the development of a molecularly targeted agent. *Cancer Cell* 2002; **1**: 31–6.

13 Pan Y *et al.* 5q11, 8p11 and 10q22 are recurrent chromosomal breakpoints in prostate cancer cell lines. *Genes, Chromosomes Cancer* 2001; **30**: 187–95.

14 Strefford JC *et al.* The use of multicolour fluorescent technology in the characterisation of prostate carcinoma cell lines: a comparison of multiplex fluorescent in-situ hybridisation and SKY data. *Cancer Genet Cytogenet* 2001; **124**: 112–21.

15 Hudson DL *et al.* Proliferative heterogeneity in the human prostate: evidence for epithelial stem cells. *Lab Invest* 2000; **80**: 1243–50.

16 Lane TM *et al.* Cytogenetics of primary prostate cultures. *Prostate and Prostatic Diseases* (2002) *in press.*

17 Knudson AG. Mutation and cancer: statistical study of retinoblastoma. *PNAS* 1971; **68**: 820–23.

18 Jones P *et al.* Cancer Epigenetics comes of age. *Nat Genet* 1999; **21**: 163–7.

19 Maruyama R *et al.* Aberrant promoter methylation profile of prostate cancers and its relationship to clinicopathological features. *Clini Cancer Res* 2002; **8**: 514–9.

20 Jermino C *et al.* Quantitation of *GSTP1* methylation in non-neoplastic prostatic tissue and organ confined prostate adenocarcinoma. *J Nat Cancer Inst* 2001; **93**: 1747–52.

21 Goessl C *et al.* DNA alterations in body fluids as molecular tumour markers for urological malignancies. *Eur Urol* 2002; **41**: 668–76.

22 Eisen M *et al.* Cluster analysis and display of genome wide expression patterns. *PNAS* 1998; **95**: 14863–8.

23 Lao J et al. Human prostate cancer and benign prostatic hyperplasia: molecular detection by gene expression profiling. *Cancer Res* 2001; **61**: 4683–8.

24 Dhanasekaran S *et al.* Delineation of prognostic biomarkers in prostate cancer. *Nature* 2001; **412**: 822–26.

25 Anderson L *et al.* A comparison of selected mRNA and protein abundances in human liver. *Electrophoresis* 1997; **18**: 533–7.

26 Guevara J *et al*. Distinctive protein
    pattern in two-dimensional
    electrophoretograms of cancerous
    prostatic tissues. *Cancer Res* 1986; **46**:
    3599–604.
27 Alaiyet AA *et al*. Identification of
    proteins in human prostate tumour
    material by two-dimensional gel
    electrophoresis and mass spectrometry.
    Cell Mol Life Sci 2001; **58**:
    307–11.
28 Cazares H *et al*. Normal, benign,
    pre-neoplastic and malignant prostate
    cells have distinct protein expression
    profiles resolved by surface enhanced
    laser desorption-ionisation spectroscopy.
    Clin Cancer Res 2002; **8**: 2541–52.
29 Bao-Ling A *et al*. Protein finger-printing
    coupled with a pattern-matching
    algorithm distinguishes prostate cancer
    from BPH and healthy men. *Cancer Res*
    2002; **62**: 3609–14.

2: What Can We Learn From Breast Cancer?

Ludger Barthelmes and Christopher A. Gateley

INTRODUCTION

Before the age of super specialisation, it was relatively easy to draw parallels between different conditions and apply insights of one disease to the management of others. Halsted is considered a pioneer of breast surgery for removing the breast, the axillary contents and pectoralis major and minor – the 'Halsted mastectomy'. In 1904, he also assisted Young in his first radical perineal prostatectomy. Incidentally, when his scrub nurse Caroline Hampton suffered from an allergic reaction to the disinfectant carbol, he asked the Goodyear Rubber Company to manufacture surgical gloves. His innovation earned him a wife and presumably the appreciation of urologists to this day when they examine the prostate.

It is perhaps timely that we do not loose sight of developments in fields other than our own. Breast cancer and prostate cancer are the two common hormone-dependant tumours. Parallels in characteristics, diagnosis and treatment of both tumours are obvious and advances in the management of one tumour has the potential to lead to progress of the other.

PROGNOSIS AND OUTCOME

Improved outcome for breast cancer has been noted since the 1980s. The reason for this improvement is multifactorial and includes the introduction of systemic therapy (tamoxifen and chemotherapy) in the 1980s and earlier diagnosis. It is difficult to measure the effect that screening has had on survival because of its relatively recent implementation and the lead-time bias. Results of the effect of breast screening on survival in the United Kingdom will not be available before another few years [1,2].

EPIDEMIOLOGY – INCIDENCE, PREVALENCE AND AGE

Incidence figures of breast and prostate cancer are similar. In the States, there are 200 000 new cases of prostate cancer and 40 000 deaths each year, compared with 180 200 new cases of breast cancer and 43 900 deaths due to breast cancer [3].

During their lifetime 1 of 11 women will be affected by breast cancer compared with a lifetime risk of prostate cancer of 1 in 9 men. The risk of breast cancer doubles every 10 years up to the age of menopause, when breast cancer incidence slows down accounting for the slope in the incidence curve. Breast cancer causes 14 000 deaths in the United Kingdom each year and is the most commone cause of death in women aged between 40–50 years [4].

The increasing incidence of prostate cancer with age is well known together with the dilemma of how to deal with it in the elderly. Whereas prostate cancer is uncommon under the age of 45 years, breast cancer is encountered in women in their late twenties. Even though the individual human tragedy of a 50-year old man suffering from prostate cancer and a 30-year old woman diagnosed with breast cancer is the same, the effect it has on possibly dependent children and the attention the wider community pays to cancer diagnosis at young age is higher. This among other reasons may be one of the causes why breast cancer enjoys a relatively high profile in the public opinion compared with prostate cancer.

GENETICS

The importance of a family history of prostate cancer is pointed out else-where with particular emphasis of the PTEN and p53 tumour-suppressor genes. DNA linkage analysis of blood samples of extended families where clusters of breast cancer were noted led to the discovery of *BRCA1* and *BRCA2* genome mutations on chromosome 17 and 13 with an autosomal dominant pattern of inheritance with partial penetrance [5,6].

Women in families with an identified mutation have a 50% chance of being a carrier. The lifetime risk of breast cancer for carriers is approxim-ately 80%. 10% of the women diagnosed with breast cancer before the age of 35 years without a family history of breast cancer have a mutation of *BRCA1* [7].

p53 is the most commonly mutated tumour-suppressor gene in breast cancer. It is rarely inherited, but mutated in almost half of all invasive breast cancers [8].

Whereas the influence of a genetic predisposition of prostate cancer is clearly recognised, this has not yet resulted in changes of clinical practice. In breast cancer, special family history clinics have been established to deal with issues of gene testing, counselling prior to testing, tracing family members and advising them on treatment options. Some women are offered screening at an age 5 years younger, before the youngest family member was diagnosed with breast cancer. A prophylactic mastectomy can significantly reduce, but not eliminate the risk of developing breast cancer. Alternatively, inclusion in a chemoprevention trial can be offered.

Since tamoxifen reduces the incidence of breast cancer in the opposite breast, its use for breast cancer prevention in women who are at increased risk has been investigated and an overview presented [9]. It confirmed that tamoxifen reduces the breast cancer incidence, but also increases the risk of endometrial carcinoma and venous thromboembolism. Newer selective estrogen receptor modulators ("SERM's") such as raloxifene may be similarly effective as tamoxifen without inducing endometrium carcinoma, but the chemoprevention of breast cancer is not yet an established practice.

SURGICAL TREATMENT AND CONCEPTS

In the nineteenth century, breast cancer served as a model for the pathogenesis of solid cancers in general. In 1860, Virchow postulated that a local cellular disturbance leads to the development of cancer in the breast. Cancer cells migrate in an orderly, centrifugal fashion along fascial planes and lymphatics to lymph nodes, which act as a circumferential barrier against the spread of breast cancer. Once they are overwhelmed with cancer cells, the tumour spreads further along the lymphatics until they reach the bloodstream.

They are then dislodged into the first capillary bed where they will form metastatic deposits [10]. Halsted's radical approach of removing the breast, the pectoralis major and minor muscles, the axillary contents and regional lymph nodes was the logical application of this concept [11]. In line with this principle, even more radical surgery was suggested for more advanced breast tumours, sometimes resulting in forequarter amputations [12].

Today, we know that the 'Halsted mastectomy' is an effective method to ensure local control of breast cancer, although less aggressive operations with preservation of the chest wall muscles are equally effective in most cases. Local control, however, does not equal cure and it has been shown over the years that 60% of women will eventually succumb to breast cancer due to distant disease without any evidence of recurrent or ongoing disease in the breast, chest wall or locoregional lymphatics [13]. Conversely, patients with local recurrence may not necessarily have worse survival. It was noted that a group of patients who refused to have their breast cancer treated survived for up to 30 years. Some had uncontrolled local disease, but this was not associated with overt distant metastasis [14]. Less aggressive, surgical approaches were introduced before World War II. Geoffrey Keynes used newly developed radium needles in advanced and inoperable breast cancer and obtained good local control [15]. Unfortunately, he was unable to pursue this approach as the radium supplies had to be dispersed during air raids on London. It was only in 1985 that randomised trials confirmed that breast conservation through a combination of wide local excision of the breast tumour plus radiotherapy is equally as effective as mastectomy for a selected group of patients [16,17].

Since it is now accepted that breast conservation by wide local excision and radiotherapy is equally effective as mastectomy, more than half of all newly diagnosed breast cancer patients have the option to choose between mastectomy and breast conservation. The psychological gain in preservation of body image by breast conservation is often paid off by anxiety for fear of recurrence, whereas depression is more often seen after mastectomy. Women are therefore faced with difficult choices at a time when the diagnosis of breast cancer can be overwhelming. Whereas surgeons have tended to focus on technical aspects of breast cancer treatment, the emotional side has not always attracted the same attention. Nurses took on an active role, being present at the time of the diagnosis, following the patient up at home to go through the diagnosis again and exploring which treatment option is most appropriate for the individual woman. Their personal knowledge of the patient is also useful after treatment to monitor the patients' adjustment. The role of specialist nurses is now well established in many specialities including urology, but breast specialist nurses were among the first to take their role further beyond traditional models of nursing. Other allied professions are currently extending their role in the management of breast disease: some radiographers receive training in reading mammograms, pathology technicians learn how to analyse fine needle aspirations in one-stop breast clinics. Given training, supervision and imagination, there may be aspects of urology care, which can safely be delegated.

Along with a varied surgical approach the concept of breast cancer has been changing. The Halsted paradigm of orderly centrifugal spread of breast cancer failed to explain why more than half of women with breast cancer succumb to their disease due to metastasis despite successful locoregional treatment. The concept of biological pre-determinism emerged: the course of breast cancer is determined by micrometastasis, which develops in the pre-clinical phase before the cancer manifests itself in the breast. The focus was directed towards systemic treatments aimed at metastatic disease already present at diagnosis and surgery stopped being the sole treatment modality.

These two concepts – orderly centrifugal spread of breast cancer versus systemic disease from the outset – are still recognised in current debates of breast cancer management.

Opponents of breast screening, point out that distant disease may have already occurred even in early screen-detected disease and improved outcome may be due to lead-time bias in line with the concept of biological pre-determinism of breast cancer.

On the other hand, the idea of centrifugal spread from the breast found new support when studies reported improved survival after mastectomy combined with radiotherapy to the chest wall. The combined approach of surgery and radiotherapy may treat local disease more effectively, preventing spread of tumour cells as postulated by Halsted [18–20].

These arguments are not unfamiliar to urological practice. With the advent of Prostate-specific antigen (PSA) testing and improved imaging, increasing number of so-called organ-defined disease are diagnosed and surgery with the curative intent to prevent the orderly spread of cancer is currently gaining popularity, whereas previously prostate cancer has been thought of as a systemic disease at the time of diagnosis.

The traditional concept of cancer is that of monoclonal, dedifferentiated cells with uncontrolled growth. Chemo- and radiotherapy interfere with cell growth and cancer cells are particularly susceptible because of their proportionally higher number of cell divisions. Cytotoxic chemotherapy regimens have been used in the management of early and advanced breast cancer since the 1980s, and the improved outcome of breast cancer treatment is partially attributed to the introduction of cytotoxic chemotherapy at that time. Attempts to circumvent the myelodepressive effects of aggressive chemotherapy regimen by bone marrow rescue have not resulted in significant improvement of survival and are only undertaken within the limits of controlled studies [21].

The survival benefit of cytotoxic chemotherapy in breast cancer is only modest as is the benefit of cytotoxic chemotherapy regimen in prostate cancer after hormone escape. Both breast and prostate cancers are prime examples of interactions between cancerous and non-cancerous tissues. The role of adjacent, non-cancerous tissues via complex messenger and receptor mechanisms on tumour growth is increasingly recognised. Skeletal seedlings are the most frequent manifestation of metastasis in prostate and breast cancer, which had been recognised by Paget in his 'seed and soil' hypothesis [22].

We know that growth factors that are released during the continuous remodelling of bone favour cancer cell proliferation and survival. Breast cancer cells have the ability to increase osteoclast proliferation and activity, which in turn promotes release of growth factors enhancing spread of metastasis. The use of bisphosphonates to treat hypercalcaemia by the inhibition of osteoclasts is well established. Evidence emerges that bisphosphonates delay the progress of bony metastasis in breast and prostate cancer and myeloma patients. Targeting the interactions between cancerous and non-cancerous tissues may prove superior to the relative indiscriminate cell kill of traditional cytotoxic chemotherapy in the treatment of breast and prostate cancer [23], but there is also evidence that bisphophonates may have a direct tumouricidal effect on breast cancer [24] and prostate cancer cell lines [25]. Generally, the use of chemotherapy in metastatic breast cancer is disappointing. The duration of responses is less than 1 year, and overall median survival of metastatic breast cancer is approximately 2 years. Similarly, chemotherapy for prostate cancer has much to wish for. Modulating the interactions on tumour growth of non-cancerous tissues with, for example, bisphosphonates may prove superior in the treatment of prostate and breast cancer, compared with the relatively indiscriminate approach of cytotoxic chemotherapy [26].

SCREENING

In 1986, Professor Sir Patrick Forrest published the findings of a committee, which was set up to evaluate breast cancer screening with mammography. At the time of the report, there was evidence from several randomised-controlled trials and case-control studies suggesting that mammographic screening reduces breast cancer mortality. The Forrest report concluded that the introduction of mammographic screening would lead to a reduction of breast cancer mortality by 25% [27]. Whereas other developments in medicine take longer to cross the sea, it just so happened that the idea of a breast screening program caught the interest and sympathy of all political parties in the United Kingdom in the run-up for the elections in 1987, and a population breast screening programme was started in 1988. The development of mammographic breast screening in the United Kingdom was controversial. Opponents considered the concept of mammographic breast screening to be flawed. This served as an incentive to breast screening supporters to define criteria of quality assurance, issue guidelines and subsequently audit the results to justify the programme. The defined, regulated treatment women received in the screening programme led to a situation of double care: women in the screening programme were treated within a defined time limit meeting set criteria of care, whereas treatment of patients with symptomatic cancers was unregulated and inconsistent. Consequently, standards for treatment of symptomatic patients were introduced and established. The multidisciplinary team approach – which is now common place in most other specialities – started off in breast screening and was soon extended to benign and malignant symptomatic breast disease to avoid dual standards for screen-detected and symptomatic disease.

The scientific basis for mammographic screening may be seen as doubtful as for PSA screening. The arguments against it will be familiar to urologists: lead-time bias, the unknown significance and potential over-treatment of carcinoma *in situ*, cost and induction of anxiety to name a few. Whenever concerns about the effectiveness of breast cancer screening are raised, a heated debate is likely to follow [28–33]. However, most will agree that breast screening has had a positive impact on the management of all breast diseases. The impact may be difficult to measure numerically, but has resulted in a profound change in the way that all breast diseases are nowadays managed. The difficulties of prostate screening have been outlined elsewhere and if a prostate screening programme is ever introduced, of whatever nature, there will be criticism about its effectiveness. This debate should be welcomed to ensure high standards of screening, and it can be anticipated that the lessons learnt from a potential prostate screening programme may be applicable to the treatment of symptomatic prostate disease.

It is no secret that funding and availability of health care in the United Kingdom is below the standards of Western Europe. However, only in the United Kingdom, the Netherlands, Sweden and Finland there have been population-based mammographic breast screening programmes in place, for a considerable period of time whereas Germany has none. Belgium, Ireland, Luxembourg, Portugal and Spain have breast screening programmes at a regional level with no intention for national coverage [34,35]. Even though the ultimate answer as to whether breast screening improves mortality is yet unknown, the consensus is that breast screening is justified and is here to stay. Nationwide registration of the population with practice lists in the NHS has been successfully exploited for targeting women for breast screening. Urologists in the United Kingdom may envy their colleagues from other countries in the Western world who are not restrained by a rigid, under-funded health system. However, prostate screening may be an area where they could have a distinct advantage over their colleagues in countries with managed health care systems, where comprehensive population screening is far more difficult.

REFERENCES

1 Botha JL, Bray F, Sankila R, Parkin DM. Breast cancer incidence and mortality trends in 16 European countries. *Eur J Cancer*. 2003; **39**: 1718–29.

2 Peto R, Borham J, Clarke M, Davies C, Beral V. UK and USA breast cancer deaths down 25% in year 2000 at ages 20–69 years. *Lancet* 2000; **355**: 1822.

3 Parker SL, Tong T, Bolden S *et al*. Cancer Statistics. *Cancer J Clin* 1997; **47**: 5–27.

4 McPherson K, Steel CM, Dixon JM. Breast cancer – epidemiology, risk factors and genetics. In: Dixon JM, Ed. ABC of Breast Disease, 2nd edn. BMJ Publishing Group, London, 2000.

5 Miki Y, Swenson J, Shattick-Eiders D. A strong candidate for the breast and ovarian cancer susceptibility gene *BRCA1*. *Science* 1994; **266**: 66–71.

6 Wooster R, Bignall G, Swift S. Identification of the breast cancer susceptibility gene *BRCA2*. *Nature* 1995; **378**: 789–92.

7 Langston AA, Malone KE, Thompson JD. BRCA1 mutations in a population-based sample of young women with breast cancer. *N Engl J Med* 1996; **334**: 137–42.

8 Ziaye D, Hupp TR, Thompson AM. *p53* and breast cancer. *Breast* 2000; **9**: 239–45.

9 Cuzick J, Powles T, Veronesi U *et al.* Overview of the main outcomes in breast-cancer prevention trials. *Lancet* 2003; **361**: 296–300.

10 Virchow R. Die krankhaften Geschwulste. Berlin, A. Hirschwald 1863–73.

11 Halsted WS. The radical operation for the cure of carcinoma of the breast. *John Hopkings Hosp Rev* 1898; **28**: 557.

12 Wangensteen OH. Remarks on extension of the Halsted operation for cancer of the breast. *Ann Surg* 1949; **130**: 315.

13 Brinkley D, Haybittle JL. The curability of breast cancer. *Lancet* 1973; **2**: 95–8.

14 Bloom HJG, Richardson WW, Harries EJ. Natural history of untreated breast cancer (1805–1933). Comparison of untreated and treated cases according to histological grade of malignancy. *Brit Med J* 1962; **I**: 213–21.

15 Keynes G. Conservative treatment of cancer of the breast. *Brit Med J*. 1937: **2**: 643–647.

16 Veronesi U, Banfi A, Del Vecchio M *et al.* Comparison of Halsted mastectomy with quadrantectomy, axillary dissection, and radiotherapy in early breast cancer: long-term results. *Eur J Cancer Clin Oncol* 1986; **22**:1085–9.

17 Fisher B, Bauer M, Margolese R *et al.* Five-year results of a randomized clinical trial comparing total mastectomy and segmental mastectomy with or without radiation in the treatment of breast cancer. *N Engl J Med* 1985; **312**: 665–73.

18 Overgaard M, Hansen PS, Overgaard J *et al.* Postoperative radiotherapy in high-risk premenopausal women with breast cancer who receive adjuvant chemotherapy. Danish Breast Cancer Cooperative Group 82b Trial. *N Eng J Med* 1997; **337**: 949–55.

19 Ragaz J, Jackson SM, Le N *et al.* Adjuvant radiotherapy and chemotherapy in node-positive premenopausal women with breast cancer. *N Engl J Med* 1997; **337**: 956–62.

20 Hellman S. Stopping metastases at their source. *N Eng J Med* 1997; **337**: 996–7.

21 Myers SE, Williams SF. Role of high-dose chemotherapy and autologous stem cell support in the treatment of breast cancer. *Haematol Oncol Clin North Am* 1993; **7**: 631–56.

22 Paget S. The distribution of secondary growth in cancer of the breast. *Lancet* 1889; **1**: 571–3.

23 Schipper H. Shifting the cancer paradigm: must we kill to cure? *J Clin Oncol* 1995; **13**: 801–7.

24 Fromigue O, Kheddoumi N, Body JJ. Bisphosphonates antagonise bone growth factors' effects on human breast cancer cells survival. *Brit J Cancer* 2003; **89**: 178–84.

25 Oades GM, Senaratne SG, Clarke IA, Kirby RS, Colston CK. Nitrogen containing bisphosphonates induce apoptosis and inhibit the mevalonate pathway, impairing RAS membrane localization in prostate cancer cells. *J Urol* 2003; **170**: 246–52.

26 Giaccone G, Pinedo HM. Novel chemotherapy agents for treatment of breast cancer. In: Tobias JS, Houghton J & Henderson IC, Eds. *Breast cancer – new horizons in research and treatment*, Arnolds, London, 2001: 81–93.

27 Breast cancer screening report to the health ministers of England, Wales, Scotland, and Northern Ireland by working group chaired by Professor Sir Patrick Forrest, 1986, London: Her Majesty's Stationary Office.

28 Gotzsche P, Olson O. Is screening for breast cancer with mammography justifiable? *Lancet* 2000, **355**: 129–34.

29 Baum M. Money may be better spent on symptomatic women. *Brit Med J* 1999; **318**: 398.

30 Baum M. Screening for breast cancer, time to think and stop? *Lancet* 1995; **346**: 436–9.

31 Goodman SN. The mammography dilemma: a crisis for evidence-based

medicine? *Ann Intern Med* 2002; **137**: 363–5.

32 Wald N. Populist instead of professional. *J Med Screen* 2000; **7**: 1.

33 Statement by the NHS breast screening programme in response to the paper in the Lancet (8 Jan, 2000). Is mammographic screening for breast cancer justified ? Press release, Julietta Patnick (National Co-ordinator) NHSBSP, 6 Jan, 2000.

34 Mullan MH, Kissin MW. Breast screening and screen-detected disease. In: Farndon JR, ed. *A companion to specialist surgical practice – breast surgery*, WB Saunders, Edinburgh, 2001: 23–65.

35 Shapiro S *et al.* Breast cancer screening programme in twenty two countries: current policies, administration and guidelines. *Int J Epidemiol* 1998; **27**: 735–42.

3: New Serum Markers for Prostate Cancer

Bernhard Brehmer, Antonios Makris and Gerhard Jakse

Biomarkers have been used to diagnose and monitor prostate cancer for more than 50 years. In particular, the discovery of the serum marker prostate-specific antigen (PSA) by Wang and co-workers (1979) significantly altered the detection and management of prostate cancer [1]. However, owing to imperfect correlation with prostate cancer activity, PSA's usefulness is limited and the established cut-off of 4 ng/mL as a valuable tool for prostate cancer detection is problematic. For example, among men with PSA of 4–10 ng/mL, the positive predictive value is only up to 25% [2]. Additionally, to distinguish between early stage prostate cancer and benign conditions like benign prostate hyperplasia, using only serum PSA is not possible. As a result, in more than 70–80% of patients with PSA from 4–10 ng/mL prostate, biopsies are performed. Another critical issue is the rising incidence of prostate cancer in <4 ng/mL PSA level. Studies have reported an incidence of up to 24.5% in PSA from 2.5–4 ng/mL [3]. Thus, it is evident that there is an urgent need for new tools to improve the specificity of PSA. The elucidation and validation of new biological markers of prostate cancer should aid detection as well as improve disease monitoring following treatment protocols. In this chapter, potential new serum markers that are current candidates for improved detection and prognostic assessment of prostate cancer are discussed (see Table 3.1), PSA derivates are not considered.

NEUROENDOCRINE MARKERS

The presence of neuroendocrine (NE) cells in prostate cancer was first described by Pretl in 1944 [4]. The physiologic role of NE cells is still unknown, but it is thought that they are involved in regulation of growth and differentiation [5]. NE cells are present in normal, hyperplastic and malignant prostate tissue, and are located in the basal layer of the acini and

Table 3.1 Serum makers in prostate cancer.

Marker	Comment
CgA	Not useful for cancer detection. Most valuable in therapy planning and prognosis. Elevated up to 48% in metastatic disease [20]. Reflects best the neuroendocrine cell presence and activity.
NSE	Contradictory results in literature whether increased, decreased or not affected by prostate cancer. No significant proven, prognostic value. No proven value in detection of prostate cancer.
IGF (I/II)/IGFBPs	Not useful in detection of or managing prostate cancer.
VEGF	Seems to be elevated in prostate cancer. Detailed investigations are still lacking.
TGF-β1	Unclear whether serum level helps to discriminate between prostate cancer and BPH. One of the most promising new serum markers. Until further prospective investigations demonstrates the significance, TGF-β1 is not for clinical routine use.
IL-6	Serum level is significantly elevated in hormone-refractory prostate cancer patients. May be a surrogate marker of the androgen-independent phenotype. Comprehensive, prospective studies are still lacking. However, IL-6 is the most promising serum marker in prostate cancer yet.
MMP/TIMP	Not useful in detection of or managing prostate cancer. Not specific for cancer. Not organ specific. Whether it is useful as a prognostic marker is unknown.
Proteomics	Proven sensitivity and specificity still lacking in prospective trials. Technology with two opportunities • diagnostic by abnormal protein fingerprint; • identification of new markers. Most promising 'marker' and simultaneously a research tool.

the ducts, being most common in the periuretheral zone [6]. The incidence of NE cells in prostatic adenocarcinoma varies from 10–100%. Aumuller (1999) demonstrated that NE cells within the prostate may represent a distinct cell lineage of their own, and differ from other prostatic cells that derive from the urogenital sinus [7].

Several primary neurocrine markers have been investigated, but till date the most frequently studied are chromogranin A (CgA) and neuron-specific enolase (NSE), either at the tissue level or in the serum from patients with prostate cancer. However, whether the histological presence of NE cells leads to an increase in serum NE markers is still a controversial point. Angelsen found that only in CgA, a positive correlation between histological findings and serum measurements could be identified. For all other examined markers, NSE, chromogranin B, serotonin and somatostatin, no correlation between serum markers and histological extent was detected [8].

Weinstein examined CgA staining in prostatectomy specimens and correlated the degree of staining with the prognosis [9]. In a multivariate analysis, the extent of NE presence indeed predicted progression of the cancer; a finding also described for CgA serum levels [10,11]. Elevated CgA values correlate with poor prognosis and are minimally influenced by either endocrine therapy or chemotherapy [12]. Cohen found an extremely high correlation between NE cells in histology and prognosis. In histology, 91% of patients with tumour-specific death showed NE cells inside the prostate cancer cell population, whereas in only 11% of survived patients, NE cells were found in the cancer [13].

Bonkhoff used immunohistochemical double label methods to evaluate the nuclear androgen receptor (AR) status in NE cells of normal, hyperplastic and neoplastic prostate cancers that recurred after hormonal and radiation therapy [14] In normal and hyperplastic glands, NE cells characterised by CgA did not reveal AR-positivity. Also co-expression of CgA and AR were very rarely detected in subsets of endocrine differentiated tumour cells. This may indicate that prostatic NE cells represent an androgen-independent cell population, whose regulatory functions are not influenced by circulating androgens. However, on the other hand, several investigators did not find any correlation between NE cells and the stage of tumour, nor did they demonstrate significant correlations between NE cells and tumour grade or prognosis [15–17].

The data regarding NSE is still more confusing. Kamiya *et al.* described in prostate cancer patients significantly *lower* NSE serum levels than in the control group [18]. Conversely, Hvamstad *et al.* observed in 33% of hormone-resistant prostate cancer patients elevated NSE in serum, and concluded that NSE is a valuable prognostic marker [19]. Other authors have failed to demonstrate any clinical significant application for serum NSE level [12,20,21].

The controversy about the serum measurements of NE markers still remains. Till date, CgA seems to be the most valuable NE marker in prostate cancer and appears to reflect the NE activity of prostate cancer better than others, for example, NSE. Overall, however, whether the NE markers are helpful in detecting prostate cancer is still not clear. A few reports of increased CgA serum level in prostate cancer compared to benign hyperplasia (BPH) can be found in literature [22]. However, CgA seems to be the most valuable of the NE markers in assessing prognoses and planning therapy. In clinical use, the measurement of NE markers is not routine as yet, even if this is postulated to be the case by some authors [23].

INSULIN-LIKE GROWTH FACTOR

Insulin-like growth factors (IGF) are important mitogenic and antiapoptotic peptides that affect the proliferation of normal and malignant cells. Two protein growth factors, IGF-I and IGF-II, have been characterised, and both demonstrate sequence similarity to insulin. Two further IGF receptors (types I and II), along with IGF-binding proteins (IGFBP-1 to -6) are both present in serum and tissue, and IGFBP proteases are involved in the IGF-network. IGFBP constitute a large protease super-family, one of the most prominent being prostate-specific antigen (PSA), a serine protease [24]. This complexity attests to the difficulty in analysing the role of IGFs in binding proteins as well as proteases in the regulatory control of both normal and abnormal prostate growth.

The validity of using IGF and IGFBPs as diagnostic and prognostic tools is still a matter of dispute. Chan observed a strong positive association between IGF-I levels and prostate cancer risk. Men in the highest quartile of IGF-I levels had a relative risk of 4.3 compared with men in the lowest quartile. This association was independent of baseline PSA levels. He suggested IGF-I as a risk factor predictor for prostate cancer [25]. A number of epidemiological studies are in conflict with his findings. In high-risk groups, for example, African Americans, decreased serum levels of IGF-I, IGF-II and IGFBP-3 were found [26]. Additionally, Woodson and co-workers performed a prospective cohort study investigating the association between serum levels of IGF-I or IGFPB-3 and their link to prostate cancer risk in Finnish men. In contrast to previous reports, he found no evidence to support a causal association between serum IGF-I or IGFBP-3 and the risk of prostate cancer [27].

Baffa measured IGF-I serum levels of 57 prostate cancer patients before and after radical prostatectomy and compared them to 39 age-matched controls. The mean serum IGF-I in cancer patients before prostatectomy (124.6 ng/mL) was significantly lower than for the healthy controls (157.5 ng/mL). He concluded that these findings indicate a significant association between low serum levels of IGF-I and prostate cancer [28]. Conversely, Peng and co-workers showed that significant increases in IGF-I serum level is associated with prostate cancer. Using patients with prostate cancer ($n = 81$), benign prostate hyperplasia ($n = 55$) and healthy male controls ($n = 84$), the specificity and sensitivity of IGF-I determination were 0.68

and 0.58, respectively [29]. However, other authors could not confirm any correlation between IGF-I and prostate cancer [30].

Elevated IGFBP-2 serum levels were found in active prostate carcinoma, and closely paralleled PSA levels. Ho and co-workers, using 16 patients, measured IGFBP-2, IGFBP-3, IGF-I, IGF-II and PSA for more than 1 year, and compared the serum levels with histologically proven BPH patients and with healthy males. The serum IGFBP-2 was significantly higher (560 mg/L) in cancer patients with high PSA than cancer patients with normal PSA (292 mg/L). Also, the serum level from PSA-normal prostate cancer patients did not differ significantly from BPH (364 mg/L) and controls (367 mg/L) [31]. The meaning of IGFBP-2 as a follow-up parameter after curative therapy is at present unclear. Yu followed-up 38 patients who developed recurrent disease 5 years after radical prostatectomy, and measured IGF-I, IGFBP-2 and IGFBP–3. These patients were compared with 40 patients after prostatectomy, who were in remission. He could not find any predictive values in the prognosis of prostate cancer [32].

Further attempts to improve the quality of IGFs and IGFBPs in the detection or prognostic assessment of prostate cancer used different ratios of PSA and different IGFs and IGFBPs. To this end, both positive[33] as well as negative [34] results can be found in the literature.

In conclusion, the importance of the IGFs and IGFBPs in the mitogenic and anti-apoptotic system of normal and malignant cells is undisputed. However, whether the measurements of the serum levels are useful in managing prostate cancer is totally unclear.

GROWTH FACTORS AND CYTOKINES

VEGF

Angiogenic cytokines like vascular endothelial growth factor (VEGF) are responsible for angiogenesis, essential for tumour growth. VEGF was first isolated from tumour ascites fluid from guinea pigs, hamsters and mice by Senger in 1983 [35]. Since then, four species of VEGF have been characterised [36]. The expression of VEGF can be induced by hypoxia, a common condition at the leading edge of a growing mass, or within a solid tumour, which leads to the sprouting of new tumour vessels [37].

VEGF expression is usually examined in immunohistochemistry in association with microvessel density, being positively correlated with it and disease-specific survival [38].

In blood, circulating VEGF has rarely been investigated. Borre and co-workers measured VEGF in plasma in a total of 51 patients. In this pilot study, elevated plasma VEGF levels were found to be associated with prostate cancer. This suggests VEGF's potential role as a marker for prostate cancer, but further investigations are required to clarify the possible extent of its role [39].

Transforming Growth Factor β

Transforming growth factor β (TGF-β) is a protein dimer encoded by two genes with 70% homology, and three possible dimer protein combinations exist to form TGF-β1, TGF-β2 and TGF-β3. TGF-β is produced as a precursor amino acid initially in an inactive or latent form, and can be activated by proteolysis (e.g. by plasminogen activator).

TGF-β1 inhibits the endothelial cell growth of the prostate [40,41], or at least the cell growth of the luminal cells as shown in cell culture experiments [42], resulting in increases in cell death and apoptosis, respectively [43].

Many investigators have measured TGF in serum of prostate cancer patients before therapy and in follow-up. Apart from detecting cancer, TGF was examined in regard to its use as a prognostic factor. Adler measured serum TGF-β1 before and after prostatectomy or antiandrogen therapy and also in 19 healthy men as control. He found a significant correlation between PSA and TGF-β1 and significantly elevated levels in patients with clinically evident metastases [44]. Other reports in the literature of elevated TGF levels in prostate cancer also support this [45].

Furthermore, the TGF-β1 serum level in combination with PSA was used for therapy control. Dipaola and co-workers assumed that 13-cis-retinoic acid (CRA) and alphainterferon (IFN-α) have anti-tumour activity in patients with early recurrence of prostate cancer after curative treatment, and found that plasma TGF-β1 correlates with changes in PSA as a result of CRA/INF-α therapy. They suggested TGF-β1 to be a useful marker for the biological effect of these agents [46].

Controversially, Lang could not find any diagnostic prediction using TGF-β1 serum levels. In 157 prostate cancer patients before and in follow-up, the serum level was measured and compared with 85 BPH patients. Neither in the follow-up in patients with progress nor in the compared BPH patients was TGF-β1 indicated to be of any use as a marker [47]. We also obtained a similar result as serum TGF-β1 was found to be non-discriminative between BPH and prostate cancer. Furthermore, no TGF-β1 increase was observed with advancing tumour stage in patients with prostate cancer [48].

The importance of TGF-β1 in the discrimination of prostate cancer and as a prognostic factor remains to be clarified. However, if the expectation as one of the most promising new serums in prostate cancer detection, as Canto indeed believes [49], does come true, this will have to be verified by further prospective studies. So far, TGF-β is not used as a routine tumour marker for prostate cancer.

Interleukin-6

Interleukin-6 (IL-6) is a pleiotropic cytokine that was first identified as a T-cell-derived lymphokine inducing maturation of B cells into antibody producing cells. The acute phase response, haematopoesis and different segments of the immune system response are affected by IL-6. In different tumours, for example, gastrointestinal tumours [50] and breast cancer [51], elevated levels of IL-6 and correlation to tumour burden were demonstrated.

Chung and co-workers measured IL-6 in three hormone refractory (DU-145, TSU and PC-3,) and in two hormone-dependent (LNCaP–ATCC and LNCaP–GW) prostate cancer cell lines. Each hormone-refractory line expressed IL-6, whereas the hormone-dependent lines did not. In addition, the effects of IL-6 on cell growth were assessed by 3-(4,5-dimethyl thiazol-2yl)-2,5-diphenyl tetrazolium bromide assay or MTT via spectrophotometric measurement of cell growth as a function of mitochondrial activity in living cells. Addition of IL-6 *in vitro* inhibited growth of hormone-dependent cells, but had no effect on hormone-refractory lines. From these cell culture experiments, Chung concluded that IL-6 appears to undergo a functional transition as a paracrine growth inhibitor to autocrine growth stimulator during the progression of prostate cancer to the hormone-refractory phenotype [52]. These cell culture results were confirmed in patients with hormone-refractory cancer. Drachenberg measured IL-6 in serum of patients with prostatitis, BPH, localised and recurrent disease and used healthy men as control. Serum levels were significantly elevated in patients with clinically evident hormone-refractory disease and statistical significance was seen when comparing the elevated serum IL-6 levels to those in normal controls, prostatitis, BPH and localised and recurrent disease [53]. IL-6 elevation in serum was also found by Adler. The serum level was measured in 5 subgroups of patients, including 19 men as control, local, local advanced and metastatic disease. IL-6 is significantly increased in cancer patients and correlated with PSA and tumour burden [44]. For 46 untreated patients (23 with and 23 without bone metastasis), Akimoto also found a correlation between metastasis and IL-6 serum level, as the IL-6 serum level were significantly higher in the patients with bone metastasis than in those without [54]. This clinical finding is supported by a cell culture report from Garcia-Moreno who evaluated the effect caused by culture medium from human prostatic carcinoma cells (PC-3) culture on human osteoblast and measured IL-6 synthesis by quantifying mRNA using reverse transcription polymerase chain reaction (RT-PCR). Human osteoblast cultured with PC-3 supernatant produced an increase in IL-6 mRNA level compared to osteoblast cultured in normal culture media. PC-3 cells seem to produce a factor that enhances the synthesis and release of IL-6, a known activator of bone resorption [55].

In literature, there is strong evidence that IL-6 correlates with prostate cancer burden and prognosis [56,57]. However, comprehensive, prospective studies to verify IL-6's benefit in prostate cancer detection and prognosis are lacking. Even so, IL-6 is the most promising serum marker candidate for prostate cancer yet.

MATRIX METALLOPROTEINASES

Matrix Metalloproteinases (MMPs) are a family of highly homologous Zn^{2+}-dependent enzymes capable of degrading the extracellular matrix (ECM) and basement membrane (BM). They are present in healthy individuals and have been shown to play an important role in physiological processes, such as wound healing [58], bone resorption [59] and pregnancy [60]. However, the main interest in MMPs relates to their role in certain pathological mechanisms, for example, rheumatoid arthritis [61,62], liver fibrosis [63] and different types of cancer.

The continuously growing MMP gene family at present contains 17 members. The MMPs have been subdivided into four groups, which are defined by the substrate-specific degradation of the ECM and BM, namely, the collagenases, stromelysins, gelatinases and matrilysin. The proteinases MMP-2 (synonym: Gelatinase A; 72 kDa) and MMP-9 (Gelatinase B; 92 kDa) belong to the group of the gelatinases. MMP-2 and MMP-9 are well known as promoters for cancer invasion and metastases in a variety of different tumours: colon [64], breast [65], brain tumours [66] and prostate cancer [67]. Also, MMP-2 and MMP-9 are expressed in benign and malignant prostate tissue [68,69]. The most important natural inhibitors of these proteinases are the tissue inhibitors of matrix metalloproteinases (TIMP). The imbalance of MMPs and natural inhibitors (TIMPs) seems to be a crucial factor that affects the progression of tumour.

In 1993, Lokeshwar first described the measurements of MMPs-2/-9 and TIMPs in condition media of primary prostate cancer cell cultures by enzyme assays [70]. The following year, Baker investigated the serum MMP and TIMP levels in 40 prostate cancer patients and a male control group. In his study, the serum TIMP-1 in combination with the collagenase level (MMP-1) was found to be as sensitive as PSA, as a marker of metastatic disease [71].

Gohji examined whether the serum MMP-2 level and MMP-2/prostate-volume density could be markers of prostate cancer. Serum samples were collected before any clinical treatment from 98 patients with prostate cancer and from 76 patients with BPH. Control sera were obtained from 70 healthy men. The serum level of MMP-2 was determined by enzyme immunoassay. A newly defined MMP-2 density parameter was determined by dividing the serum level of MMP-2 by the prostate volume, which was measured by ultrasonography. The mean serum level of MMP-2 in prostate cancer patients was significantly higher than in the control and BPH groups. Furthermore, the serum MMP-2 levels in prostate cancer patients with metastasis were highly elevated when compared with those without metastases. The MMP-2 density in pathologically organ-confined prostate cancer was significantly higher than that in BPH [72]. Gohji's work was corroborated by other studies [73,74]. However, these first enthusiastic reports were dampened by the study from Jung. He found that the sampling process has great influences on the MMP level, and therefore also the diagnostic validity of MMPs [75].

As mentioned above, MMPs also play an important role in physiologic processes like wound healing as well as in many different non-malignant pathological processes. Furthermore, MMP and TIMP imbalance is a phenomenon of many different types of cancer and not specific for prostate cancer. Because of that, MMPs and TIMPs seem, at the present time, not to be so useful in the initial diagnosis for prostate cancer; however, whether they could be employed in follow-up is unknown.

SERUM PROTEOMICS

When in February 2001, the human genome project was published, it became obvious that gene sequences alone cannot predict cell function or activity, and that ultimately the proteomics, the protein content and activity of the cells, has to be resolved. Recently, it has been shown that there is not necessarily any direct correlation between mRNA expression and protein level [76]. Emerging proteomic technology allows for the direct scanning of cellular proteins. Each organ and tissue perfused by blood can modify circulating proteins or peptides. Consequently, the serum proteom may reflect the abnormality or pathologic state of the organs and tissue [77].

Till date, the most commonly used proteomic tools for studying the disease-associated changes in serum is the combination of two-dimensional electrophoresis (2D-PAGE) with mass spectrometric or the protein-chip technology in combination with mass spectrometric analysis of deregulated proteins [78]. In contrast to existing screening methods, which focus on single proteins and genes such as PSA or p53, a specific protein fingerprint is produced [79]. These protein fingerprints can be correlated to standard protein fingerprints and the single peaks can be prepared for further analyses. Apart from defining significant and typical fingerprints for particular disease, another key area of the proteomic technology is the identification of potential diagnostic markers [80]. Serum, homogenised cells or any other kind of protein mixtures can be used for proteomic analysis.

Most investigations of the proteomics in prostate cancer are still on the tissue level or in cell lines [81]. Abraham and colleagues analysed cellular proteomic fingerprints from prostate cancer cells and benign epithelial prostatic epithelium, as control, isolated by microdissection. Of the over 700 proteins assessed, 40 tumour-specific changes were identified and 33 of these proteins were determined by mass spectrometry. In all malignant-benign cell proteomics comparisons, the protein profiles were highly similar [82]. In 34 radical prostatectomy specimens, Meehan generated proteomic fingerprints from malignant and benign epithelial cells and identified 20 proteins, which were lost in malignant transformation including PSA, alpha-1 antichymotrypsin (ACT), haptoglobin [83].

Banez generated the proteomic spectra from 106 prostate cancer patients and 56 healthy controls using two chip-systems and biomarker pattern software. Combined spectral data from both chips generated, achieved 85% sensitivity and 85% specificity for the detection of prostate cancer [84]. This finding is in agreement with Petricoin who found a specificity of 71% in 137 patents with PSA 4–10 ng/mL [77].

A new chapter in the early detection of prostate cancer has been started with the advent of proteomic technology. Initially, the proteomic fingerprint itself may be useful as a marker for malignancy, and additionally this technology offers the possibility for direct identification of specific proteins in malignant sera.

CONCLUSION

In conclusion, many different serum proteins have been suggested as adequate serum markers for prostrate cancer detection or as a prognostic assessment tool. Currently, two different approaches are in process to replace PSA as the gold standard prostate cancer serum marker:

1   The search for 'classic' tumour markers. Single serum proteins are investigated for diagnostic use and prognostic assessment tool. Particularly, more recent NE markers and IGF/IGFBP are under investigation.

2   Cellular and serum proteomics seem to be a new and promising technology for diagnostic use as well as for further research for new 'classic' serum markers. At present, it is too early to assess the capability of this technology, but we do expect improvements in detection, staging and monitoring of prostate cancer to result from research in this area.

However, PSA still remains the first line test for prostate cancer screening, until future investigations elucidate a more reliable candidate.

REFERENCES

1 Wang MC, Valenzuela LA, Murphy GP et al. Purification of a human prostate specific antigen. *Invest Urol* 1979; 17: 159.

2 Catalona WJ, Smith DS, Ratliff TL et al. Detection of organ-confined prostate cancer is increased through prostate-specific antigen-based screening. *JAMA* 1993; 270: 948.

3 Babaian RJ, Johnston DA, Naccarato W et al. The incidence of prostate cancer in a screening population with a serum prostate specific antigen between 2.5 and 4.0 ng/mL: relation to biopsy strategy. *J Urol* 2001; 165: 757.

4 Pretl K. Zur Frage der Endokrinie der menschlichen Vorsteherdrüse. *Virchows Arch* 1944; 312: 393.

5 di Sant'Agnese PA. Neuroendocrine differentiation in human prostatic carcinoma. *Hum Pathol* 1992; 23: 287.

6 Cussenot O, Villette JM, Cochand-Priollet B et al. Evaluation and clinical value of neuroendocrine differentiation in human prostatic tumors. *Prostate Suppl* 1998; 8: 43.

7 Aumuller G, Leonhardt M, Janssen M et al. Neurogenic origin of human prostate endocrine cells. *Urology* 1999; 53: 1041.

8 Angelsen A, Syversen U, Haugen OA et al. Neuroendocrine differentiation in carcinomas of the prostate: do neuroendocrine serum markers reflect immunohistochemical findings? *Prostate* 1997; 30: 1.

9 Weinstein MH, Partin AW, Veltri RW et al. Neuroendocrine differentiation in prostate cancer: enhanced prediction of progression after radical prostatectomy. *Hum Pathol* 1996; 27: 683.

10 Deftos LJ, Nakada S, Burton DW et al. Immunoassay and immunohistology studies of chromogranin A as a neuroendocrine marker in patients with carcinoma of the prostate. *Urology* 1996; 48: 58.

11 Chuang CK, Wu TL, Tsao KC et al. Elevated serum chromogranin A precedes prostate-specific antigen elevation and predicts failure of androgen deprivation therapy in patients with advanced prostate cancer. *J Formos Med Assoc* 2003; 102: 480.

12 Berruti A, Dogliotti L, Mosca A et al. Circulating neuroendocrine markers in patients with prostate carcinoma. *Cancer*, 2000; 88: 2590.

13 Cohen RJ, Glezerson G, Haffejee Z. Neuroendocrine cells – a new prognostic parameter in prostate cancer. *Br J Urol* 1991; 68: 258.

14 Bonkhoff H, Stein U, Remberger K. Androgen receptor status in endocrine-paracrine cell types of the normal, hyperplastic, and neoplastic human prostate. *Virchows Arch A Pathol Anat Histopathol*, 1993; 423: 291.

15 Aprikian AG, Cordon-Cardo C, Fair WR et al. Characterization of neuroendocrine differentiation in human benign prostate and prostatic adenocarcinoma. *Cancer* 1993; 71: 3952.

16 Bubendorf L, Sauter G, Moch H et al. Ki67 labelling index: an independent predictor of progression in prostate cancer treated by radical prostatectomy. *J Pathol* 1996; 178: 437.

17 Noordzij MA, van der Kwast TH, van Steenbrugge GJ et al. The prognostic influence of neuroendocrine cells in prostate cancer: results of a long-term follow-up study with patients treated by radical prostatectomy. *Int J Cancer* 1995; 62: 252.

18 Kamiya N, Akakura K, Suzuki H et al. Pretreatment serum level of neuron specific enolase (NSE) as a prognostic factor in metastatic prostate cancer patients treated with endocrine therapy. *Eur Urol* 2003; 44: 309.

19 Hvamstad T, Jordal A, Hekmat N et al. Neuroendocrine serum tumour markers in hormone-resistant prostate cancer. *Eur Urol* 2003; 44: 215.

20 Kadmon D, Thompson TC, Lynch GR et al. Elevated plasma chromogranin-A concentrations in prostatic carcinoma. *J Urol* 1991; 146: 358.

21 Tarle M, Frkovic-Grazio S, Kraljic I et al. A more objective staging of advanced prostate cancer–routine recognition of malignant endocrine structures: the assessment of serum TPS, PSA, and NSE values. *Prostate* 1994; 24: 143.

22 Yu DS, Hsieh DS, Chen HI et al. The expression of neuropeptides in hyperplastic and malignant prostate

tissue and its possible clinical implications. *J Urol* 2001; **166**: 871.

23 Ahel MZ, Kovacic K, Tarle M. Cross-correlation of serum chromogranin A, %-F-PSA and bone scans in prostate cancer diagnosis.Anticancer Res 2001; **21**: 1363.

24 Peehl DM, Cohen P, Rosenfeld RG. The insulin-like growth factor system in the prostate. *World J Urol* 1995; **13**: 306.

25 Chan JM, Stampfer MJ, Giovannucci E *et al.* Plasma insulin-like growth factor-I and prostate cancer risk: a prospective study. *Science* 1998; **279**: 563.

26 Winter DL, Hanlon AL, Raysor SL *et al.* Plasma levels of IGF-1, IGF-2, and IGFBP-3 in white and African-American men at increased risk of prostate cancer. *Urology* 2001; **58**: 614.

27 Woodson K, Tangrea JA, Pollak M *et al.* Serum insulin-like growth factor I: tumor marker or etiologic factor? A prospective study of prostate cancer among Finnish men. *Cancer Res* 2003; **63**: 3991.

28 Baffa R, Reiss K, El Gabry EA *et al.* Low serum insulin-like growth factor 1 (IGF-1): a significant association with prostate cancer. *Tech Urol* 2000; **6**: 236.

29 Peng L, Tang S, Xie J *et al.* [Quantitative analysis of IGF-1 and its application in the diagnosis of prostate cancer]. *Hua Xi Yi Ke Da Xue Xue Bao* 2002; **33**: 137.

30 Cutting CW, Hunt C, Nisbet JA *et al.* Serum insulin-like growth factor-1 is not a useful marker of prostate cancer. *BJU Int* 1999; **83**: 996.

31 Ho PJ, Baxter R. Insulin-like growth factor-binding protein-2 in patients with prostate carcinoma and benign prostatic hyperplasia. *Clin Endocrinol (Oxf)* 1997; **46**: 145.

32 Yu H, Nicar MR, Shi R *et al.* Levels of insulin-like growth factor I (IGF-I) and IGF binding proteins 2 and 3 in serial postoperative serum samples and risk of prostate cancer recurrence. *Urology* 2001; **57**: 471.

33 Miyata Y, Sakai H, Hayashi T *et al.* Serum insulin-like growth factor binding protein-3/prostate-specific antigen ratio is a useful predictive marker in patients with advanced prostate cancer. *Prostate* 2003; **54**: 125.

34 Stattin P, Stenman UH, Riboli E *et al.* Ratios of IGF-I, IGF binding protein-3,

and prostate-specific antigen in prostate cancer detection. *J Clin Endocrinol Metab* 2001; **86**: 5745.

35 Senger DR, Galli SJ, Dvorak AM *et al.* Tumor cells secrete a vascular permeability factor that promotes accumulation of ascites fluid. *Science* 1983; **219**: 983.

36 Ferrara N, Houck KA, Jakeman LB *et al.* The vascular endothelial growth factor family of polypeptides. *J Cell Biochem* 1991; **47**: 211.

37 Liu, Y, Cox SR, Morita T *et al.* Hypoxia regulates vascular endothelial growth factor gene expression in endothelial cells. Identification of a $5'$ enhancer. *Circ Res* 1995; **77**: 638.

38 Borre M, Nerstrom B, Overgaard J. Association between immunohistochemical expression of vascular endothelial growth factor (VEGF), VEGF-expressing neuroendocrine-differentiated tumor cells, and outcome in prostate cancer patients subjected to watchful waiting. *Clin Cancer Res* 2000; **6**: 1882.

39 Kohli M, Kaushal V, Spencer HJ *et al.* Prospective study of circulating angiogenic markers in prostate-specific antigen (PSA)-stable and PSA-progressive hormone-sensitive advanced prostate cancer. *Urology* 2000; **61**: 765.

40 Byrne RL, Leung H, Neal DE. Peptide growth factors in the prostate as mediators of stromal epithelial interaction. *Br J Urol* 1996; **77**: 627.

41 Miniati DN, Chang Y, Shu WP *et al.* Role of prostatic basal cells in the regulation and suppression of human prostate cancer cells. *Cancer Lett* 1996; **104**: 137.

42 Salm SN, Koikawa Y, Ogilvie V *et al.* Generation of active TGF-beta by prostatic cell cocultures using novel basal and luminal prostatic epithelial cell lines. *J Cell Physiol* 2000; **184**: 70.

43 Ilio KY, Sensibar JA, Lee C. Effect of TGF-beta 1, TGF-alpha, and EGF on cell proliferation and cell death in rat ventral prostatic epithelial cells in culture. *J Androl* 1995; **16**: 482.

44 Adler HL, Mccurdy MA, Kattan MW *et al.* Elevated levels of circulating interleukin-6 and transforming growth factor-beta1 in patients with metastatic

prostatic carcinoma. *J Urol* 1999; **161**: 182.

45 Perry KT, Anthony CT, Case T *et al.* Transforming growth factor beta as a clinical biomarker for prostate cancer. *Urology* 1997; **49**: 151.

46 Dipaola RS, Weiss RE, Cummings KB *et al.* Effect of 13-cis-retinoic acid and alpha-interferon on transforming growth factor beta1 in patients with rising prostate-specific antigen. *Clin Cancer Res* 1997; **3**: 1999.

47 Lange I, Hammerer P, Knabbe C *et al.* [Plasma TGF-beta1 concentrations in patients with prostate carcinoma or benign prostatic hyperplasia] *Urologe A* 1998; **37**: 199.

48 Wolff JM, Fandel TH, Borchers H *et al.* Serum concentrations of transforming growth factor-beta 1 in patients with benign and malignant prostatic diseases. *Anticancer Res* 1999; **19**: 2657.

49 Canto EI, Shariat SF, Slawin KM. Biochemical staging of prostate cancer. *Urol Clin North Am* 2003; **30**: 263.

50 De Vita F, Romano C, Orditura M *et al.* Interleukin-6 serum level correlates with survival in advanced gastrointestinal cancer patients but is not an independent prognostic indicator. *J Interferon Cytokine Res* 2001; **21**: 45.

51 Salgado R, Junius S, Benoy I *et al.* Circulating interleukin-6 predicts survival in patients with metastatic breast cancer. *Int J Cancer* 2003; **103**: 642.

52 Chung TD, Yu JJ, Spiotto MT *et al.* Characterization of the role of IL-6 in the progression of prostate cancer. *Prostate* 1999; **38**: 199.

53 Drachenberg DE, Elgamal AA, Rowbotham R *et al.* Circulating levels of interleukin-6 in patients with hormone refractory prostate cancer. *Prostate* 1999; **41**: 127.

54 Akimoto S, Okumura A, Fuse H. Relationship between serum levels of interleukin-6, tumor necrosis factor-alpha and bone turnover markers in prostate cancer patients. *Endocr J* 1998; **45**: 183.

55 Garcia-Moreno C, Mendez-Davila C, de La PC *et al.* Human prostatic carcinoma cells produce an increase in the synthesis of interleukin-6 by human osteoblasts. *Prostate* 2002; **50**: 241.

56 Nakashima J, Tachibana M, Horiguchi Y *et al.* Serum interleukin 6 as a prognostic factor in patients with prostate cancer. *Clin Cancer Res* 2000; **6**: 2702.

57 Twillie DA, Eisenberger MA, Carducci MA *et al.* Interleukin-6: a candidate mediator of human prostate cancer morbidity. *Urology* 1995; **45**: 542.

58 Wysocki AB, Staiano CL, Grinnell F. Wound fluid from chronic leg ulcers contains elevated levels of metalloproteinases MMP-2 and MMP-9. *J Invest Dermatol* 1993; **101**: 64.

59 Mikuni TY, Cheng YS. Metalloproteinases in endochondral bone formation: appearance of tissue inhibitor-resistant metalloproteinases. *Arch Biochem Biophys* 1987; **259**: 576.

60 Huppertz B, Kertschanska S, Demir AY *et al.* Immunohistochemistry of matrix metalloproteinases (MMP), their substrates, and their inhibitors (TIMP) during trophoblast invasion in the human placenta. *Cell Tissue Res* 1998; **291**: 133.

61 Mikuni TY, Cheng YS. Metalloproteinases in endochondral bone formation: appearance of tissue inhibitor-resistant metalloproteinases. *Arch Biochem Biophys* 1987; **259**: 576.

62 Ahrens D, Koch AE, Pope RM *et al.* Expression of matrix metalloproteinase 9 (96-kd gelatinase B) in human rheumatoid arthritis. *Arthritis Rheum* 1996; **39**: 1576.

63 Arthur MJ. Collagenases and liver fibrosis. *J Hepatol* 1995; **22**: 43.

64 Karakiulakis G, Papanikolaou C, Jankovic SM *et al.* Increased type IV collagen-degrading activity in metastases originating from primary tumors of the human colon. *Invasion Metastasis* 1997; **17**: 158.

65 Bachmeier BE, Nerlich AG, Lichtinghagen R *et al.* Matrix metalloproteinases (MMPs) in breast cancer cell lines of different tumorigenicity. *Anticancer Res* 2001; **21**: 3821.

66 Pagenstecher A, Wussler EM, Opdenakker G *et al.* Distinct expression patterns and levels of enzymatic activity of matrix metalloproteinases and their inhibitors in primary brain tumors. *J Neuropathol Exp Neurol* 2001; **60**: 598.

67 Brehmer B, Biesterfeld S, Jakse G. Expression of matrix metalloproteinases (MMP-2 and -9) and their inhibitors (TIMP-1 and -2) in prostate cancer tissue. *Prostate Cancer Prostatic Dis* 2003; **6**: 217.

68 Wilson MJ, Sellers RG, Wiehr C *et al.* Expression of matrix metalloproteinase-2 and -9 and their inhibitors, tissue inhibitor of metalloproteinase-1 and -2, in primary cultures of human prostatic stromal and epithelial cells. *J Cell Physiol* 2002; **191**: 208.

69 Varani J, Hattori Y, Dame MK *et al.* Matrix metalloproteinases (MMPs) in fresh human prostate tumour tissue and organcultured prostate tissue: levels of collagenolytic and gelatinolytic MMPs are low, variable and different in fresh tissue versus organ-cultured tissue. *Br J Cancer* 2001; **84**: 1076.

70 Lokeshwar BL, Selzer MG, Block NL *et al.* Secretion of matrix metalloproteinases and their inhibitors (tissue inhibitor of metalloproteinases) by human prostate in explant cultures: reduced tissue inhibitor of metalloproteinase secretion by malignant tissues. *Cancer Res* 1993; **53**: 4493.

71 Baker T, Tickle S, Wasan H *et al.* Serum metalloproteinases and their inhibitors: markers for malignant potential. *Br J Cancer* 1994; **70**: 506.

72 Gohji K, Fujimoto N, Hara I *et al.* Serum matrix metalloproteinase-2 and its density in men with prostate cancer as a new predictor of disease extension. *Int J Cancer* 1998; **79**: 96.

73 Kanoh Y, Akahoshi T, Ohara T *et al.* Expression of matrix metalloproteinase-2 and prostate-specific antigen in localized and metastatic prostate cancer. *Anticancer Res* 2002; **22**: 1813.

74 Zucker S, Hymowitz M, Conner C *et al.* Measurement of matrix metalloproteinases and tissue inhibitors of metalloproteinases in blood and tissues. Clinical and experimental applications. *Ann N Y Acad Sci* 1999; **878**: 212.

75 Jung K, Lein M, Laube C *et al.* Blood specimen collection methods influence the concentration and the diagnostic validity of matrix metalloproteinase 9 in blood. *Clin Chim Acta* 2001; **314**: 241.

76 Anderson L, Seilhamer J. A comparison of selected mRNA and protein abundances in human liver. *Electrophoresis* 1997; **18**: 533.

77 Petricoin EF, III, Ornstein DK, Paweletz CP *et al.* Serum proteomic patterns for detection of prostate cancer. *J Natl Cancer Inst* 2002; **94**: 1576.

78 Paweletz CP, Liotta LA, Petricoin EF, III. New technologies for biomarker analysis of prostate cancer progression: laser capture microdissection and tissue proteomics. *Urology* 2001; **57**: 160.

79 Conrads TP, Veenstra TD. The utility of proteomic patterns for the diagnosis of cancer. *Curr Drug Targets Immune Endocr Metabol Disord* 2004; **4**: 41.

80 Issaq HJ, Veenstra TD, Conrads TP *et al.* The SELDI-TOF MS approach to proteomics: protein profiling and biomarker identification. *Biochem Biophys Res Commun* 2002; **292**: 587.

81 Griffin TJ, Lock CM, Li XJ *et al.* Abundance ratio-dependent proteomic analysis by mass spectrometry. *Anal Chem* 2003; **75**: 867.

82 Ahram M, Best CJ, Flaig MJ *et al.* Proteomic analysis of human prostate cancer. *Mol Carcinog* 2002; **33**: 9.

83 Meehan KL, Holland JW, Dawkins HJ. Proteomic analysis of normal and malignant prostate tissue to identify novel proteins lost in cancer. *Prostate* 2002; **50**: 54.

84 Banez LL, Prasanna P, Sun L *et al.* Diagnostic potential of serum proteomic patterns in prostate cancer. *J Urol* 2003; **170**: 442.

4: The History of Tissue Recombination Technology: Current and Future Research

Kenichiro Ishii and Simon Hayward

INTRODUCTION

This chapter outlines the historical applications of tissue recombination technology with particular reference to prostatic research. Techniques used to examine the molecular mechanisms of stromal-epithelial interactions are described. Recent examples are used to illustrate and provide references for these methods. New technological innovations have increased the flexibility of tissue recombination allowing us to experimentally manipulate specific molecular pathways. These methods include developments in transgenic and gene knockout mouse technology and new efficient gene delivery and expression systems. A development with profound implications for future work is the use of small interfering RNA molecules (siRNA) to silence gene expression, an area that historically has been more problematic than the overexpression of genes in a controlled manner. Combinations of these approaches have the potential to transform our understanding of the basis of intercellular communication and to point the way towards new approaches with which to manage benign and malignant proliferative conditions.

The prostate, like most visceral organs, is composed of epithelial and stromal tissue layers, which communicate with each other to provide instructive and permissive information. Interactions between the stromal/mesenchymal and epithelial tissue layers of organs have long been recognised as critical determinants of development [1]. Stromal changes are also believed to be involved in non-malignant proliferative conditions such as benign prostatic hyperplasia (BPH) [2] and to play a role in the regulation of tumour progression [3–7]. The complex interactions between tissues and their interactions with the whole animal in an *in vivo* environment cannot be approached in any *in vitro* system. Thus, *in vivo* models have played a key role in expanding our understanding of the complex pathways involved in development and malignancy. An important contribution to this knowledge base has been provided by the use of tissue recombinations, which allow the manipulation of individual tissues to determine their overall effect on the organ.

In Vivo Modelling of Stromal-Epithelial Interactions

In vivo studies of the interactions between stromal and epithelial cells date back at least three decades. The methods that have been developed reflect the interests of the biologists who were working in this area. *In vivo* approaches can be subdivided according to the type of graft. Direct grafting of epithelial cells and structures to hosts allows interactions between the host stroma and epithelial cells of interest, while grafting of tissue fragments allows continued tissue-specific interactions. Such approaches do not, however, allow for manipulations of the interactions between epithelial and stromal cells. In contrast, tissue recombination allows an investigator to bring together defined epithelial and mesenchymal cell populations, and to determine how these cells respond to each other.

A number of graft sites have been utilised for *in vivo* studies, these include the developing chick chorio-allantoic membrane as well as the intra-ocular, sub-renal capsule, sub-cutaneous and orthotopic sites in rodents. Currently, the most commonly used are the sub-cutaneous and sub-renal capsule sites. Grafting to these locations is well tolerated by the hosts. Sub-cutaneous grafting is not very efficient, presumably because the site is poorly vascularised, but can be improved by using the extracellular matrix extract Matrigel, which encourages the growth of blood vessels towards the graft. The renal capsule is a highly vascularised and much more efficient graft site, however surgery to the renal capsule is technically more demanding. The prostatic orthotopic site is also technically difficult to access and additionally has limited capacity, however, this is the graft site of choice for investigating specific processes such as metastasis.

Graft site efficiency is an important consideration in many applications. For example, it is difficult to undertake translational studies if the graft site is not efficient. A recent communication compared the efficiency of grafting human prostate cancer tissues to the renal capsule and sub-cutaneous sites of severe combined immunodeficient (SCID) mice and, determined that in the hands of a skilled investigator the take rate of human prostate tissue samples was 58% (50/86) in sub-cutaneous grafts, 72% (41/57) at the anterior prostate orthotopic site and 93% (114/122) when tissue from the same patients was grafted to the renal capsule of the same mice [8]. This study illustrates the reason for using the renal capsule site and, along with other technical improvements has given rise to the development of a new, highly efficient model with which to pursue translational studies on human prostate cancer tissues in an *in vivo* environment.

Tissue Recombination

Tissue recombination has been widely applied to the developmental biology of the urogenital tract. Tissue recombinants are made by mixing stromal or mesenchymal cells as tissues or separated by enzymic digestion into single cells [9–13]. The recombinants are then grafted beneath the renal capsule of a rodent host. The choice of host is determined by a number of considerations. Recombinants that use tissues derived exclusively from an inbred strain can be grafted back to syngeneic hosts. However, recombinants using tissues from outbred animals or from humans require the use of immunocompromised (nude or SCID) hosts. Human prostatic tumours have long been known to be immunogenic in nude mice [14]. Therefore, samples containing human cells with malignant potential are best grafted to SCID hosts. The *in vivo* environment provided by the rodent host can be modified, for example, by treating hosts with androgens or anti-androgens to manipulate the hormonal environment or with systemic drugs. After a period of growth and development the host is sacrificed and the graft harvested for analysis.

In general, recombinants can be made using mesenchymal and epithelial cells from the same tissue (homotypic) or from different tissues (heterotypic). Mesenchymal and epithelial cells can be derived from the same species (homospecific) or from different species (heterospecific). Conceptually, it is important to note that epithelial and stromal tissues communicate in ways that can be 'understood' across species barriers. Thus, as an example, embryonic rat urogenital sinus mesenchyme can reprogram adult human bladder epithelium to undergo prostatic differentiation, demonstrating a strong level of conservation in the signalling mechanisms between humans and rats [15]. A major advantage of heterospecific recombinants is easy confirmation that epithelial or stromal tissue is derived from a particular source by testing its species of origin. Heterospecific recombinants also allow experimental manipulation of stromal cells. Thus it is possible, for example, to explore the effects of specific pathways on human epithelium by recombining mesenchyme from a transgenic mouse with human epithelial cells, allowing an investigation of the effects of specific paracrine pathways on human cells. A generalised summary of the tissue recombination technique is presented in Fig. 4.1.

Interactions between epithelial and mesenchymal cells are classified as permissive or instructive [16]. A permissive effect supports a previously executed developmental program. An example would be the support of differentiation and secretory activity of human prostatic epithelial organoids by

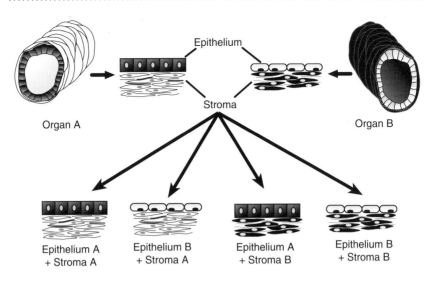

Fig. 4.1 Summary of the technique of tissue recombination. Stromal and epithelial tissues are separated from each other and isolated. The tissues are then recombined in either homotypic (stromal and epithelial cells from the same organ) or heterotypic (stromal and epithelial cells from different organs) combinations.

rodent sub-cutaneous fibroblasts [17]. In contrast, an instructive effect elicits a new program of differentiation. Instructive interactions were first described in the context of normal development [18]. However, it is now clear that foetal mesenchyme is capable of reprogramming the developmental profile of adult epithelia, for example, urogenital sinus mesenchyme can induce prostatic differentiation in adult bladder epithelium [19,20].

In the context of prostatic research, and indeed for all sex-steroid target organs in the male and female genital tract, one of the most important findings to emerge from tissue recombination studies is an understanding of the mechanistic basis for the action of sex-steroid hormones. For many years, there was a tacit assumption that androgenic, oestrogenic and progestogenic effects on epithelial cells resulted directly from the action of these hormones on receptors located in the epithelial cells. A classical series of experiments using testicular feminised (Tfm) mice (that cannot express a functional androgen receptor) demonstrated that gland morphogenesis depends on mesenchymally localised androgen receptor and is independent of the presence of epithelial androgen receptor [21,22]. Prostatic epithelial cells that could not express the androgen receptor also did not express any characteristic secretory markers [23], underlining the role for epithelial receptors in differentiated function.

Oestrogen receptor-α and progesterone receptor deficient strains, have been used more recently in tissue recombination models to perform a detailed examination of the role of oestrogens and progestins in the male and female urogenital tracts. These studies have demonstrated that in these organs, sex-steroid hormones exert control of epithelial proliferation (in a positive and a negative manner) and also control epithelial apoptosis via paracrine mechanisms resulting from effects on mesenchymally located receptors [24–26]. In contrast, control of differentiated epithelial functions (e.g. cornification of vaginal epithelium) seems to be a result of the action of steroid hormones on receptors located in the epithelial cells.

Recent *in vivo* studies using a sub-cutaneous grafting model have confirmed that control of benign prostatic epithelial differentiation, requires the presence of stromal androgen receptors. By using a Tfm nude mouse, the authors were able to demonstrate that prostate cancer can respond directly to androgenic stimulation by increasing its proliferation [27]. Thus, one of the important differences between benign and malignant prostate is the manner in which androgenic signalling is processed into regulation of proliferation.

Tissue Recombination and Prostate Cancer

The use of tissue recombination experiments to investigate prostate cancer falls into two types of experiments. First, those aimed at examining the nature of the interactions between stromal and epithelial cells in prostate tumours; and, second, recombination experiments aimed at generating models of prostatic carcinogenesis.

The nature of stromal cells surrounding prostate tumours has been observed to be somewhat different from that seen in the normal prostate. Adult human prostatic stroma is composed of a fibromuscular matrix surrounding the prostatic ducts. These stromal cells express androgen receptors (AR) and respond to androgens by restraining prostatic epithelial proliferation [28]. In contrast, the stromal cells surrounding a prostate tumour are more typically of a fibroblastic or myofibroblastic nature [4,6,29–31]. This change in the stromal microenvironment gives rise to what has been termed 'carcinoma-associated fibroblasts' or a 'reactive stroma'. These stromal cells do not appear to restrict epithelial cell proliferation. Thus when an immortalised human prostatic epithelial cell line is recombined with urogenital sinus mesenchyme from a foetal rat there is a brief period of growth giving rise to glandular structures, which become effectively growth quiescent over a long period [32]. In contrast, tissue recombinants composed of the same prostatic epithelial cell line and carcinoma-associated fibroblasts derived from human prostate tumours give rise to large poorly differentiated tumours [33]. Thus, rather than acting to repress epithelial proliferation (as would be expected of normal prostatic stroma) the stromal cells surrounding a human prostate tumour seem able to enhance the process of carcinogenesis in a tissue recombination model. Our most recent data suggest that interactions between carcinoma-associated fibroblasts and genetically initiated human prostatic epithelial cells give rise to permanent and characteristic genetic changes in the epithelium, which are associated with malignant transformation of the epithelial cells [34,35].

One of the first sets of experiments to test the idea that stromal cells may facilitate prostatic carcinogenesis was performed in a tissue recombination system by Thompson and colleagues. In these experiments either the urogenital sinus (prostatic anlagen) or its individual mesenchymal (UGM) or epithelial (UGE) components were transfected using a virus carrying the *myc* and *ras* oncogenes. In tissue recombinants containing un-infected UGM and infected UGE, epithelial hyperplasias were detected. Similarly, in prostatic reconstitutions composed of infected UGM plus un-infected UGE, stromal desmoplasias were observed. Carcinomas were found only in recombinants in which both UGM and UGE were infected [12,36,37]. These findings demonstrated that in this model changes were required in both the epithelium and in stromal microenvironment for prostatic carcinogenesis to occur. These experiments are also important because they illustrate the use of viral vectors to introduce genes of interest into either epithelial or stromal cells in tissue recombinants. In more recent studies, we and others have demonstrated that over expression of myc in benign adult human epithelium is sufficient to immortalise the cells [38,39] and to elicit malignant transformation allowing us to generate a metastatic tumour model from a tissue recombinant [39].

Cell rescue by tissue recombination

In many cases the use of transgenic and gene knockout technology has resulted in the generation of a perinatal or embryonic-lethal phenotype. Quite commonly this is not due to problems in the tissue of interest, but results in such tissues being unavailable because of loss of the foetus. In such cases, it is often possible to rescue tissues of interest or their embryonic precursors. These tissues can be grown as sub-renal capsule grafts in athymic mouse hosts and then used as a source of tissue for the manufacturing of tissue recombinants to amplify cells of interest. A recent example of the rescue of adult tissue from a perinatally lethal mutation resulted in the characterization of the Fox A null prostate demonstrating the critical role that forkhead box transcription factors play in prostatic development and differentiation [40]. More technically complex is the rescue of adult tissues from mutants that die embroynically even before the organ rudiments have formed. An example of such a problem is the rescue of cloacal tissue from retinoblastoma (*Rb*) gene null foetuses. Rb-deficient foetuses die at about 14 days of gestation before the formation of the prostate [41]. Cloacal tissue dissected from the foetuses and grafted beneath the renal capsule of male athymic mice, gives rise to Rb-deficient prostate, bladder, seminal vesicle and a range of other tissues [42]. Such tissues can then be used in tissue recombinants to examine the role of the *Rb* gene in processes such as organ development and carcinogenesis [42]. These studies established that Rb is not required for prostate formation and Rb-deficient prostate is extremely sensitive to hormonal carcinogens, producing a model that follows the human pattern of prostate cancer progression. Tissue recombinants were also used as a source from which to generate the first Rb-deficient epithelial cell line [43]. Such work highlights the idea that tissue recombinations can be used to examine mesenchyma and epithelia from the huge variety of gene knockout and transgenic sources now available.

Current Practice and Future Directions

The role of tissue microenvironment in cancer progression is starting to receive increased attention. Thus, there will be fresh impetus to develop new methods with which to examine and manipulate interactions between stromal and epithelial cells. Many of these methods will also have applications in the study of development and of the biology of benign disease.

As described above, the availability of transgenic and gene knockout technologies add to the flexibility of the tissue recombination technique. Genetic manipulation of cells in culture through traditional transfection methods or by the increasingly popular and highly efficient retroviral and adenoviral approaches lend the ability to manipulate the various cell populations at will (summarised in Fig. 4.2). Gene expression in target cells can be controlled by constitutively active promoters such as cytomegalovirus or by conditional promoters. Conditional promoters fall into two main groups; cell-type specific promoters, which are reasonably well developed for these applications. These include the various forms of the probasin promoter, the Prostate specific antigen (PSA) promoter and cytokeratin promoters targeted at luminal or basal epithelial cells. Stromal cell promoters are less common, although some, such as the various smooth muscle protein promoters, are well characterised. Newer promoters, such as ps20 (Rowley, personal communication) and mts1/S100A4/FSP [44], may become available in the foreseeable future. The second group of promoters are inducible. Examples would include the metallothionein system, in which gene expression is triggered by the presence of metal ions. This system has been used for many years. *In vivo*, this promoter is activated by adding zinc to drinking water. The metallothionein system is not organ specific and it is leaky in the sense that cellular concentrations of zinc can trigger metallothionein promoter activity. It should be noted

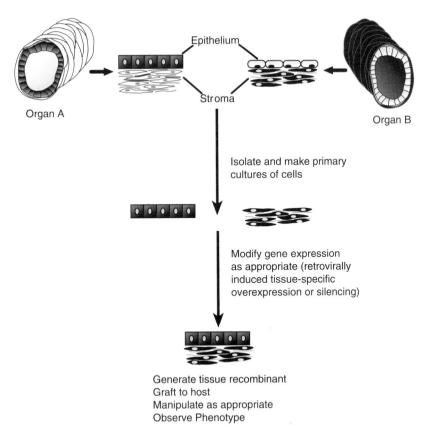

Fig. 4.2 Generic scheme for genetic manipulation in a tissue recombinant. Stromal and epithelial cells or tissues from either human or rodent sources are separated from each other and isolated. The cells can then be genetically modified *in vitro* and recombined to examine the effects of the overexpression or silencing of specific genes.

that the prostate contains high concentrations of zinc that can trigger the metallothionein promoter in the absence of an external stimulus. A number of other regulatable systems are available, including the tet-on/tet-off system, in which gene expression can be induced or suppressed by tetracycline or its analogue doxycycline [45,46]. The main disadvantage of this system is the need to insert the gene of interest and the tet-regulatable element. Another interesting and more tightly regulated promoter is the RU486 inducible system [47]. Ecdysone-based regulatable promoters are also available. These are extremely tightly regulated but are prohibitively expensive for *in vivo* models.

Molecular manipulation of cells in tissue recombinants has been used in the past to investigate the role of oncogenes in prostatic carcinogenesis [12] and the role of growth factors in prostatic development [48,49]. The advent of new retroviral and lentiviral systems is set to allow the development of new

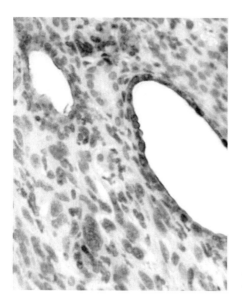

Fig. 4.3 Immunohistochemical localisation of a retrovirally infected cell line demonstrating the ability to detect expression of green fluorescent protein when co-expressed with a gene of interest within a tissue recombinant.

models of carcinogenesis, using tested approaches such as the introduction of oncogenic proteins, such as SV40 T antigen, or the introduction of proteins believed, on the basis of expression patterns, to play a role in carcinogenesis *in vivo*. This approach will also allow the dissection of the role of specific mitogens and morphogens in development, carcinogenesis and in tumour progression. One of the refinements allowed by the present generation of vectors is the use of an internal ribosomal entry sequence (IRES), which allows the co-expression of reporter proteins along with the gene of interest. The use of fluorescent protein markers, such as green fluorescent protein (GFP), allows for detection and selection of cells in culture expressing the virally introduced gene of interest and further allows for simple immunohistochemical detection of such infected cells following harvesting and fixation of grafts as shown in Fig. 4.3.

Silencing of genes has historically proven to be more problematic than their overexpression. Recent developments in the use of siRNA molecules have the potential for rapid developments in this area. Short hairpin RNA sequences 21–23 nucleotides in length can be used to efficiently downregulate gene expression *in vitro*, a process that goes by the unfortunate acronym of SHAGging (short-hairpin-activated gene silencing) [50]. Expression of siRNA molecules is driven by the U6 promoter (pSHAG1) or the H1-RNA promoter (pSUPER) [51] to generate double stranded RNA molecules, which can specifically downregulate gene expression. A number of laboratories have developed these promoter systems for use with retroviral gene delivery systems containing other selectable markers with which to modify gene expression in tissue recombinants.

As with retroviral introduction of genes, gene silencing allows a detailed dissection of molecular pathways involved in a variety of developmental and disease processes. A particular advantage of this technique is that it has the potential to be used to examine the biology of metastasis promoters in *in vivo* systems, thus allowing all phases of cancer progression from initiation to metastasis to be examined within a single *in vivo* model system.

An application of tissue recombinants that is currently being discussed but which, to our knowledge, has not been applied at the time of writing, is the use of this technology as a rapid screening tool with which to establish the value of making transgenic or gene knockout mice. Since it is now possible to either overexpress or to silence genes of interest in particular tissue types, it is possible to use tissue recombinants as a means to rapidly determine whether a given genetic modification is likely to give rise to a phenotype of interest in an organ. Thus, tissue recombination could be used to pre-validate the generation of transgenic or gene knockout mice, thus saving valuable resources by selecting the most likely successes and screening out the likely failures. We have recently described proof of principle experiments demonstrating the feasibility of this approach [52].

SUMMARY

Tissue recombination has many advantages. A major incentive to use this method is that cells can grow in an experimentally manipulatable *in vivo* environment. Another incentive is that epithelial and stromal cells have normal interactions with each other (or interactions modified according to the experimental design). Thus, for example this technique allows, prostatic epithelium to grow in the context of a prostatic stromal environment, to some extent obviating the appeal of using an orthotopic graft site, which in many cases is technically far more challenging than the sub-renal capsule site normally used for recombinants. A third major advantage is the enormous flexibility of the system. Mesenchymal and epithelial cells from a huge range of sources can be used. The availability of transgenic and gene knockout mice allows molecular pathways to be dissected. Cells can also be modified in culture and then used in recombinants.

A number of important biological principles have been established and confirmed by the technique of tissue and cell recombination. These include the concept that the differentiation of epithelial cells is dictated and supported by the local mesenchymal environment, the idea that adult epithelial cells retain an ability to respond to foetal inductive influences and the idea that steroid hormones elicit control of proliferation of benign epithelia via paracrine mechanisms, while differentiated functions of the epithelial cells rely on stimulation of receptors within the epithelium.

Rapid advances in molecular biology and in genetic control systems are continuing to expand the scope of the various *in vitro* and *in vivo* methods. Therefore, at this time we are limited only by our ability to devise informative experiments.

ACKNOWLEDGEMENTS

We are grateful to Dr David Rowley (Baylor College of Medicine) for permission to comment on unpublished data and to Dr Karin Williams for Fig. 4.3. This work was supported in part by NIH grant CA96403 and Department of Defense Prostate Cancer Research Program Grant DAMD 17-02-1-0151.

REFERENCES

1 Cunha GR, Chung LWK, Shannon JM, Reese BA. Stromal-epithelial interactions in sex differentiation. *Biol Reprod.* 1980; **22**: 19–43.

2 McNeal JE. Prostate anatomy and BPH morphogenisis. *Prog Clin Biol Res* 1984; **145**: 27–54.

3 Hodges GM, Hicks RM, Spacey GD. Epithelial-stromal interactions in normal and chemical carcinogen-treated adult bladder. *Cancer Res* 1977; **37**: 3720–30.

4 Tuxhorn JA, Ayala GE, Rowley DR. Reactive stroma in prostate cancer progression. *J Urol* 2001; **166**: 2472–83.

5 Ronnov-Jessen L, Petersen OW, Bissell MJ. Cellular changes involved in conversion of normal to malignant breast: importance of the stromal reaction. *Physiol Rev* 1996; **76**: 69–125.

6 Hayward SW, Rosen MA, Cunha GR. Stromal-epithelial interactions in normal and neoplastic prostate. *Br J Urology* 1997; **79**: 18–26.

7 Chung LW. The role of stromal-epithelial interaction in normal and malignant growth. *Cancer Surv* 1995; **23**: 33–42.

8 Wang Y, Revelo MP, Sudilovsky D, *et al.* Development and characterization of efficient xenograft models for benign and malignant human prostate tissue. *Prostate* 2005; **64**: 149–59.

9 Cunha GR, Donjacour AA. Mesenchymal-epithelial interactions: Technical considerations. In: Coffey DS, Bruchovsky N, Gardner WA, Resnick MI & Karr JP, eds. *Assessment of Current Concepts and Approaches to the Study of Prostate Cancer.* New York: AR Liss, 1987: 273–82.

10 Hayward SW, Haughney PC, Rosen MA, *et al.* Interactions between adult human prostatic epithelium and rat urogenital sinus mesenchyme in a tissue recombination model. *Differentiation* 1998; **63**: 131–40.

11 Haughney PC, Hayward SW, Dahiya R, Cunha GR. Species-specific detection of growth factor gene expression in developing prostatic tissue. *Biol of Reprod* 1998; **59**: 93–9.

12 Thompson TC, Southgate J, Kitchener G, Land H. Multistage carcinogenesis induced by *ras* and *myc* oncogenes in a reconstituted organ. *Cell* 1989; **56**: 917–30.

13 Hayward SW, Haughney PC, Lopes ES, Danielpour D, Cunha GR. The rat prostatic epithelial cell line NRP-152 can differentiate *in vivo* in response to its stromal environment. *Prostate* 1999; **39**: 205–12.

14 Reid LM, Minato N, Gresser I, Holland J, Kadish A, Bloom BR. Influence of anti-mouse interferon serum on the growth and metastasis of tumor cells persistently infected with virus and of human prostatic tumors in athymic nude mice. *Proc Natl Acad Sci* USA 1981; **78**: 1171–5.

15 Aboseit S, El-Sakha A, Young P, Cunha G. Mesenchymal reprogramming of adult human epithelial differentiation. *Differentiation* 1999; **65**: 113–8.

16 Haffen K, Kedinger M, Simon-Assmann P. Mesenchyme-dependent differentiation of epithelial progenitor cells in the gut. *J Pediatr Gastroenterol. Nutr.* 1987; **6**: 14–23.

17 Hayward SW, Del Buono R, Hall PA, Deshpande N. A functional model of human prostate epithelium: the role of androgens and stroma in architectural organisation and the maintenance of differentiated secretory function. *J Cell Sci* 1992; **102**: 361–72.

18 Cunha GR, Alarid ET, Turner T, Donjacour AA, Boutin EL, Foster BA. Normal and abnormal development of the male urogenital tract: role of androgens, mesenchymal-epithelial interactions and growth factors. *J Androl* 1992; **13**: 465–75.

19 Cunha GR, Fujii H, Neubauer BL, Shannon JM, Sawyer LM, Reese BA. Epithelial-mesenchymal interactions in prostatic development. I. Morphological observations of prostatic induction by urogenital sinus mesenchyme in epithelium of the adult rodent urinary bladder. *J Cell Biol.* 1983; **96**: 1662–70.

20 Neubauer BL, Chung LWK, McCormick KA, Taguchi O, Thompson TC, Cunha GR. Epithelial-mesenchymal interactions in prostatic development. II. Biochemical observations of prostatic induction by urogenital sinus mesenchyme in epithelium of the adult rodent urinary bladder. *J Cell Biol* 1983; **96**: 1671–6.

21 Cunha GR, Chung LWK. Stromal-epithelial interactions: I. Induction of prostatic phenotype in urothelium of testicular feminized (Tfm/y) mice. *J Steroid Biochem* 1981; **14**: 1317–21.

22 Cunha G, Lung B. The possible influences of temporal factors in androgenic responsiveness of urogenital tissue recombinants from wild-type and androgen-insensitive (Tfm) mice. *J Exp Zool* 1978; **205**: 181–94.

23 Donjacour AA, Cunha GR. Assessment of prostatic protein secretion in tissue recombinants made of urogenital sinus mesenchyme and urothelium from normal or androgen-insensitive mice. *Endocrinology* 1993; **131**: 2342–50.

24 Kurita T, Young P, Brody J, Lydon JP, O'Malley BW, Cunha GR. Stromal progesterone receptors mediate the inhibitory effects of progesterone on estrogen-induced uterine epithelial cell (UtE) proliferation. *Endocrinology* 1998; **139**: 4708–13.

25 Buchanan DL, Kurita T, Taylor JA, Lubahn DL, Cunha GR, Cooke PS. Role of stromal and epithelial estrogen receptors in vaginal epithelial proliferation, stratification and cornification. *Endocrinology* 1998; **139**: 4345–52.

26 Kurita T, Wang YZ, Donjacour AA, et al. Paracrine regulation of apoptosis by steroid hormones in the male and female reproductive system. *Cell Death Differ* 2001; **8**: 192–200.

27 Gao J, Arnold JT, Isaacs JT. Conversion from a paracrine to an autocrine mechanism of androgen-stimulated growth during malignant transformation of prostatic epithelial cells. *Cancer Res* 2001; **61**: 5038–44.

28 Hayward SW, Cunha GR. The prostate: development and physiology. *Radiol Clin North Am* 2000; **38**: 1–14.

29 Hayward SW, Cunha GR, Dahiya R. Normal development and carcinogenesis of the prostate: a unifying hypothesis. *Ann N Y Acad Sci* 1996; **784**: 50–62.

30 Arnold JT, Isaacs JT. Mechanisms involved in the progression of androgen-independent prostate cancers: it is not only the cancer cell's fault. *Endocr Relat Cancer* 2002; **9**: 61–73.

31 Rowley DR. What might a stromal response mean to prostate cancer progression? *Cancer Metastasis Rev* 1998; **17**: 411–9.

32 Wang YZ, Sudilovsky D, Zhang B, et al. A Human prostatic epithelial model of hormonal carcinogenesis. *Cancer Res* 2001; **61**: 6064–72.

33 Olumi AF, Grossfeld GD, Hayward SW, Carroll PR, Tlsty TD, Cunha GR. Carcinoma-associated fibroblasts direct tumor progression of initiated human prostatic epithelium. *Cancer Res.* 1999; **59**: 5002–11.

34 Phillips JL, Hayward SW, Wang Y, et al. The consequences of chromosomal aneuploidy on gene expression profiles in a cell line model for prostate

carcinogenesis. *Cancer Res* 2001; **61**: 8143–9.

35 Hayward SW, Wang Y, Cao M, *et al.* Malignant transformation in a nontumorigenic human prostatic epithelial cell line. *Cancer Res* 2001; **61**: 8135–42.

36 Thompson TC. Growth factors and oncogenes in prostate cancer. *Cancer Cells* 1990; **11**: 345–54.

37 Thompson TC, Timme TL, Kadmon D, Park SH, Egawa S, Yoshida K. Genetic predisposition and mesenchymal-epithelial interactions in ras+myc-induced carcinogenesis in reconstituted mouse prostate. *Molec Carcinogenesis* 1993; **7**: 165–79.

38 Gil J, Kerai P, Lleonart M, *et al.* Immortalization of primary human prostate epithelial cells by c-Myc. *Cancer Res* 2005; **65**: 2179–85.

39 Williams K, Fernandez S, Stien X, *et al.* Unopposed c-MYC expression in benign prostatic epithelium causes a cancer phenotype. *Prostate* 2005; **63**: 369–84.

40 Gao N, Ishii K, Mirosevich J, *et al.* Forkhead box A1 regulates prostate ductal morphogenesis and promotes epithelial cell maturation. *Development* 2005; **132**: 3431–43.

41 Jacks T, Fazeli A, Schmitt EM, Bronson RT, Goodell MA, Weinberg RA. Effects of an *Rb* mutation in the mouse. *Nature* 1992; **359**: 295–300.

42 Wang Y, Hayward S, Donjacour A, *et al.* Sex hormone-induced carcinogenesis in Rb-deficient prostate tissue. *Cancer Res* 2000; **60**: 6008–17.

43 Day K, McCabe M, Zhao X, *et al.* Rescue of embryonic epithelium reveals that the Rb-/- genotype confers growth factor independence and immortality, but does not influence epithelial differentiation or tissue morphogenesis. *J Biol Chem* 2002; **277**: 44475–84.

44 Cohn MA, Hjelmso I, Wu LC, Guldberg P, Lukanidin EM, Tulchinsky

EM. Characterization of Sp1, AP-1, CBF and KRC binding sites and minisatellite DNA as functional elements of the metastasis-associated mts1/S100A4 gene intronic enhancer. *Nucleic Acids Res* 2001; **29**: 3335–46.

45 Furth P, St Onge L, Boger H, *et al.* Temporal control of gene expression in transgenic mice by a tetracycline-responsive promoter. *Proc Natl Acad Sci* USA 1994; **91**: 9302–6.

46 Schockett PE, Schatz DG. Diverse strategies for tetracycline-regulated inducible gene expression. *Proc Natl Acad Sci* USA 1996; **93**: 5173–6.

47 Oligino T, Poliani PL, Wang Y, *et al.* Drug inducible transgene expression in brain using a herpes simplex virus vector. *Gene Ther* 1998; **5**: 491–6.

48 Yang G, Timme TL, Park SH, Wu X, Wyllie MG, Thompson TC. Transforming growth factor beta 1 transduced mouse prostate reconstitutions: II. Induction of apoptosis by doxazosin [see comments]. *Prostate* 1997; **33**: 157–63.

49 Yang G, Timme TL, Park SH, Thompson TC. Transforming growth factor beta 1 transduced mouse prostate reconstitutions: I. Induction of neuronal phenotypes [see comments]. *Prostate* 1997; **33**: 151–6.

50 Paddison PJ, Caudy AA, Bernstein E, Hannon GJ, Conklin DS. Short hairpin RNAs (shRNAs) induce sequence-specific silencing in mammalian cells. *Genes Dev* 2002; **16**: 948–58.

51 Brummelkamp TR, Bernards R, Agami R. A system for stable expression of short interfering RNAs in mammalian cells. *Science* 2002; **296**: 550–3.

52 Ishii K, Shappell SB, Matusik RJ, Hayward SW. The use of tissue recombination to predict phenotypes of transgenic mouse models of prostate carcinoma. *Lab Invest* 2005; **85**: 1086–103.

5: Why We Cannot Use the Results of Non-Randomised Trials to Inform Us About Treatment for Early Prostate Cancer

Malcolm Mason and John Staffurth

THE NATURAL HISTORY OF PROSTATE CANCER IS UNCLEAR

The Finasteride Study

Nothing illustrates the dilemma of early prostate cancer better than the Finasteride prevention study [1]. The intention of this trial was to prevent prostate cancer using the 5-alpha reductase inhibitor, Finasteride. To do this, using a double-blind randomised trial, routine biopsies were taken in men who did not develop clinically or biochemically evident disease. The trial was powered on the expectation of a 6% incidence of prostate cancer in the control arm, over a 7-year period. In fact, 24% of the patients were diagnosed by the end of the study – a four-fold excess. Beyond doubt, the majority of the prostate cancers detected in this way were clinically 'insignificant' – no one could claim that 24% of the male population will develop clinically significant disease. Yet, was that study population so very different from men in our current clinical practice? An increasing number are presenting with marginally elevated Prostate-specific antigens (PSAs), and are then going on to prostatic biopsy. Admittedly, the men in the Finasteride study were biopsied in the face of a normal PSA, but patients today are very different from their counterparts a decade ago.

The point is that there has been an increase in the number of *men with early incidental prostate cancers that do not need any treatment* [2,3]. Because these men have a very high prostate cancer-specific survival rate without intervention, the results of any intervention will be coloured by the proportion of such men included; were it possible to select a population of men, all of whom had 'insignificant' cancer, their prostate cancer-specific survival would be 100%, irrespective of their treatment. The Finasteride prevention study showed that it might be more difficult than one might think to avoid selecting men in that category.

Connecticut Data

The results of 'watchful waiting' in the Connecticut cancer registry have been widely (and rightly) cited [4]. They indicate two facets of the disease: first, they show the outcome in men diagnosed up to 20 years ago – hence, arguably, a population different from today's. Even so, substantial numbers of men achieve long-term survival after an initial policy of 'watchful waiting'. Second, they show graphically the two competing agents of fate – death from prostate cancer, and death from other causes. The relative contributions of each to an individual's expectation of death depend on the age (and hence fitness) of the individual, and on the tumour grade and presenting PSA. It is hard to escape the observation that due to the modern selection of younger, fitter patients with lower PSAs, and smaller volume PSA-detected disease, today's competing survival curves might indicate a lesser contribution of prostate cancer to overall mortality, at least for lower-grade disease, and these data can only be a guide to advising patients in 2004 [3].

Active Monitoring

The term 'watchful waiting' carries with it a number of implications, which create a picture of the clinician in a 'back seat' role; in its purest form, intervention of any sort is withheld unless it is absolutely necessary. This approach, or something like it, has been broadly adopted in the United States 'PIVOT' study [5], for which it has to be said, the study organisers had sometimes been vilified even before a single result was published, And confident statements about the efficacy of radical treatment abound [6]. Why? There is not a shred of evidence from any randomised trial that intervention improves overall survival, even in the context of disease progression on 'watchful waiting'. It has to be said, though, that the concept of watchful waiting is a difficult one for patients and physicians alike ('you watch, while I wait to die' was how one patient put it to the ProtecT study team – see next section for details). In response to this, a modified concept, now popularly called 'active monitoring', has arisen, in which disease progression will be more carefully documented, and specific action taken on such progression [7–9]. This carries with it a number of new challenges:

- What are the criteria for disease progression?
- A rise in PSA?
- By how much?
- What action should be taken?
- Should routine re-biopsies be performed?
- How are they interpreted?

   This approach certainly generates a framework whereby it seems likely that a high proportion of patients will be guaranteed the outcome of not dying of prostate cancer, either following a documented lack of disease progression, or following intervention for disease progression. We must, however, remember that such good outcomes, assuming them to be confirmed, *do not prove that the intervention for disease progression was necessary in terms of survival*. This is not arguing against the concept of 'active monitoring' – far from it – we practice it enthusiastically in our centre. Rather, it is a plea to remember the limitations on what it can tell us. We do, meanwhile, applaud the bravery and scientific integrity of the PIVOT team. Their study will be a vital addition to the literature, and critics should be challenged to prove that they are compromising survival in any way (whether 'watchful waiting' compromises other aspects, such as morbidity or quality of life is admittedly a valid question).

A similar approach has been adopted by the CapSURE team in the United States [9]. The philosophy is firmly in the camp of 'active monitoring', with routine re-biopsy as part of the protocol. It is undeniable that, by using this approach, it is possible to define a group of men at extremely low risk of disease progression – itself a worthwhile and important goal. Although such policies of active monitoring including re-biopsies are clearly the right approach for some patients, they cannot improve the prostate cancer-specific survival for either individual patients or the population at whole. It must, therefore, be remembered that all of the 'active' treatments available at present are associated with some degree of late toxicity that have an impact on quality of life: any attempt to identify patients who do not need such interventions should be strongly encouraged. However, the important message from these active monitoring programmes is to underline the existence of such men at a very low risk of progression. Proving that radical therapy of any kind actually 'cures' such men is impossible without a randomised trial, and probably impossible even with a randomised trial, unless it were to enrol a huge number of men. Within some active monitoring programmes, the percentage of men who undergo definitive treatment is actually quite high [10]; but this fact does not, however, mean that they actually needed the treatment.

The UK ProtecT study

The ProtecT study will be the only randomised trial comparing radical surgery, radical external beam radiotherapy and active monitoring, in asymptomatic men diagnosed with organ-confined prostate cancer via PSA testing [11]. It aims to recruit 600 000 men for testing, resulting in a study population of around 1500 men with localised prostate cancer. Importantly, the feasibility study has already demonstrated that men will agree to such a randomisation [11], and throws down the gauntlet to challenge our profession to develop other, necessary randomised trials in difficult areas, and not to hide behind the shield of asserting that 'patients would not agree to be randomised'. Importantly, this trial is overseen by an international steering committee, whose role is to ensure that it remains scientifically valid and ethical to continue the trial in the face of current and new data. That they have continued to support it to date (March 2005) says something!

The Results of Modern Unrandomised Case Series are Superb

Surgery and external beam radiotherapy

Patients, who search the internet for advice on treatment, are often struck by the excellence of the results of radical prostatectomy. Indeed, it is not difficult to find case series with cause-specific survival rates of close to 95% [12–14], though overall survival is more difficult to find. If it is an acceptable statement that progression-free survival rates of 80% can be achieved with modern surgery, what does this mean? It would be better to say that 'progression-free survival rates of 80% can be achieved with the combination of modern surgery plus modern case selection'. How much of the excellent outcome is due to the surgery, and how much to the case selection? It is impossible to say, and yet this aspect of the equation is frequently overlooked in scientific reports, let alone in the routine counselling of patients with prostate cancer [15]. This is fundamental to the argument against the over-interpretation of unrandomised data. When the Surveillance, Epidemiology and End Results (SEER) group published their important study showing overall survival rates in a large population database of men managed initially with surgery, radiotherapy, or 'surveillance' [16], one of their observations was that the results of surgery were substantially 'improved' by analysing the 'treatment received', rather than by the 'intent to treat'. A personal observation is that these data, although unrandomised, are often used to imply that surgery is superior to radiotherapy, an assertion that simply cannot be justified. The 'intent to treat' scenario just described, clearly shows something of the impact of case selection, and yet it is impossible to judge, from the SEER data, what factors led to the selection of radiotherapy rather than surgery, *except* that, as a whole, the radiotherapy patients were older. Lest the reader interpret this as a parochial defence of radiotherapy, read on! In the meantime, what *can* be said with some justification is that the data from surgical case series are generally more mature than those from modern, high-dose conformal radiotherapy (MHDCRT for simplicity) case series. This is understandable so, since the technological advances in the last 10–15 years render external beam radiotherapy a 'moving target' [17]. The undisputed technical excellence of modern radiotherapy is to be applauded, but exactly similar outcomes are reported after MHDCRT to those of surgery, at least within the limitations of the available follow-up times, and it has to be said that exactly the same criticisms of surgical case series apply to radiotherapy case series [18]. Many of the reports of improvements in outcome associated with MHDCRT are from single-centre non-randomised case series and are therefore subject to the same inherent biases; the case for higher radiation doses delivered by increasingly complicated techniques is not by any means proven, although randomised trials are underway in the United States, across Europe and in the United Kingdom.

Let us propose that no future case series reports will be accepted for publication unless they contain an extensive analysis of patient factors such as performance status, co-morbid conditions, urinary and gastrointestinal organ function (e.g. rectal and bladder physiology) as well as precise tumour factors! They will, however, still never be as good as a randomised trial at eliminating bias in comparisons of treatment efficacy!

What should we make of the single randomised trial (the Scandinavian Prostate Cancer Collaborative (SPCC) comparison of radical prostatectomy with watchful waiting) [19], which includes a 'watchful waiting' arm? It would be easy to say that as yet it shows no overall survival benefit for radical prostatectomy. This is true, and is an important reason why the fundamental question remains an open one. However, the trial also, currently, shows a significant difference in metastasis-free survival, and prostate cancer-specific survival in favour of the surgical arm. What does this mean? On the one hand, one has to advocate caution (there are relatively few events, and the magnitude of the difference is more than one would expect from contemporaneous data on disease progression with 'active monitoring'). On the other hand, a significant survival benefit *could* emerge with longer follow-up: a multitude of non-randomised studies would be unlikely to show this; and a real benefit to future patients would have been missed. Equally, although it is conceptually compelling to assume that metastasis-free survival is a valid surrogate for overall survival, even this is unproven, and could yet be wrong. This study will continue to yield important data, but the case is far from closed!

Brachytherapy

If something of the uncritical enthusiasm for radical prostatectomy has waned somewhat in recent years, as the arguments for a randomised trial have gained ground, there is a depressing feeling of '*déjà vu*' in relation to brachytherapy. A brief visit to the internet should convince those who doubt this point. Yes, the results of unrandomised case series are superb [20], if

comparable to the best series using other modalities [21]. Uncritical enthusiasts for this form of therapy do themselves, their modality, their more
critical colleagues, and ultimately their patients, no service. How often have
we been wrong in the annals of oncology history?

A randomised trial (American College of Surgeons Oncology Group trial
Zoo70 – SPIRIT) was set up to compare brachytherapy with radical surgery with 'favourable' prostate cancer (low PSA, small volume disease, no
high-grade histology). Despite continued enthusiasm from UK centres, only
56 of the necessary 1980 patients were recruited and the central administration in the United States closed the trial. The failure of this trial may simply
reflect the lack of certainty regarding the need for any treatment for these
patients. Inclusion of an 'active monitoring' arm, akin to ProtecT, would
surely have made the trial more scientifically relevant. It is extremely encouraging, and a credit to the United Kingdom, that a randomised controlled
trial, evaluating the use of a brachytherapy boost in addition to external
beam radiotherapy, is due for completion soon.

Cryotherapy

Interestingly, there are case series of radical treatment using cryotherapy,
with impressive outcomes, and a worldwide experience now totalling several thousand patients [22–24]. Why has it not achieved the popularity of,
say, brachytherapy, with which it shares a number of logistical and technological challenges? While this situation is probably set to change, it is also
an interesting insight into the effects of human nature on the planning of
therapeutic resources! What prospects a randomised trial?

A further cautionary note for perusers of websites advertising the success
of treatment (increasingly patients themselves) is the tendency to use biochemical control as the end point of choice. One seminal study adhered to
a strict policy of observation for men with a rising PSA after surgery [25].
A total of 1997 men underwent a radical retropubic prostatectomy, with
315 developing PSA greater than 0.2 ng/mL. Of these, 304 were followed,
with no adjuvant treatment, to the development of objective metastatic disease. The median actuarial time to metastatic disease was 8 years from
the time of PSA elevation, and the median time to death following the
development of metastatic disease was 5 years.

THE RATIONALE FOR RANDOMISATION APPLIES TO PROSTATE CANCER, TOO

The arguments for randomisation as a way of establishing treatment efficacy
have been widely accepted across the whole of medicine. In oncology, these

arguments have been particularly strong; the list of things about which we might have been (or were) wrong about is impressive, and includes:

• Radical mastectomy or conservative treatment for breast cancer, overturning the belief that radical surgery improved survival [26].

• Adjuvant chemotherapy for breast cancer, overturning the belief that it did not improve survival [27].

• Post-operative radiotherapy for lung cancer, which proved, unexpectedly, to worsen survival [28].

• Chemotherapy for lung cancer, which proved, unexpectedly, to improve survival albeit modestly [29].

• Aspirin for preventing repeated myocardial infarction, which was considered controversial, and not universally introduced until after a meta-analysis [30].

• Statins in the reduction of coronary disease, where the same was true [31].

This is true, even if some of these questions required a meta-analysis of randomised trials. Nonetheless, for all of these questions, randomisation is the most powerful tool that we have for eliminating bias, and bias is unquestionably present in our evaluation of treatment for early prostate cancer. How could it be otherwise? This cannot be stated too strongly. Let those who argue that they can adequately infer treatment efficacy from unrandomised trials defend themselves. Why would early prostate cancer be different from any other area of medicine? How can such a stance be maintained when there are examples, from the SEER data as well as from elsewhere, that bias does indeed exist in early prostate cancer. Neither can the argument that 'it can't be done' hold credence in the face of the ongoing recruitment into the ProtecT study. This does not detract from the need to understand the biological basis for the diversity of disease behaviour in prostate cancer – this is vital if we are to understand the factors associated with disease progression – and which of these are associated with prostate cancer deaths. Neither should we under-estimate the value of observational studies. They are what they are, and they may have strengths as well as limitations. Let us, however, swing the pendulum, just a little!

REFERENCES

1 Thompson IM, Goodman PJ, Tangen CM et al. The Influence of Finasteride on the Development of Prostate Cancer. N Engl J of Med 2003; 349: 215–24.

2 Chodak GW. The role of watchful waiting in the management of localized prostate cancer. J Urol 1994; 152: 1766–8.

3 Kessler B, Albertsen P. The natural history of prostate cancer. Urol Clin North Am 2003; 30: 219–26.

4 Schwartz E, Albertsen P. Nomograms for clinically localized disease. Part III: watchful waiting. Semin Urol Oncol 2002; 20: 140–5.

5 Wilt TJ, Brawer MK. The Prostate Cancer Intervention Versus Observation

Trial (PIVOT). *Oncology (Huntingt)* 1997; **11**: 1133–9.

6 Frohmuller HG, Theiss M. Radical prostatectomy in the management of localized prostate cancer. *Eur J Surg Oncol* 1995; **21**: 336–40.

7 Klotz L. Expectant management with selective delayed intervention for favorable risk prostate cancer. *Urol Oncol* 2002; **7**: 175–9.

8 Klotz L. Active surveillance with selective delayed intervention: a biologically nuanced approach to favorable-risk prostate cancer. *Clin Prostate Cancer* 2003; **2**: 106–10.

9 Cooperberg MR, Broering JM, Litwin MS *et al.* The contemporary management of prostate cancer in the United States: lessons from the cancer of the prostate strategic urologic research endeavor (CapSURE), a national disease registry. *J Urol* 2004; **171**: 1393–401.

10 Carter CA, Donahue T, Sun L *et al.* Temporarily deferred therapy (watchful waiting) for men younger than 70 years and with low-risk localized prostate cancer in the prostate-specific antigen era. *J Clin Oncol* 2003; **21**: 4001–8.

11 Donovan J, Hamdy F, Neal D *et al.* Prostate Testing for Cancer and Treatment (ProtecT) feasibility study. *Health Technol Assess* 2003; **7**: 1–88.

12 Moul JW, Wu H, Sun L *et al.* Epidemiology of radical prostatectomy for localized prostate cancer in the era of prostate-specific antigen: an overview of the Department of Defense Center for Prostate Disease Research national database. *Surgery* 2002; **132**: 213–9.

13 Oberpenning F, Hamm M, Schmid HP, Hertle L, Semjonow A. Radical prostatectomy: survival outcome and correlation to prostate-specific antigen levels. *Anticancer Res* 2000; **20**: 4969–72.

14 Gerber GS, Thisted RA, Scardino PT *et al.* Results of radical prostatectomy in men with clinically localized prostate cancer. *JAMA* 1996; **276**: 615–9.

15 Fowler FJ, Jr., McNaughton Collins M, Albertsen PC, Zietman A, Elliott DB, Barry MJ. Comparison of recommendations by urologists and radiation oncologists for treatment of clinically localized prostate cancer. *JAMA* 2000; **283**: 3217–22.

16 Lu-Yao GL, Yao SL. Population-based study of long-term survival in patients with clinically localised prostate cancer. *Lancet* 1997; **349**: 906–10.

17 Kupelian PA, Buchsbaum JC, Elshaikh MA, Reddy CA, Klein EA. Improvement in relapse-free survival throughout the PSA era in patients with localized prostate cancer treated with definitive radiotherapy: year of treatment an independent predictor of outcome. *Int J Radiat Oncol Biol Phy* 2003; **57**: 629–34.

18 Peschel RE, Colberg JW. Surgery, brachytherapy, and external-beam radiotherapy for early prostate cancer. *Lancet Oncol* 2003; **4**: 233–41.

19 Holmberg L, Bill-Axelson A, Helgesen F, Salo JO, Folmerz P, Haggman M, et al. A randomized trial comparing radical prostatectomy with watchful waiting in early prostate cancer. *N Engl J Med* 2002; **347**: 781–9.

20 Grimm PD, Blasko JC, Sylvester JE, Meier RM, Cavanagh W. 10-Year biochemical (prostate-specific antigen) control of prostate cancer with 125I brachytherapy. *Int J Radiat Oncol Biol Phy* 2001; **51**: 31–40.

21 Norderhaug I, Dahl O, Hoisaeter PA *et al.* Brachytherapy for prostate cancer: a systematic review of clinical and cost effectiveness. *Eur Urol* 2003; **44**: 40–6.

22 Fahmy WE, Bissada NK. Cryosurgery for prostate cancer. *Arch Androl* 2003; **49**: 397–407.

23 Shinohara K. Prostate cancer: cryotherapy. *Urol Clin North Am* 2003; **30**: 725–36, viii.

24 Bahn DK, Lee F, Badalament R, Kumar A, Greski J, Chernick M. Targeted cryoablation of the prostate: 7-year outcomes in the primary treatment of prostate cancer. *Urology* 2002; **60**: 3–11.

25 Pound CR, Partin AW, Eisenberger MA, Chan DW, Pearson JD, Walsh PC. Natural history of progression after PSA elevation following radical prostatectomy. *JAMA* 1999; **281**: 1591–7.

26 Fisher B, Anderson S, Bryant J *et al.* Twenty-year follow-up of a randomized trial comparing total mastectomy, lumpectomy, and lumpectomy plus

irradiation for the treatment of invasive breast cancer. *N Engl J Med* 2002; **347**: 1233–41.

27 Anonymous. Effects of adjuvant tamoxifen and of cytotoxic therapy on mortality in early breast cancer. An overview of 61 randomized trials among 28,896 women. Early Breast Cancer Trialists' Collaborative Group. *N Engl J Med* 1988; **319**: 1681–92.

28 Anonymous. Postoperative radiotherapy for non-small cell lung cancer. PORT Meta-analysis Trialists Group. *Cochrane Database Syst Rev* 2000(2): CD002142.

29 Anonymous. Chemotherapy for non-small cell lung cancer. Non-small Cell Lung Cancer Collaborative Group. *Cochrane Database Syst Rev* 2000(2): CD002139.

30 Anonymous. Collaborative meta-analysis of randomised trials of antiplatelet therapy for prevention of death, myocardial infarction, and stroke in high risk patients. *BMJ* 2002; **324**: 71–86.

31 LaRosa JC, He J, Vupputuri S. Effect of statins on risk of coronary disease: a meta-analysis of randomized controlled trials. *JAMA* 1999; **282**: 2340–6.

Part 2: Diagnosis and Evaluation

6: Equivocal PSA Results and Free Total PSA Ratio

Bob Djavan, Michael Dobrovits and Michael Marberger

Prostate cancer is the first male malignancy and the second leading cause of cancer related death [1–3]. In order to reduce the mortality, urologists mainly focused on early detection of this disease. Since its discovery in 1979, prostate-specific antigen (PSA) has unequivocally proved its usefulness as a serum marker for prostate cancer. However, in patients with a PSA below 10 ng/mL an important and large overlap exists between benign prostatic hyperplasia (BPH) and prostate cancer. Indeed, PSA is not prostate cancer specific and develops at an age when the prevalence of BPH is high. Previous reports indicate that two-thirds of the patients who undergo biopsies based on a PSA of 4–10 ng/mL have no histological evidence of prostate cancer [4]. In this PSA range – also referred to as the grey zone – several concepts have been introduced, all aiming to optimise the clinical use of PSA by improving its sensitivity and specificity, and trying to decrease the number of unnecessary biopsies in men with benign disease. These concepts include PSA density (relating the serum PSA to the volume of the prostate), age adjusted PSA reference ranges (adjusting the PSA level with patient age), PSA velocity (evaluating the rate of change of PSA values with time) and determination of PSA molecular forms (free versus protein bound molecular forms of PSA).

Undoubtedly the most exciting advance in PSA testing has been the recognition that PSA circulates not in one form, but complexed to protease inhibitors [5,6]. This is due to the fact that PSA, like other serine proteases, should not occur in an enzymatically active form in blood. Therefore, regulation of enzymatic action of PSA is controlled by different means. First, PSA is produced as an inactive protease, which is converted to the active enzyme by release of a small propeptide [7]. This activation is suggested to be dependent on the action of human glandular kallikrein (hK2) [7–10], a closely related homologous protein. It is, like PSA, exclusively expressed by the prostate [11]. Second, no candidate enzyme has been proposed to be responsible for the internal peptide bond cleavages, for example, at Lys145–Lys146 and at Lys182–Ser183, which results in a different three-dimensional structure and loss of enzymatic activity and the production of a PSA-form often referred to as 'nicked PSA' [5,12]. Finally, the enzymatic action may also be inactivated by the reaction of PSA with several abundant extracellular protease inhibitors, such as alpha-2-macroglobulin (AMG), the AMG homologous inhibitor called pregnancy zone protein, alpha-1-antichymotrypsin (ACT), alpha-1-antitrypsin (API) or protein C inhibitor (PCI) [5,6,13,14].

PSA, FREE PSA AND FREE TO TOTAL PSA RATIO

Most of the PSA that is in circulation is complexed to ACT and other inhibitor complexes, including the PSA–AMG complex. The latter one is complicated to measure and only occurs at low or very low levels in blood, *in vivo* [6,14–17]. On the contrary free or non-complexed PSA compromises a much smaller amount in the circulation although this is the major form found in the ejaculate, but free PSA in blood differs from enzymatically active PSA in the ejaculate. Free PSA in blood is enzymatically inactive and, hence, unreactive with the large excess of inhibitors in blood [5,15,17,18]. PSA is also bound toAMG, but this fraction is present at very low levels in blood, *in vivo* [16,17]. Its forms are not detected by commercial immunoassays, and can only be measured by complicated relatively insensitive assays used for research purpose only [16,17]. This may be aggravated due to non-optimised storage of samples *in vitro*.

Information is rare about the actual site of complexation of PSA to the protease inhibitors. This knowledge would be essential to understand such basic apparent dilemmas as the fact that the PSA complexed with ACT occurs in a much smaller amount than the PSA–AMG complex in blood, when in fact, enzymatically active PSA reacts much faster with AMG than with ACT *in vitro* [16,17,19]. This would suggest that PSA produced from benign prostatic tissue mainly would bind to AMG – being undetectable – and consequently total PSA has a higher free total ratio as only a minority is bound to ACT. It has been suggested that ACT may be present to a greater degree in normal and transformed prostatic epithelium as compared to that represented by benign prostatic hyperplasia [20]. Thus, complexation could conceivably occur within the prostate itself as opposed to formation of PSA–ACT complex in the systemic blood circulation. We know that the free form of PSA is present in a greater proportion in men without carcinoma and by contrast, the PSA–ACT complex comprises a greater proportion of the total PSA in men with malignancy. Still, we do not know why the amount of PSA complexed to ACT is larger in blood from cancer patients than those with BPH.

In 1991, Stenman and associates demonstrated a correlation between a high level of complexed PSA and prostate cancer in order to differentiate between benign and malignant disease [6]. Subsequently, Christensson

Table 6.1 Sensitivity, specificity and positive predictive and negative values at different cut-off values. Free to total PSA and PSA 4.0–10 ng/mL (521 patients).

%Free to total PSA cut-off	%Sensitivity	%Specificity	Positive predictive value	Negative predictive value
10	33.690	92.308	0.74118	0.68041
15	54.545	79.021	0.62963	0.72669
20	68.984	69.930	0.60000	0.77519
30	87.701	54.196	0.55593	0.87079
40	96.257	32.168	0.48128	0.92929

Source: Djavan et al. [1]

Table 6.2 Specificity of F/T PSA level at various sensitivity levels.

Sensitivity (%)	Cut-off	Specificity (%)
90	22	29
95	25	20
98	32	6

Source: Catalona et al. [25]

demonstrated that the ratio of free to total PSA was lower in men with cancer [21]. Luderer et al. [22] demonstrated that – over the truncated range of total PSA between 4.0 and 10.0 ng/mL – the total PSA did not differ between men with and without carcinoma. However, free PSA was significantly lower in men with cancer. Similar results have been reported also by Higashihara [23], Chen [24] and Djavan [1] (Table 6.1).

Perhaps the most definitive trial of the usefulness of measuring free to total PSA was recently reported by Catalona and colleagues [25]. In this seven-institution prospective trial, 773 men aged 50 to 75 with a total PSA between 4.0–10.0 ng/mL with no evidence of cancer at digital rectal examination were included and evaluated. Utilising the Hybritech method, the authors observed that when the free to total PSA ratio was less than 25%, the sensitivity was 95% and the specificity enhanced by 20%. Consequently, if the clinician is willing to miss 5% of cancers, one out of five negative biopsies could be avoided (Table 6.2).

The trial also determined that with a 22% free to total ratio, the sensitivity dropped to 90% but the specificity increased to 29%, and therefore avoiding almost one-third of unnecessary biopsies.

Another trial performed by Hugosson et al. during 1995–96 [26] in Sweden included 5853 of almost 10 000 (about 60%) invited, randomly selected men, aged 50 to 66 years, who were tested for free and total PSA levels in blood [26]. There were 145 men diagnosed with cancer among 612 biopsied men with total PSA >3.0 ng/mL. 24% of the men diagnosed with cancer (i.e. 36/145 men) had total PSA levels from 3.0–4.0 ng/mL using the EG&G Wallace Dual Prostatus assay. Only 5/36 of these men had abnormal findings at digital rectal exam (DRE) [27].

The large number of men with benign biopsy findings (466/611 biopsied men) could have been reduced by 44% using a cut-off ≤18% free PSA. This would have occurred at the expense of not detecting 11% (16/145) of men with cancer, who had >18% free PSA mainly resulting from an enlarged prostate gland [26]. The usefulness of analysing the percentage of free PSA in men with total PSA levels <3.0 ng/mL is also shown by another trial undertaken in 1988–89, of 1748 of 2400 invited men aged 55–70 years who were examined by DRE, TRUS and PSA. The carefully stored samples (−70°C) were analysed for percent free PSA in 1995 [28]. In total, 367 of the 1748 examined men were biopsied and in 64 men prostate cancer was diagnosed. In 9/9 cancer patients with total PSA levels below 3.0 ng/mL, ≤18% free PSA was indicative for cancer as opposed to no cancer detected in 159 biopsied men with >18% free PSA [28].

While measuring the free to total PSA ratio is significantly beneficial to cancer detection, several concerns exist. First, the detailed molecular nature of the free form has yet to be clarified. Further, it is urgently necessary to stress the vital importance of introducing pre-analytical handling instructions, as the levels of free PSA and percent free PSA may decrease during sample storage *in vitro* [18]. This may, at least in part, be due to protease activity in the sample released by blood clotting and/or granulocytes. This might account for inferior stability of free PSA in serum compared to samples collected as EDTA- or heparin-anticoagulated plasma [18,29]. Further the PSA–ACT complex may also decompose and increase the free PSA levels in serum [30], though the dissociation rate of the complex is insignificant under optimal storage conditions [31]. For further details, the reader is referred to the excellent summary by Woodrum and associates [32]. Perhaps of greatest concern is the fact, that different manufacturer assays may give different results on the same sera with respect to the free to total PSA ratio. The use of measurement of two analytes, potentially compounds the bias between different manufacturer assays. We have observed considerable bias in total PSA [33,34] and also free PSA [34]. More recently, we have demonstrated significant bias when the free assays of different manufacturers are compared and when the free/total PSA assays from the same manufacturers are contrasted [33]. In this latter investigation, 240 sera referred for routine PSA testing were compared utilising three different manufacturers' free and their corresponding total assays. Tables 6.3 and 6.4 demonstrate the significant

Table 6.3 Variation in results from different manufacturer assay.

Assay	Cut-off for 95% sensitivity (%)	Specificity (%)
Hyb. F/Hyb. T	22	38
Dia. F/Hyb. T	35	19
Chi. F/Hyb. T	35	33
DELFIA/WALLAC	37	36

Source: Djavan *et al.* [1] and Nixon *et al.* [34]
Hyb.=Hybritech
Dia.=Dianon
Chi.=Chiron
F=Free PSA
T=Total PSA

Table 6.4 Sensitivity and specificity of total PSA and the free to total PSA ratio.

Assay	Sensitivity (%)	Specificity (%) total PSA	Specificity (%) F/T PSA	Cut-point total PSA (ng/mL)	Cut-point F/T PSA (%)
ACS:180 PSA2	100	0	0	0.02	90
and free PSA	95	10	17	1.7	25
	90	25	54	3.3	15
Enzymun PSA	100	0	0	0.02	100
and free PSA	95	5	7	1.1	43
	90	24	32	3.0	23
Tandem-R PSA	100	1	1	0.4	52
and free PSA	95	7	22	2.1	25
	90	17	31	3.4	21

Source: Data from Roth *et al.* [33]

findings. We observed similarity with the Chiron ACS-180 and Tandem-R assays, but different results with the Enzymum assay.

These data show marked variability when different manufacturer assays are employed. Clinicians should be aware of the assays used in their institution and the laboratorian should define the performance of each free to total PSA assay in their patient setting prior to utilising this test clinically.

Free to Total PSA and Repeat Biopsy

Prostate cancer on repeat biopsy is not an uncommon finding and will be encountered in 10–20% of cases. Free to total PSA is one of the most accurate predictors of prostate cancer in these subjects, being a significantly better predictor of repeat biopsy malignancy than total PSA, PSA density and transition zone PSA density. Repeat biopsy should be performed in men with free to total PSA less than 30% [35].

Certain issues remain with respect to understanding the proper utilisation of the free to total PSA ratio. First of all, the most important question is on whom to use this test. Should it's use be general – as the total PSA –, or only on those within a more restricted PSA range, say 4.0–10.0 ng/mL? Another possible cohort would be those men with a PSA <4.0 ng/mL where approximately 25% of carcinomas are detected. Finally, it may be beneficial using it in those patients who have undergone a previous negative prostate needle biopsy. It is widely recognised that 20–30% of such men harbour malignancy, which is detected on repeat biopsy. Recently, we have demonstrated that free to total PSA may help to stratify those men who have carcinoma despite an initial negative biopsy [36].

Complexed PSA

Although utilisation of serum PSA testing for early detection of prostate cancer is generally accepted, the specificity PSA assays show is low. Thus, improvement of specificity in early detection of prostate carcinoma is needed to avoid costly and unnecessary biopsies. It has been recognised that the majority of PSA found in men with cancer is complexed to ACT as opposed to PSA found in healthy men [6,21]. However, early work to measure PSA–ACT complexes encountered difficulties demonstrating non-specific binding or over-recovery due to technical problems in accurate measurement of complexed PSA [21]. Indeed, the reason we used free to total PSA is because such assays were not available despite the fact that it was recognised that complexed PSA was the most important moiety to measure. This derives from the fact that this form is in greater proportion in men with carcinoma. The previous technical problems in designing specific PSA–ACT complex assay procedures have largely been overcome [31]. However, decomposition of the PSA–ACT complex during storage at unfavourable conditions may release enzymatically active PSA *in vitro* [31]. *In vitro*, this may result in formation of either AMG–PSA complexes, or false elevation of free PSA, if the AMG fraction in blood has become inactivated. This could explain some of the data reported on samples stored at −20°C for more than 20 years [30].

Recently, the Bayer Corporation has developed a specific PSA assay directed against complexed PSA. We performed an initial evaluation of this assay utilising a series of men who previously underwent ultrasound-guided needle biopsy for whom archival serum was available. We compared the results of the Bayer Immuno-1 cPSA assay (Bayer Corporation,

Tarrytown, New York) and the Hybritech-Tandem-R free and total assays (Hybritech, Incorporated, San Diego, CA). As expected, the mean to total PSA and complexed PSA were higher in those men with carcinoma and the free to total PSA was lower. A good correlation between total PSA and the sum of free and complexed PSA was observed. At 95% sensitivity, specificity for total PSA was 22%. A complexed PSA cut-off of 2.52 demonstrated an enhanced specificity of 26.7%. The free to total PSA ratio at 28% resulted in a specificity of only 15.6%.

COMBINATION OF PSA AND PSA DERIVATIVES

Prostate-specific antigen based parameters can be combined to improve Prostate cancer (CaP) detection. In a recent study by Djavan *et al.* [37], the ability of PSA density (PSAD), PSA transition zone (PSA-TZ), PSA velocity, percent free PSA and their combination to improve the detection of CaP were evaluated with univariate and multivariate analysis as well as receiver operating characteristic (ROC) curves. The combination of PSA-TZ and f/t PSA significantly increased the area under the curve (AUC) as compared to the use of any other combination ($p = 0.020$, Mc Nemar test). In fact, PSA-TZ + f/t PSA showed an AUC of 88.1% followed by PSA-TZ + PSAD (82.9%), PSA-TZ + PSA (82.4%), PSAD + PSA (78.4%) and f/t PSA + PSAD (73.4%). Obviously, volume dependent PSA parameters such as PSAD and PSA-TZ were crucial when PSA parameters were combined. However, if volume independent PSA combinations are to be considered, f/t PSA + PSA clearly outperformed all other possible combinations.

HUMAN GLANDULAR KALLIKREIN 2

Prostate-specific antigen and Human glandular kallikrein 2(hK2) are proteases that, along with human kallikrein 1 (hK1), comprise the kallikrein family, a subgroup of a large family of serine proteases [38–42].

The hK2 protein has approximately 79% identity in primary structure to PSA [43], shares several important properties with PSA, such as tissue-restricted expression pattern, though hK2 has markedly different enzymatic properties [44–46]. Several of these properties suggest that hK2 may also be useful in diagnosis of prostate cancer.

The majority of hK2 in serum is free, only about 5–20% of hK2 is believed to be present in complexed form, mainly as a complex with ACT [47–49]. The serum levels of hK2 are very low in females and in prostate cancer patients following radical prostatectomy, whereas the hK2 levels are significantly higher in men with benign prostatic disease than in young healthy men. Further, the levels are significantly elevated in men with localised prostate cancer compared to those with BPH [50,51]. Recently, it has been proposed that hK2 measurements in combination with free and total PSA can improve the sensitivity and specificity of cancer detection and avoid unnecessary biopsies, also in total PSA levels from 2.5 to 4.0 ng/mL. Certainly, larger studies are needed to confirm the utility of the hK2 measurements in serum and the interpretations hK2 with free and total PSA may require appropriate algorithms, such as logistic regression and artificial neural networks. Overall, hK2 seems to offer complimentary information to PSA. Its potential for replacing the latter however, is doubtful.

CONCLUSION

In summary, PSA, free PSA and lately complexed PSA have evolved our management of men with prostate cancer. Several drawbacks, however, limit their broad use: variations in sample handling and assay manufacturer, as well as uncertainties with respect to free to total PSA ratio cut-offs and the resultant sensitivities and specificities. Significant advances particularly in the realm of increased specificity and sensitivity of the total PSA assay will undoubtedly continue to unfold. Novel markers such as human kallikrein type 2, prostate-specific membrane antigen, and complexed PSA will surely aid clinicians and their patients.

However, no complete agreement exists regarding the appropriate cutpoint for free to total PSA ratio, especially for an individual patient for whom the presence or absence of cancer is more important than a percentage of risk of cancer.

According to the existing data, clinicians mainly focus on total PSA when determining whether to perform an initial biopsy or not. If the first biopsy shows no sign of malignancy, free to total PSA ratio will aid, in combination with other factors, such as family history, digital rectal examination, PSA velocity and complexed PSA, whether to perform a repeat biopsy or not.

REFERENCES

1 Djavan B, Zlotta AR, Byttebier G et al. Prostate specific antigen density of the transitional zone for early detection of prostate cancer. J Urol 1998; 160: 411–9.

2 Parker SL, Tong T, Bolden S, Winog PA. Cancer statistics,1996. CA Cancer J 1996; 46: 5–27.

3 Dijkman GA, Debruyne FM. Epidemiology of prostate cancer. Eur Urol 1996; 30: 281–95.

4 Brawer MK. Prosate-specific antigen: critical issues. Urology 1994; 44: 9.

5 Christensson A, Laurell CB, Lilja H. Enzymatic activity of prostate-specific antigen and its reaction with extracellular serine proteinase inhibitors. Eur J Biochem 1990; 194: 755.

6 Stenman U, Leinonen J, Alfthan H, Rannikko S, Tuhkanen K, Althan O. A complex between PSA and a

1-antichymotrypsin is the major form of PSA in serum of patients with prostatic cancer: Assay of the complex improves clinical sensitivity for cancer. *Cancer Res* 1991; **51**: 222.

7 Lundwall A, Lilja H. Molecular cloning of human prostate-specific antigen cDNA. *FEBS Lett* 1987; **214**: 317–22.

8 Lovgren J, Rajakoski K, Karp M, Lundwall A, Lilja H. Activation of the zymogen form of prostate-specific-antigen by human glandular kallikrein 2. *Biophys Res Comm* 1997; **238**: 549–55.

9 Takayama TK, Fujikawa K, Davie EW. Characterization of the percurser of prostate-specific antigen-activation by trypsin and by human glandular kallikrein. *J Biol Chem* 1997; **272**: 21582–8.

10 Kumar A, Mikolajczyk SD, Goel AS, Millar LS, Saedi M. Expression of form of prostate-specific antigen by mammalian cells and its conversion to mature, active form by human kallikrein2. *Cancer Res* 1997; **57**: 3111–4.

11 Chapdelaine P, Paradis G, Temblay RR, Dube JY. High level of expression in the prostate of a human glandular kallikrein mRNA related to prostate-specific antigen. *FEBS Lett* 1998; **236**: 205–8.

12 Zhang WM, Leinonon J, Kalkkinen N, Dowell B, Stenman UH. Purification and characterization of different molecular forms of prostate-specific antigen in human seminal fluid. *Clin Chem* 1995; **41**: 1567–73.

13 Espana F, Sanchez CJ, Vera CD, Estelles A, Gilabert J. A quantitative ELISA for a measurement of complexes of prostate-specific antigen with a protein C inhibitor when using a purified standard. *J Lab Clin Med* 1993; **122**: 709–711.

14 Christensson A, Lilja H. Complex formation between protein C inhibitor and prostate-specific antigen *in vitro* and in human semen. *Eur J Biochem* 1994; **220**: 45–53.

15 Lilja H, Christensson A, Dahlen U *et al*. Prostate-specific antigen in human serum occurs predominantly in complex with alpha-1 antichymotrypsin. *Clin Chem* 1991; **37**: 1618–25.

16 Zhang WM, Finne P, Leinonen J *et al*. Characterization and immunological determination of the complex between prostate-specific antigen and alpha-2-macroglobulin. *Clin Chem* 1998; **44**: 2471–9.

17 Lilja H, Haese A, Bjork T *et al*. Significance and metabolism of complexed and non-complexed prostate-specific antigen (PSA) forms and human glandular kallikrein 2 (hK2) in localized prostate cancer before and after radical prostatectomy. *J Urol* 1999; **162**: 2029–34.

18 Piironen T, Pettersson K, Suonpaa M *et al*. *In vitro* stability of free prostate-specific antigen (PSA) and prostate-specific antigen (PSA) complexed to alpha-1-antichymotrypsin in blood samples. *Urology* 1996; **48**: 81–7.

19 Leinonen J, Stenman UH. Complex formation between PSA isoenzymes and prostate inhibitors. *J Urol* 1996; **155**: 1099–103.

20 Bjork T, Bjartell A, Abrahamsson PA, Hulkko S, diSant'Agnese A, Lilja H. Alpha 1-antichymotrypsin production in PSA-producind cells is common in prostate cancer but rare in benign prostatic hyperplasia. *Urology* 1994; **43**: 427–34.

21 Christensson A, Bjork T, Nilsson O *et al*. Serum prostate-specific antigen complexed to alpha 1-antichymotrypsin as an indicator of prostate cancer. *J Urol* 1993; **150**: 100–5.

22 Luderer AA, Chen Y, Thiel R *et al*. Measurement of the proportion of free to total PSA improves diagnostic performance of PSA in the diagnostic gray zone of total PSA. *Urology* 1995; **46**: 187–94.

23 Higashihara E, Nutahara K, Kojima M *et al*. Significance of serum free prostate-specific antigen in the screening of prostate cancer. *J Urol* 1996; **156**: 1964–8.

24 Chen Y, Luderer AA, Thiel RP, Carlson G, Cuny CL, Soriano TF. Using proportions of free to total prostate-specific antigen, age, and total prostate-specific antigen to predict the probability of prostate cancer. *Urology* 1996; **47**: 518–24.

25 Catalona WJ, Partin AW, Slawin KM *et al.* Use of the percentage of free prostate-specific antigen to enhance differentiation of prostate cancer from benign prostatic disease: A prospective multicenter clinical trial. *JAMA* 1998; **279**: 1542–7.

26 Hugosson J, Aus G, Berdahl S *et al.* Population based screening for prostate cancer by measurements of free and total concentration of prostate-specific antigen (PSA). *Urology* 2001 (submitted).

27 Lodding P, Luderer AA, Thiel RP, Carlson G, Cuny CL, Soriano TF. Characteristics of screening detected prostate cancer in men 50–65 years old with 3 to 4 ng/ml prostate-specific antigen. *J Urol* 1998; **159**: 899–903.

28 Tornblom M, Norming U, Adolfsson *et al.* Diagnostic value of percent free-PSA: Retrospective analysis of a population- based screening study with emphasis on men with PSA less than 3.0 ng/ml. *Urology* 1999; **53**: 945–50.

29 Woodrum D, French C, Shamel LB. Stability of free prostate-specific antigen in serum samples under a variety of sample collection and storage condition. *Urology (Suppl)* 1996; **33**: 9.

30 Stenman UH, Hakama M, Knekt P, Aromaa A, Teppo L, Leinonen J. Serum concentrations of prostate specific antigen and its complex with alpha 1-antichymotrypsin before diagnosis of prostate cancer. *Lancet* 1994; **344**: 1594–8.

31 Pettersson K, Piironen T, Seppala M *et al.* Free and complexed prostate-specific antigen (PSA): *In vitro* stability, epitop map, and development of immunoflurometric assays for specifc and sensitive detection of free PSA and PSA-alpha-1-antichymotrypsin complex. *Clin Chem* 1995; **41**: 1480–8.

32 Woodrum DL, Brawer MK, Partin AW, Catalona WJ, Southwick PC. Interpretation of free prostate-specific antigen clinical research studies for the detection of prostate cancer. *J Urol* 1998; **159**: 5–12.

33 Roth HJ, Christensen-Stewart S, Brawer MK. A comparison of three free and total PSA assays. *PCPD* 1998; **1**: 326–31.

34 Nixon RG, Gold MH, Blase AB, Meyer GE, Brawer MK. Comparison of three investigative assays for the free form of prostate-specific antigen. *J Urol* 1998; **160**: 420–5.

35 Djavan B, Zlotta A, Remzi M *et al.* Optimal predictors of prostate cancer on repeat prostate biopsy: a prospective study of 1051 men. *J Urol* 2000; **163**: 1144–9.

36 Letran JL, Blase AB, Loberiza FR, Meyer GE, Ransom SD, Brawer MK. Repeat ultrasound-guided prostate needle biopsy: The utility of free to total PSA ratio in predicting those men with or without prostatic carcinoma. *J Urol* 1998; **160**: 426–9.

37 Djavan B, Remzi M, Zlotta AR *et al.* Combination and multivariate analysis of PSA-based parameters for prostate cancer. *Tech Urol* 1999; **5**: 71–6.

38 Lilja H: A kallikrein-like prostate protease in prostatic fluid cleaves the predominant seminal vesical protein. *J Clin Invest* 1985; **76**: 1899–1903.

39 Watt KW, Lee PJA, Timkulu T *et al.* Human prostate-specific antigen: structural and functional similarity with serine proteases. *Proc Natl Acad Sci USA* 1986; **83**: 3166–70.

40 Berg T, Bratshaw RA, Carretero OA *et al.* A common nomenclature for members of the tissue (glandular) kallikrein gene families. *Agents Actions Suppl* 1996; **38**: 19–25.

41 Lilja H. Structure, function and regulation of the enzyme activity of prostate-specific antigen. *World J Urol* 1993; **11**: 188–91.

42 Ban Y, Wang MC, Watt KW *et al.* The proteolytic activity of human prostate-specific antigen. *Biochem Biophys Res Commun* 1984; **123**: 482–8.

43 Schedlich LJ, Bennetts BH, Morris BJ. Primary structure of human glandular kallikrein gene. *DNA* 1987; **6**: 429–37.

44 Mikolajczyk SD, Millar LS, Kumar A, Saedi MS. Human glandular kallikrein 2, hK2, shows arginine-restricted specificity and forms complexes with plasma protease inhibitors. *Prostate* 1998; **34**: 44–50.

45 Lovgren J, Airas K, Lilja H. Enzymatic action of human glandular kallikrein 2 (hK2): Substrate specificity and regulation by Zn^{2+} and extracellular protease inhibitors. *Eur J Biochem* 1999; **262**: 781–9.

46 Denmeade SR, Lou W, Lovgren J,
    Malm J, Lilja H, Issacs JT. Specific and
    efficient peptide substrates for assaying
    the proteolytic activity of
    prostate-specific antigen. *Cancer Res*
    1997; **57**: 4924–30.

47 Piironen T, Lovgren J, Karp M *et al.*
    Immunofluorometric assay for sensitive
    and specific measurement of human
    prostatic glandular kallikrein (hK2)
    in serum. *Clin Chem* 1996; **42**:
    1034–41.

48 Becker C, Piironen T, Kiviniemi J,
    Lilja H, Petersson K. Sensitive and
    specific immunodetection of human
    glandular kallikrein 2 (hK2) in serum.
    Clin Chem 2000; **46**: 198–206.

49 Grauer LS, Finlay JA, Mikolajczyk SD,
    Pusateri KD, Wolfert RL. Detection of
    human glandular kallikrein hK2 as its
    precursor form, and in complex with
    protease inhibitors in prostate carcinoma
    serum. *J Androl* 1998; **19**: 407–11.

50 Charlesworth MC, Young Cyf, Klee GG
    et al. Detection of a prostate-specific
    protein, hK2, in sera of patients with
    elevated prostate-specific antigen levels.
    Urology 1997; **49**: 487–93.

51 Becker C, Piirone T, Pettersson K *et al.*
    Discrimination of men with prostate
    cancer from those with benign disease by
    measurements of human glandular
    kallikrein (hK2) in serum. *J Urol* 2000;
    163: 311–16.

7: Equivocal Prostate Needle Biopsies

Murali Varma and David Griffiths

Why biopsy? – a self evident question, perhaps; however, examination of this particular question may help to determine what information is required from a biopsy and also give some clues as to how to reduce ambiguity in biopsies. Biopsy of the prostate, usually digitally guided, was first used to confirm a clinical diagnosis of carcinoma. While occasional cases of suspected carcinoma could be shown to be due to granulomatous prostatitis or some other rare benign condition, the expectation was that cancer would be confirmed, the biopsy being largely of confirmatory value although it may also give some prognostic value by virtue of the grade. Stage of the tumour would be given clinically – indeed treatment might progress without formal histological diagnosis.

Biopsy is now often used to sample glands that show no clinical or ultrasonographic evidence of prostate cancer. It is thus important to know what one can expect to find in a clinically normal prostate gland. Autopsy studies and studies of prostate cancer in radical cystoprostatectomies demonstrate that 30–50% of men between the ages of 55 and 75 have histopathologically detectable prostate cancer, if the whole gland is examined [1]. However, only about 2% of age-matched men would be expected to die of prostate cancer. It is thus clear that a large proportion of these tumours are of no clinical significance. Studies that have analysed the likely characteristics of clinically significant prostate cancer suggest that cases that are low grade (Gleason score <7) and below 0.2–0.5 mL in volume may be of no clinical importance [2,3], although an age-related volume threshold may be more relevant [4]. Fortunately, there is reliable information that by far the majority of prostate-specific antigen (PSA)-detected prostate cancers are clinically significant by these criteria [5].

Now that serum PSA is used as a screening tool, the purpose of the biopsy has become substantially different than its purpose in the pre-PSA era; with much greater demands on the information the biopsy gives to the clinician. Biopsies taken in patients with only elevated PSA have a much lower risk of carcinoma; (30–60%) – the primary purpose of the biopsy is to make the diagnosis rather than confirm a diagnosis. Thus, it is desirable that if the patient has cancer then the biopsy should show this and conversely if the patient does not have cancer then it would be advantageous if the biopsy demonstrates this fact with some confidence. In practice, this is sometimes not possible. Reported frequencies of equivocal biopsies – typically when the pathologist reports 'atypical suspicious for cancer' – vary widely from 0.4–23% with a median of 4.5%. This variation in frequency may reflect a number of variables, ranging from the experience of the pathologist to patient population and quality of the histopathological processing and availability of immunocytochemistry.

The presence of even a few atypical glands in a prostate needle biopsy is potentially significant, as minimal cancer in the biopsy does not necessarily equate to low volume, clinically insignificant cancer in the prostate gland. Patients with limited cancer in needle biopsy (variously defined as a single core with less than 2 mm or 3 mm aggregate length, or less than 10% core involvement) have been reported to have a 26–52% risk of extraprostatic extension [6–8]. The proportion of cancers identified by prostate needle biopsy would depend on tumour size as well as the location of the tumour within the prostate gland. Small tumours, increasingly encountered in the era of PSA screening, are often poorly represented in the biopsies particularly if these have been obtained from the standard sextant sites. About 20% of tumours in radical prostatectomy specimens are located predominantly in the anterior prostate gland [9], which is poorly sampled by trans-rectal biopsies particularly in patients with large gland volumes. Moreover, standard sextant biopsies are obtained in a mid-lobe parasagittal plane and tumours that are predominantly lateral may not be adequately sampled [10].

For all the above reasons, the histopathologist must make every effort to avoid equivocal prostate needle biopsy reports by taking extreme care with the technical aspects of processing needle cores and in the interpretation of the biopsies. It has been demonstrated that the cancer detection rate in needle biopsies is directly proportional to the microscopic length of needle cores examined [11,12], 18-gauge needle biopsies are very thin and fold easily, so sub-optimal embedding would result in parts of the biopsy remaining unrepresented in the histological sections examined with the potential for missing small cancers or the malignant focus being under-represented leading to a diagnosis of 'suspicious for adenocarcinoma, but not diagnostic due to paucity of atypical glands'. Submitting and processing cores separately makes accurate cutting of individual cores easier [13]. It has also been shown that clinically relevant diagnostic information would be missed if the biopsies are not routinely examined through multiple levels [14]. The Pathology Committee of the European Randomised Study of Screening for Prostate Cancer recommend that at least two levels of each core must be examined [11].

Further levels are indicated in diagnostically equivocal biopsies as this simple procedure may resolve a difficult differential diagnosis.

In our centre, cores are routinely submitted in separate cassettes and examined through at least three levels with unstained sections from each level saved on treated slides for immunohistochemical studies if required. In our experience, this protocol permits optimal embedding of the 18-gauge needle cores. It is important to save unstained sections at the time of initial processing, as small atypical foci are often not represented in additional levels and the chance to render a definite diagnosis with the aid of immunohistochemistry may be lost [14].

Attention to section thickness and quality of haematoxylin and eosin staining is also important. Presence of prominent nucleoli in the atypical glands is one of the principal cytologic criteria for diagnosis of prostate cancer and histopathologists tend to be reluctant to make a definite diagnosis of adenocarcinoma in the absence of nucleolar prominence [15]. Nucleoli may not be apparent in malignant glands if the sections are thick or overstained with haematoxylin.

While high-grade prostate cancer usually does not pose any diagnostic difficulty, well to moderately differentiated tumours can mimic and be mimicked by a wide variety of benign conditions (Table 7.1). Detailed discussion of the histological criteria for the diagnosis of prostate cancer and the differential diagnosis of atypical small glandular proliferations in needle biopsies is beyond the scope of this chapter and the reader is referred to recent textbooks dealing with these issues in depth [16–18].

Table 7.1 Histological differential diagnosis of prostate cancer.

Benign mimickers of prostate cancer	Prostate cancer variants that mimic benign conditions
Atrophy	Pseudo-atrophic carcinoma
Post-atrophic hyperplasia	Pseudo-hyperplastic carcinoma
Adenosis (atypical adenomatous hyperplasia)	Foamy gland carcinoma
Cribriform hyperplasia	Cribriform adenocarcinoma
Basal cell hyperplasia	Cancer with hormonal effect
Cowpers gland	
Verumontanum mucosal gland hyperplasia	
Hyperplasia of mesonephric remnants	
Nephrogenic adenoma	
Seminal vesicle/ejaculatory duct	
Radiation atypia	
Granulomatous prostatitis[a]	
Prostatic paraganglia[a]	

[a] Mimics high-grade cancer.

The diagnosis of prostate cancer in needle biopsies is based on a combination of architectural and cytological features [19]. The architectural features that are assessed at low to medium power magnification include an infiltrative pattern, glandular crowding, variation in glandular size, irregular acinar outlines and perineural invasion. These architectural features are more difficult to appreciate in needle biopsies with a small number of atypical glands as compared to trans-urethral resection specimens. The most important cytological features of prostate cancer are nuclear enlargement, nuclear hyperchromasia, nucleolar prominence and the absence of a basal cell layer. However, none of these features are entirely specific for malignancy. For example, a pseudo-infiltrative pattern is often evident in atrophy and post-atrophic hyperplasia, glandular crowding is a feature of adenosis, benign glands may closely abut nerves mimicking perineural invasion and nuclear abnormalities described above may be present in benign glands adjacent to inflammation.

When several of the features of cancer and none of the features of benignity are present, the diagnosis of prostate adenocarcinoma can be made with confidence. However, in other cases the degree of atypia may be insufficient to permit a definitive diagnosis of prostate cancer on morphologic grounds alone. These diagnostically equivocal biopsies fall into two groups.

In the first, and most common situation, the changes are quantitatively insufficient to permit definite diagnosis of cancer. These biopsies contain only a few glands lined by markedly atypical epithelial cells with all the cytological features of malignancy. However, it is recognised that larger glands with high-grade prostatic intraepithelial neoplasia (PIN) may be associated with smaller acini lined by atypical epithelial cells. These 'outpouchings of PIN' are more easily identified in radical prostatectomy specimens in which the low power architecture can be appreciated. However, in needle biopsies the small acini may be difficult to distinguish from infiltrating cancer (Plate 5, facing page 84). Unless the small atypical glands are too numerous or too crowded to represent outpouchings, such biopsies with only a few atypical glands would be reported as 'atypical small acinar proliferation suggestive of malignancy but outpouchings of high-grade PIN cannot be excluded'.

In the other scenario, the atypical changes are qualitatively insufficient for a definite diagnosis of cancer. In these biopsies, there may be relatively larger foci with significant architectural distortion but lacking convincing cytological features of malignancy or associated with prominent inflammation that makes interpretation of the significance of cytological atypia difficult.

In both the above described scenerios, the pathologist often resorts to immunohistochemistry using basal cell markers that are positive in benign glands but negative in prostate cancer. The most commonly used basal cell marker is the high molecular weight cytokeratin antibody, 34betaE12 but other markers such as cytokeratin 5/6, LP34 and p63 may also be used either alone or in combination. A basal cell pattern of immunoreactivity with these markers in the atypical glands would generally preclude a definitive diagnosis of malignancy as basal cells are rarely present in prostate cancer [20,21]. However, absence of basal cell immunoreactivity must be interpreted with caution, as a small but significant proportion of benign glands appear negative on immunostaining with these markers [22]. Moreover, immunoreactivity is often patchy in non-cancerous conditions such as adenosis and high-grade PIN, and some gland outlines may lack immunoreactivity in the tissue planes examined. Hence, immunohistochemical findings must always be interpreted in conjunction with morphology. Basal cell markers are most useful in biopsies that contain suspicious foci composed of several architecturally atypical glands showing insufficient cytological atypia to allow a definite diagnosis of malignancy. In such cases, the absence of immunoreactivity in the entire focus would permit a confident diagnosis of cancer. In small foci composed of more than a few glands showing morphological features very suspicious for carcinoma, absence of immunoreactivity would provide further support for a diagnosis of cancer. In contrast, the absence of immunoreactivity in foci composed of only a few atypical glands is not diagnostic, as benign glands may not be uniformly positive with basal cell markers and outpouchings of high-grade PIN may also lack immunoreactivity (Plate 5, facing page 84). The other drawback of basal cell immunohistochemistry is that the diagnosis of cancer is based on the absence of immunoreactivity and the possibility of spurious negativity related to technical problems would have to be excluded. Recently, a new immunohistochemical marker α-methylacyl CoA racemase (AMACR/P504S) that is positive in prostate cancer and negative in benign glands has been described [23,24]. The clinical utility of this marker remains to be established but it could be very useful as part of an immunohistochemical panel including one or more basal cell marker. However, AMACR/P504S is often positive in glands of high-grade PIN [25] and adenosis [26], and generally weak immunoreactivity has been reported in upto 29% of benign biopsies [27]. Hence, like basal cell markers, AMACR/P504S immunoreactivity must be interpreted in conjunction with morphology and positivity in a few atypical glands would not be diagnostic of cancer as adenosis and outpouchings of high-grade PIN would not be excluded. AMACR/P504S may be most useful in trans-urethral resection specimens with diathermy artefact and atypical glands negative for basal-cell markers on immunostaining. In this situation, AMACR/P504S positivity in the atypical focus would favour cancer rather than diathermy related false negative basal-cell immunoreactivity in benign glands.

Patients with equivocal prostate biopsies are at high risk of prostate cancer with up to 49% incidence on repeat biopsy; there appears to be no correlation between the histological level of suspicion and the likelihood of cancer on repeat biopsy [12,28]. Hence, all patients with equivocal biopsies should undergo repeat biopsies irrespective of clinical and pathological findings. As a significant proportion of patients with histological diagnosis of atypia have prostate cancer at the time of initial biopsy, prompt re-biopsy is indicated. The optimal protocol for repeat biopsy is uncertain and various strategies have been recommended. It is clear that repeat biopsies limited to the site of atypical biopsy are inadequate as the cancer identified on repeat biopsy is often at a site other than that with the atypical glands on initial biopsy. Allen *et al.* found cancer in the same sextant site as the initial atypical biopsy in only 48% of the positive repeat biopsies, while 85% of cancers were identified in either the same sextant as the atypical core, adjacent ipsilateral sextant or adjacent contralateral sextant [29]. They suggest a repeat biopsy protocol that includes three cores from the site of atypical biopsy, two cores from adjacent sites and one core from every other sextant site. This protocol would require submission all prostate cores separately to permit localisation of atypical biopsy cores.

However, it should be noted that the data regarding the incidence of cancer on re-biopsy following a histological diagnosis of atypia have largely been obtained from studies in which the biopsies (both initial and repeat) were taken from the standard sextant sites. It is unclear whether the risk of cancer is the same after atypia diagnosed following extended biopsy protocols (including lateral, medial and transitional cores) for initial and repeat biopsies.

Thus accurate diagnosis on the needle cores that are submitted to the pathologist require a high standard of technical processing and the availability of carefully quality-controlled immunocytochemistry as well as appropriate diagnostic skills. With these facilities, most atypical foci on needle biopsies can be resolved by careful morphological examination in conjunction with judicial interpretation of immunocytochemistry. Even under these favourable circumstances a small proportion of biopsies – typically 2 to 4% – from a screening population will remain equivocal. At this stage, the pathologist can be of no further help as grading the degree of suspicion does not appear to be of any value predicting the incidence of cancer on re-biopsy.

Most of this chapter has been focused on the problem of making a diagnosis of prostate cancer. The second and in some ways more challenging purpose of the prostate biopsy is to contribute to an assessment of the clinical significance of any tumour present. This is an issue that will become increasingly important with the expansion of PSA screening and the realisation that some of the tumours identified by biopsy offer no significant risk to those harbouring them. The patients with these low risk tumours will either have PSA elevated for other reasons or will have tumours producing quantities of PSA disproportionate to their size. Using the criteria outlined previously the proportion of 'clinically insignificant tumours' in radical prostatectomy specimens is variously estimated to be from 2% to 10%. However it may be as high as 30% in patients with minimal tumour on biopsy [30]. Few are likely to want radical treatment for a tumour that can be shown to have no clinical importance. In addition, even if a clinically significant tumour is identified it may be at such an early stage that it may be safe to defer treatment. The historical data showing that small amounts of tumour on biopsy may be associated with advanced disease in a relatively high proportion of cases may have little relevance in the context of extended biopsy protocols in combination with scrupulous attention to histological procedures. Biopsy findings (usually taken in combination with PSA levels) can make a significant contribution to predicting whether pT3 disease or nodal disease is present [31,32]. Steriometric modelling shows that if a consistent extended biopsy protocol is used then the biopsy findings should provide accurate information on the tumour size. Previous studies have shown a good correlation between biopsy findings and tumour size in radical prostatectomy specimens. However these studies, most commonly based on biopsies from sextant protocols, have usually concluded that the correlation is not sufficiently strong to make judgments on tumour size in individual cases. Most studies on extended protocols have emphasised their greater efficiency at detecting carcinoma; there being little information yet on correlating biopsy findings with tumour size.

There may be some grounds for optimism; repeat biopsies following an extended protocol will more commonly have the same findings as the first biopsy [33,34] when compared to repeat biopsy following sextant biopsies. This illustrates that extended protocols are a more reliable way to assess the gland. Our own experience supports this: re-biopsy of 32 cases with high-grade PIN found following an extended protocol has resulted in only two cases with cancer; both involving only a small part of one core. Nor have we found any advanced cancers on radical prostatectomy when only a small part of one core has been invaded by cancer.

In conclusion, even with the best facilities it will be impossible to eliminate the equivocal biopsy; indeed attempts to predict the clinical significance of tumours identified following extended protocol biopsies may present the urologist with a whole new class of equivocal biopsies – those with cancer but in which it is uncertain if the tumour fulfils criteria for being clinically significant.

REFERENCES

1 Montie JE. Observations on the epidemiology and natural-history of prostate-cancer. *Urology* 1994; **44**: 2–8.

2 Stamey TA, Freiha FS, McNeal JE, Redwine EA, Whittemore AS, Schmid HP. Localized prostate cancer. Relationship of tumor volume to clinical significance for treatment of prostate cancer. *Cancer* 1993; **71**: 933–8.

3 Carter HB, Sauvageot J, Walsh PC, Epstein JI. Prospective evaluation of men with stage T1C adenocarcinoma of the prostate. *J Urol* 1997; **157**: 2206–9.

4 Dugan JA, Bostwick DG, Myers RP, Qian J, Bergstralh EJ, Oesterling JE. The definition and preoperative prediction of clinically insignificant prostate cancer. *Jama* 1996; **275**: 288–94.

5 Smith DS, Humphrey PA, Catalona WJ. The early detection of prostate carcinoma with prostate specific antigen: the Washington University experience. *Cancer* 1997; **80**: 1852–6.

6 Cupp MR, Bostwick DG, Myers RP, Oesterling JE. The volume of prostate cancer in the biopsy specimen cannot reliably predict the quantity of cancer in the radical prostatectomy specimen on an individual basis. *J Urol* 1995; **153**: 1543–8.

7 Bruce RG, Rankin WR, Cibull ML, Rayens MK, Banks ER, Wood DP, Jr. Single focus of adenocarcinoma in the prostate biopsy specimen is not predictive of the pathologic stage of disease. *Urology* 1996; **48**: 75–9.

8 Weldon VE, Tavel FR, Neuwirth H, Cohen R. Failure of focal prostate cancer on biopsy to predict focal prostate cancer: the importance of prevalence. *J Urol* 1995; **154**: 1074–7.

9 Bott SR, Young MP, Kellett MJ, Parkinson MC. Anterior prostate cancer: is it more difficult to diagnose? *BJU Int* 2002; **89**: 886–9.

10 Eskew LA, Bare RL, McCullough DL. Systematic 5 region prostate biopsy is superior to sextant method for diagnosing carcinoma of the prostate. *J Urol* 1997; **157**: 199–202; discussion 202–3.

11 van der Kwast TH, Lopes C, Santonja C, *et al.* Guidelines for processing and reporting of prostatic needle biopsies. *J Clin Pathol* 2003; **56**: 336–40.

12 Iczkowski KA, Chen HM, Yang XJ, Beach RA. Prostate cancer diagnosed after initial biopsy with atypical small acinar proliferation suspicious for malignancy is similar to cancer found on initial biopsy. *Urology* 2002; **60**: 851–4.

13 Kao J, Upton M, Zhang P, Rosen S. Individual prostate biopsy core embedding facilitates maximal tissue representation. *J Urol* 2002; **168**: 496–9.

14 Green R, Epstein JI. Use of intervening unstained slides for immunohistochemical stains for high molecular weight cytokeratin on prostatic needle biopsies. *Am J Surg Pathol* 1999; **23**: 567–70.

15 Epstein JI. Diagnostic criteria of limited adenocarcinoma of the prostate on needle biopsy. *Human pathology* 1995; **26**: 223–9.

16 Bostwick DG, Dundore PA. *Biopsy Pathology of the Prostate*. London: Chapman & Hall, 1997.

17 Young RH, Srigley JR, Amin MB, Ulbright TM, Cubilla AL. *Tumours of the Prostate Gland, Seminal Vesicles, Male Urethra and Penis*. Washington: AFIP Press, 2000.

18 Epstein JI, Yang XJ. *Prostate biopsy interpretation*. 3rd edn. Lippincott Williams and Wilkins, Philadelphia, 2002.

19 Varma M, Lee MW, Tamboli P, *et al.* Morphologic criteria for the diagnosis of prostatic adenocarcinoma in needle biopsy specimens. A study of 250 consecutive cases in a routine surgical pathology practice. *Arch Pathol Lab Med* 2002; **126**: 554–61.

20 Yang XJ, Lecksell K, Gaudin P, Epstein JI. Rare expression of high-molecular-weight cytokeratin in adenocarcinoma of the prostate gland: a study of 100 cases of metastatic and locally advanced prostate cancer. *Am J Surg Pathol* 1999; **23**: 147–52.

21 Oliai BR, Kahane H, Epstein JI. Can basal cells be seen in adenocarcinoma of the prostate? an immunohistochemical study using high molecular weight cytokeratin (clone 34 betaE-12)

antibody. *Am J Surg Pathol* 2002; **26**: 1151–60.

22 Goldstein NS, Underhill J, Roszka J, Neill JS. Cytokeratin 34 beta E-12 immunoreactivity in benign prostatic acini. Quantitation, pattern assessment, and electron microscopic study. *Am J Clin Pathol* 1999; **112**: 69–74.

23 Jiang Z, Woda BA, Rock KL, *et al.* P504S: a new molecular marker for the detection of prostate carcinoma. *Am J Surg Pathol* 2001; **25**: 1397–404.

24 Rubin MA, Zhou M, Dhanasekaran SM, *et al.* alpha-Methylacyl coenzyme A racemase as a tissue biomarker for prostate cancer. *Jama* 2002; **287**: 1662–70.

25 Yang XJ, Wu CL, Amin MB, Young RH, Fanger GR, Jiang Z. P504S in diagnosis of prostate cancer; a multi-institutional analysis. *Mod Pathol* 2002; **15**: 187A.

26 Yang XJ, Wu CL, Woda BA, *et al.* Expression of alpha-methylacyl-CoA racemase (P504S) in atypical adenomatous hyperplasia of the prostate. *Am J Surg Pathol* 2002; **26**: 921–5.

27 Beach R, Gown AM, De Peralta-Venturina MN, *et al.* P504S immunohistochemical detection in 405 prostatic specimens including 376 18-gauge needle biopsies. *Am J Surg Pathol* 2002; **26**: 1588–96.

28 Chan TY, Epstein JI. Follow-up of atypical prostate needle biopsies suspicious for cancer. *Urology* 1999; **53**: 351–5.

29 Allen EA, Kahane H, Epstein JI. Repeat biopsy strategies for men with atypical diagnoses on initial prostate needle biopsy. *Urology* 1998; **52**: 803–7.

30 Terris MK, McNeal JE, Stamey TA. Detection of clinically significant prostate cancer by transrectal ultrasound-guided systematic biopsies. *J Urol* 1992; **148**: 829–32.

31 Partin AW, Kattan MW, Subong EN, *et al.* Combination of prostate-specific antigen, clinical stage, and Gleason score to predict pathological stage of localized prostate cancer. A multi-institutional update. *Jama* 1997; **277**: 1445–51.

32 Bostwick DG, Cupp MR, Oesterling JE. Tumor volume in prostate-cancer-correlation of needle-biopsy and radical prostatectomy findings. *Lab Invest* 1993; **68**:57.

33 San Francisco IF, DeWolf WC, Rosen S, Upton M, Olumi AF. Extended prostate needle biopsy improves concordance of Gleason grading between prostate needle biopsy and radical prostatectomy. *J Urol* 2003; **169**: 136–40.

34 Mian BM, Naya Y, Okihara K, Vakar-Lopez F, Troncoso P, Babaian RJ. Predictors of cancer in repeat extended multisite prostate biopsy in men with previous negative extended multisite biopsy. *Urology* 2002; **60**: 836–40.

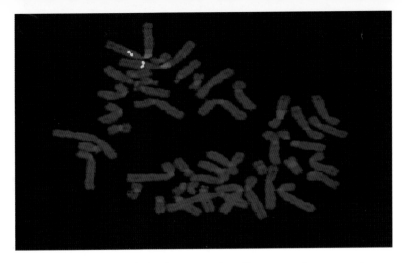

Plate 1 BAC-derived FISH probe binding to a region of interest on chromosome 1.

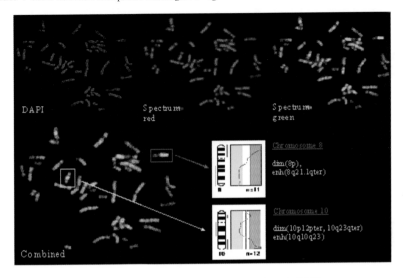

DAPI

Spectrum red

Spectrum green

Chromosome 8

dim(8p),
enh(8q21.1qter)

Chromosome 10

dim(10p12pter, 10q23qter)
enh(10q10q23)

Combined

Plate 2 Images acquired during conventional (chromosome-based) CGH.

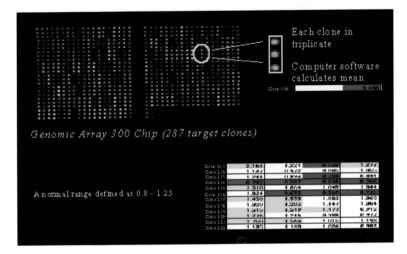

Each clone in triplicate

Computer software calculates mean

Genomic Array 300 Chip (287 target clones)

A normal range defined as 0.8 - 1.25

Plate 3 Image acquisition in array-based CGH demonstrating loss and gain of genomic material.

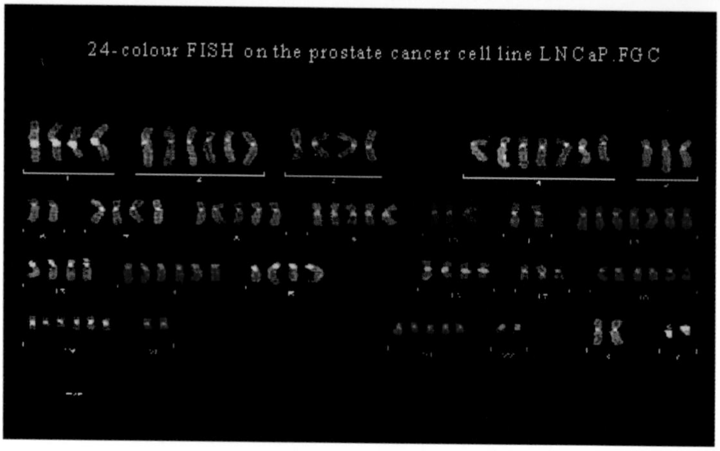

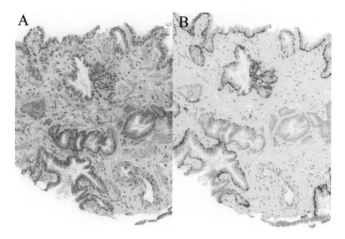

Plate 4 Multiplex FISH of the prostate cancer cell line LNCaP.FGC.

A

B

Plate 5 (a) Atypical glandular proliferation adjacent to high grade PIN (H&E). (b) 34beta E-12 immunostaining reveals absence of immunoreactivity in some of the small glands. However these immunonegative glands are in continuity with high-grade PIN showing a discontinuous basal layer and hence represent outpouchings of high-grade PIN.

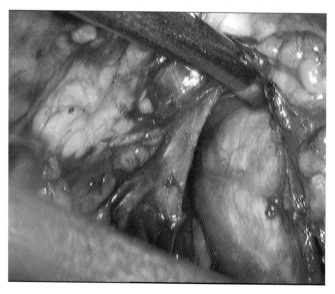

Plate 6 Preparation of the apex for dorsal venous complex suture ligation.

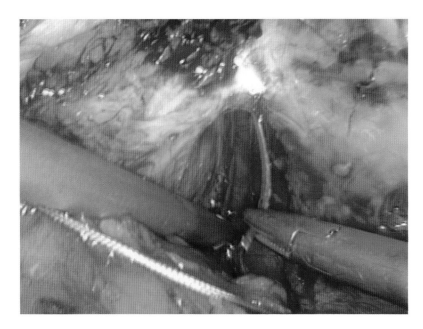

Plate 7 Dorsal venous complex ligation.

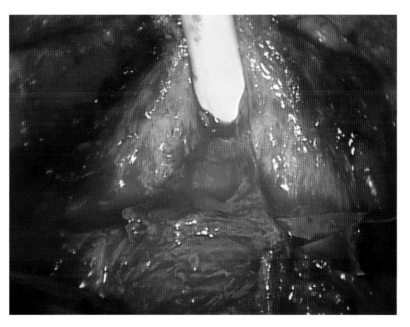

Plate 8 Posterior bladder-neck dissection.

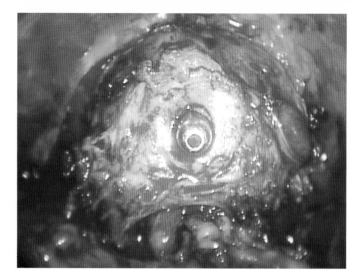

Plate 9 Posterior dissection demonstrating ampullae.

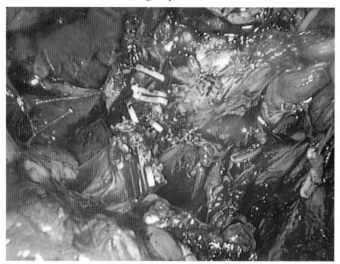

Plate 10 Preservation of the left neuro-vascular bundle.

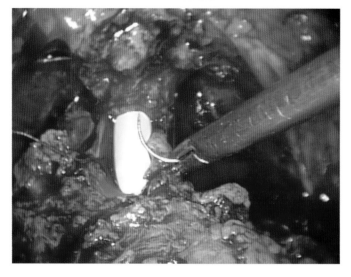

Plate 11 Urethro-vesical anastomosis demonstrating the Van Velthoven technique.

8: Prostate Biopsy: How Many Cores and Where From?

Richard Clements

INTRODUCTION

The incidence of prostatic cancer is anticipated to increase significantly with the increasing age of the population throughout the Western world and this has major workload implications for health-care systems in Europe and the United States. Prostate cancer is now the most common tumour of the adult male, and it has been estimated that there will be 232 090 new cancers diagnosed in the United States by 2005 [1]. Major progress has been made in the diagnosis of prostate cancer in the last 20 years, with the introduction of prostate-specific antigen (PSA) screening and trans-rectal ultrasound (TRUS). These developments have caused stage migration in prostate cancer diagnosis and a marked increase in the incidence of localised prostate cancer. The advent of PSA testing has led to the diagnosis of cancers at an earlier stage; such early prostate cancer is, however, a clinical enigma as the need for active treatment remains unclear. Biopsy of the gland is necessary to confirm or exclude cancer within the prostate gland. Digitally guided prostate biopsy has been largely abandoned, and replaced by TRUS guided systematic biopsy, performed as an outpatient, with a spring-loaded biopsy needle device. Ultrasound-guided prostate biopsy has now become one of the most common diagnostic biopsy procedures undertaken in Radiology and Urology Departments. Even with modern high-frequency transducers and colour Doppler imaging, TRUS has limited ability to distinguish benign from malignant disease within the prostate, as many cancers are isoechoic and not apparent on grey scale imaging. TRUS remains central in prostate cancer diagnosis, however, as it has the ability to enable effective, accurate and objective needle sampling of the prostate, and it can provide additional information to the discerning radiologist or urologist. It has been reported that only about 20% of urologists perform targeted biopsy based on sonographic findings; most biopsies are undertaken by a systematic technique without reference to specific ultrasonic appearances [2].

There is still significant controversy about the sampling technique to be used in prostate biopsy, but recent protocols have demonstrated the importance of obtaining systematic samples from the lateral part of both lobes to complement the traditional para-sagittal cores. It is essential that the biopsy is undertaken under cover of antibiotic prophylaxis, as there is potential morbidity from the procedure. Local anaesthetic agents are increasingly used to minimise the discomfort of the procedure; these may cause a slight increase in the infective complications of TRUS sampling [3].

INDICATIONS FOR PROSTATE BIOPSY

1   Abnormal digital rectal examination (DRE) – any nodular or firm area of the prostate needs to be sampled regardless of the PSA level.
2   Elevated PSA – the traditional upper limit of a normal serum PSA level has been 4 ng/mL, and patients with a serum PSA level above this range justify biopsy. About 25% of cancers may be detected in men with a PSA below this level. The PSA level may be refined through the use of derivative indices listed below, or through the use of percent free PSA.
3   Age-related PSA – where the PSA level is related to the patients' age. The American Urological Association (AUA) best practice policy gives age specific reference ranges for white men, African American men and Asian men [4].
4   Increased PSA density – where the serum PSA level is divided by the prostate volume. (This index requires a TRUS volume determination.)
5   Increased PSA transition zone density – where the serum PSA level is divided by the transition zone volume. (This index also requires a TRUS volume determination, this time of the transition zone (TZ) volume.)
6   Increased PSA velocity – where the PSA rises significantly with time, for example, 0.75 ng/mL/year.

TRUS GUIDED BIOPSY – PATIENT PREPARATION

1 *Antibiotic prophylaxis.* TRUS-guided prostate biopsy must be undertaken with the administration of prophylactic antibiotics. Many different antibiotic regimens have been used including gentamycin, quinalones, cephalosporins and metronidazole. The use of antibiotics has been studied in a randomised study [5], where patients either received a 1 or 3-day course of antibiotics or placebo. This study reported an increased rate of urinary infection in patients receiving placebo, but no particular advantage from the use of a 3-day regimen over a 1-day regimen. It is the author's current practice to use Ofloxacin 200 mg twice daily for 3 days, with the first dose given 30 min

prior to the biopsy, together with Metronidazole 400 mg three times for 1 day.

2 *Bowel preparation.* It has been the traditional practice in the United States to administer a cleansing enema prior to trans-rectal prostate biopsy; the initial rationale of this was to improve the visualisation of the prostate with TRUS by avoiding faecal artefacts. The usual practice in the United Kingdom has been to omit this cleansing enema. Recent studies have compared the complication rate with and without the enema, and have demonstrated an increase in bacteraemia and infective complications with the use of a cleansing enema [6]. In a separate study, Carey & Korman [7] found no advantage in the use of a pre-biopsy enema. It would thus seem appropriate to avoid the use of the cleansing enema.

3 *Bleeding tendency.* It has been thought important that a biopsy should not be performed in a patient with a bleeding tendency. Traditionally this has been assessed by checking that the patient is not taking anticoagulant medication, for example, warfarin, or anti-platelet medication such as clopidrogel and asking if there have been any history of previous untoward bleeding with surgery or trauma. Anticoagulants are usually stopped prior to a trans-rectal prostate biopsy, but there are reported series of prostate biopsies without stopping anticoagulant where there have been no increased complications [8]. Many older men are now taking low does of aspirin as a cardiovascular prophylactic measure; many radiologists and urologists, including the author, stop this treatment for a few days prior to prostate biopsy, but the literature is unclear whether this is needed [9–11]. Non-steroidal anti-inflammatory agents may also alter the patient's normal clotting and such medication may be also stopped for a few days prior to the procedure [12].

LOCAL ANAESTHESIA?

Patients vary considerably in the discomfort and pain they report with TRUS-guided biopsy. Trans-rectal prostate biopsies were traditionally taken without the use of local anaesthetics. Pain is however a frequent side effect of the procedure, with 10–25% of men reporting moderate to severe pain [13]. With the current trend towards an increase in the number of cores taken at systematic biopsy, attempts have been made to decrease any pain associated with the procedure, either through the use of endorectal topical anaesthetic gel, or by local anaesthetic infiltration around the prostate. Topical administration of gel is of doubtful value, as a randomised study reported no difference in pain reported with the use of 2% lidocaine gel [14]. Current techniques have centred on infiltration of anaesthetic agents at three sites around the prostate – the apex of the prostate, the neurovascular bundles or lateral to the seminal vesicles. A comparison of these different approaches has been reported [15], and infiltration of the prostatic capsule at the apex of the prostate appears to be the most effective technique. Wu and colleagues [16] compared an injection of 1% lidocaine and placebo (normal saline) injected lateral to the seminal vesicles under TRUS guidance, and found that an injection of local anaesthesia did not diminish biopsy-associated pain. Obek and colleagues [3] have reported a study looking at the potential complications of peri-prostatic local anaesthetic infiltration. In 100 consecutive patients, local anaesthetic infiltration caused no change in post-biopsy haematuria, but did decrease post-biopsy rectal bleeding. The incidence of bacteruria was significantly higher in patients receiving anaes-thesia: there was an increase in post-biopsy infective complications but this was not statistically significant. Further studies on the complications associ-ated with the use of local anaesthetic infiltration are warranted. Studies have also been reported using a mixture of short-and long-acting local anaes-thetic agents (bupivacaine and lidocaine) with apparent longer-term pain relief [17].

SAMPLING TECHNIQUE

Systematic Biopsy

Current biopsy strategies are centred on the use of TRUS-guided systematic biopsy. The systematic biopsy approach was first proposed by Hodge and Stamey in 1989 [18] taking a 6-core 'sextant' biopsy in the para-sagittal planes at the base, mid-gland and apex of both lobes of the prostate. At the time the sextant approach was first advocated, there was a feeling that 6 cores might be excessive and that a 4 core 'quadrant' approach would be adequate. Enthusiasm for the 'quadrant' approach was short lived and the 'sextant' biopsy became widely accepted, because of its higher detection rate; it has been the basis of the systematic biopsy approach throughout the 1990s. There are numerous reports in the literature on the yield of sextant biopsies, and most authors report a cancer detection rate of between 20–30% for men with a PSA between 4–10 ng/mL and a palpably normal gland. This sextant approach gave a higher detection rate than previous biopsy strategies based on digitally guided biopsy, or TRUS guided biopsy of hypoechoic areas. More recently, there has been the realisation that this 6-core approach under-estimates larger glands and that a higher diagnostic yield of cancer could be obtained by taking both additional cores and cores placed more later-ally. Bauer et al. [19] undertook three-dimensional reconstructions of the specimens obtained at radical prostatectomy and demonstrated that most prostate cancers are located postero-laterally in the prostate. Liu et al. [20]

performed rebiopsy of 187 men after negative sextant biopsy and found cancer in 28% in the lateral peripheral zone (PZ); from this and other studies, it was appreciated that lateral PZ cores should be obtained. Initially a modified 6-core approach was proposed, with the mid-gland cores taken more laterally, thereby sampling a greater volume of peripheral zone tissue. Various strategies taking additional cores have been subsequently reported. Additional mid-gland cores were reported by Salomon *et al.* [21], as a means to improve the local staging. One hundred and seventy seven men underwent sextant biopsy plus three mid-line additional cores prior to radical prostatectomy. Of these, 59 men had one positive biopsy and 13 of these also had 1–3 positive mid-biopsies. Positive surgical margins were more likely in those men (54%) with positive mid-gland cores, compared to 19% in the 46 men with only a single positive focus at sextant biopsy. Supplementing the sextant biopsy with lateral cores into a 10-core biopsy was suggested by Presti *et al.* [22]; in a series of 483 consecutive patients, lateral biopsies were added to the routine sextant biopsy. In this series, patients with a prostate volume greater than 50 cc in size also underwent systematic TZ cores in addition to cores from the mid-lobar para-sagittal plane. Overall, 202 of the 483 men had cancer on biopsy (42%). Traditional sextant biopsies missed 20% of cancers, while a 6-core sextant biopsy of lateral PZ cores missed 11% of cancers. The combination of sextant and lateral PZ biopsies as a 10-core biopsy, detected 194 cancers (96%). The eight-missed cancers were detected by lesion directed (five), or TZ (three) biopsies. Eliminating the mid-lobar base biopsies from the PZ 10-core biopsy approach gave an 8-core PZ regimen, that would detect 95% rather than 96% of the cancers. This study concluded that a traditional sextant approach was inadequate and that a minimum 8-core biopsy including the apex, mid-lobar mid-gland, lateral mid-gland and lateral base should routinely be performed. This important study has been widely adopted and 10-core biopsy forms the basis of many contemporary biopsy protocols.

Further evidence in favour of such an approach came from Eskew [23] who proposed a five region biopsy. About 119 patients underwent biopsy using a scheme that added lateral and mid-line PZ cores to the basic sextant scheme giving a total of 13 cores. Of the 48 patients with cancer, 17 (35%) had cancer only in these additional regions; this approach was found to be of particular benefit to patients with a PSA in the 4–10 ng/mL range. Subsequently a saturation biopsy approach has been proposed [24] taking over 14 cores; this latter approach has not gained widespread acceptance as it is associated with a higher morbidity and also requires some form of intravenous sedation or general anaesthesia. Other biopsy approaches in a fan starting laterally and extending towards the centre have also been reported [25].

The 10-core approach as proposed by Presti *et al.* [22] is now the standard approach advocated in most academic centres involved in studies to detect prostate cancer, for adequate sampling of the palpably normal gland in a man with an elevated PSA level. It should be emphasised that the prostate biopsy protocol needs to be tailored to the individual patient, based on their age, general tolerance of the procedure and the findings on digital rectal examination; patients with a clinically obvious advanced cancer would not need the full series of 10 cores to obtain histological proof of the diagnosis. Rectal bleeding has been found to be more prevalent after prostate biopsy, when the number of cores has been increased from 6 to 8 or 12 cores but the duration of bleeding did not increase [26].

Transition Zone

The policies described above have concentrated on peripheral zone biopsy and have given relatively little attention to the TZ. Small TZ cancers cannot be identified separately by TRUS from the hyperplastic nodules of benign prostatic hyperplasia (BPH). Primary TZ cancer does however occur in about 20% of cases of prostate cancer [27] and various studies have investigated whether TZ biopsies should be performed at an initial diagnostic biopsy assessment or at a subsequent repeat biopsy procedure after negative initial systematic biopsy. In particular, the work of Bauer and colleagues [19] and Presti [22] has demonstrated that TZ biopsies were rarely required if laterally orientated cores were taken. It should be noted that anterior TZ biopsies have a higher complication rate and are more likely to be associated with heavy haematuria and clot retention.

The current conclusion is that TZ biopsies should not be performed at the initial biopsy procedure but that the taking of anterior TZ cores using a longer needle if necessary to reach the anterior TZ should be considered in a patient with persistent elevated PSA and negative systematic biopsy. Trans-urethral resection of the prostate has been advocated by some urologists as a means of sampling the transition zone where previous biopsies are negative [28] but this approach is not widely used. Furthermore magnetic resonance imaging (MR) may be used as a means of detecting areas for targeted biopsy [29,30].

TARGETED BIOPSY

Peripheral Zone Hypoechoic Areas

It was recognised for many years that the predominant sonographic abnormality of prostate cancer is a PZ hypoechoic area [31]; indeed in the early days of TRUS with digitally palpated prostate nodules, this was the most common appearance of cancer. From an *in vitro* analysis of prostatectomy specimens, it was appreciated that cancer was hypoechoic or subtly hypoechoic. With the stage migration that has followed the use of PSA screening, most prostate cancers are now isoechoic and thus not visible on TRUS; they can only be detected by systematic biopsy. The introduction of the systematic biopsy approach caused a tendency to disregard the assessment of PZ focal hypoechoic areas. Nonetheless, it should be appreciated that hypoechoic areas do represent cancer in about 30% of cases [32] and thus systematic biopsy cores should be directed through such areas or additional cores taken to ensure thorough sampling. Many of these hypoechoic areas are subtle and may not be visible on lower specification equipment, or sub-optimally set focal length or transducer frequency but an experienced sonologist will appreciate the alteration in the sonographic architecture. A useful additional sign of an extensive diffusely infiltrating carcinoma may cause an alteration in the overall echotexture of the gland; in these cases, a loss of the differentiation between the PZ and TZ may be an important feature of prostate cancer.

Peripheral Zone Hypervascular Foci

It has almost been 10 years since the development of trans-rectal colour Doppler but its utility in prostate cancer diagnosis still remains unclear. It was initially hoped that colour Doppler might demonstrate changes in prostate vascularity (tumour angiogenesis) that would enhance the detection of cancers that were isoechoic on grey scale imaging. Colour Doppler may demonstrate prostate cancer as hypervascular foci but this is usually in lesions that are already visible on grey scale imaging as hypoechoic areas; only rarely does it demonstrate tumours that are isoechoic on grey scale imaging [33]. Nonetheless, it is often valuable to use colour Doppler during a TRUS scanning procedure as it may help draw attention to an area requiring biopsy that might otherwise be overlooked. This is particularly true in the antero-lateral peripheral zone. Prostate cancer has been shown to be associated with hypervascular foci on colour Doppler [34,35], and such foci may be sought during a TRUS scan and sampled. This may be undertaken as part of the systematic biopsy, ensuring that one of the cores is directed through the hypervascular focus. Use of colour Doppler does not however obviate a systematic biopsy [35].

Sonographic Contrast Agents

A few sonographic contrast agents are now commercially available; these agents consist of a suspension of gas microbubbles. They have a role both

Table 8.1 Ultrasound contrast agents.

Ultrasound contrast agent	Manufacturer	Gas
Levovist	Schering	Air
Sonovue	Bracco	Sulphur hexafluoride
Imavist[a]	Alliance Pharmaceuticals	Perfluorohexane
Definity[a]	Dupont	Perfluoropropane
Echogen[a]	Sonus Pharmaceuticals	Dodecafluorpentane
Optison[a]	Tyco	Perfluorohexane
Sonazoid[a]	Nycomed Amersham	Perfluorocarbon

[a]Under development: Not currently licensed in United Kingdom.

in cardiology, and in radiology in the assessment of certain liver pathology, and their potential use in prostate cancer detection is under evaluation in research units. The agents that are now available in the United Kingdom, or under development are listed in Table 8.1. These agents vary in their physical properties and half-life, and may be administered as either a bolus or infusion; they may be scanned with grey scale imaging or colour Doppler. The different agents achieve the gas suspension in different ways. In Levovist – (Schering AG, Berlin), there are microparticles of molecular aggregates of air and galactose. In other agents, the microbubbles are low solubility gases. These change from the liquid state into the gaseous state following injection into the body. Examples of such agents are sulphur hexa-flouride in Sonovue – (Bracco, Milan, Italy), perfluoropropane – Definity (Dupont Pharmaceuticals, Billerica, MA, United States) and dodecaflouropentane – Echogen (Sonus Pharmaceuticals, Bothel, WA, Unites States).

There have been few reports on their value in prostate cancer diagnosis; these have been predominantly derived from one US institution – the Ultrasound Department of Thomas Jefferson University in Philadelphia, United States. Observations on the value of these agents in prostate cancer diagnosis are conflicting and current experience indicate that they will have a limited role in prostate cancer diagnosis. In an early presentation, Rickards and colleagues [36] used sextant biopsies following intravenous contrast injection in 22 patients and found that the use of the agent increased the sensitivity but decreased the specificity of the prostate sextant biopsy. A subsequent report [37] has suggested that direct biopsy of focally enhancing hypervascular areas yields a better detection rate than systematic sextant biopsy, and was cost-effective because of the low pathological processing costs. A further report from the same group [38] evaluated the value of targeted biopsy using TRUS with contrast enhancement with a different contrast agent. Forty patients were evaluated by a harmonic imaging technique with an infusion and bolus of Definity (perfluoropropane microbubbles) (Dupont Pharmaceuticals, Billerica, MA, United States). A sextant biopsy was performed and these sextant biopsy sites were scored for their level of contrast enhancement. Targeted biopsy of other sites of contrast enhancement was also undertaken. A suspicious site on contrast enhancement was five times more likely to be positive for cancer than a standard sextant biopsy site. No specific advantage was found with the bolus technique compared with the infusion technique.

These reports have so far failed to show a major improvement in the diagnostic accuracy of prostate cancer diagnosis with sonographic contrast agents. The development of these agents has occurred contemporaneously with the developments in the systematic biopsy described earlier; with the increased diagnostic accuracy of the 10-core systematic biopsy, it is difficult to currently envisage the widespread use of expensive sonographic contrast agents in routine prostate cancer diagnosis. This assessment could change however if these agents, through their ability to depict neo-vascularity of prostate cancers, were shown to give additional prognostic information, for example, if they were able to help to differentiate high-grade from low-grade cancers, and were able to predict the biological potential of an individual cancer. There is some preliminary evidence to support this proposition [39]. In 230 patients investigated with both contrast-enhanced targeted biopsy and systematic biopsy reported by Frauscher and colleagues, the cancers identified by targeted contrast-enhanced biopsy were of significantly higher Gleason score than those detected by systematic biopsy. New serum tests are being developed for prostate cancer diagnosis and these may improve our identification of patients requiring TRUS-guided biopsy; in those circumstances the optimum method of prostate cancer detection, whether 10-core systematic biopsy or targeted biopsy of contrast-enhanced cancer vascularity will need to be re-evaluated.

MANAGEMENT OF THE BIOPSY CORE SPECIMEN

Relatively little attention has so far been given by radiologists, urologists or histopathologists to the optimum management of the histological cores obtained at contemporary prostate biopsy. Research studies have concentrated on the number and position of the cores and have tended to disregard both the needle design, or handling of the biopsy specimen once it has been obtained and placed in formalin solution. The traditional needle used with a spring-loaded biopsy device has an inner needle, which is advanced first and followed immediately by an outer cannula, which cuts off the tissue lying within the notch of the inner needle. Recently, a needle that uses an end core technique has been proposed [40]; use of this needle gave a greater tissue yield but tissue was not obtained in 20% of firings. In future, further refinements in needle design may give a more reliable improvement in cancer diagnosis. There is now an appreciation that improvements in diagnostic accuracy can also be obtained by using a pre-embedding technique for the tissue cores. Placing the core in a plastic cassette within formalin, immediately at the time of obtaining the core, results in a straighter core, which is both easier and cheaper for the histopathologist to process. This technique is being used by histopathologists in the handling of breast biopsy cores and more recently has been used in the prostate [41]. Results reported from Innsbruck show that this technique improved the tissue per section level [41]. It led to a 100% decrease in the number of tissue sections necessary for complete work-up and to a higher percentage of tissue per section level. Another recent development from the Stanford group has looked at reducing histopathological costs by colour coding the cores [42]. Various different colours were tried in developing a strategy to decrease pathology costs. By marking all cores from the right side in green ink, and those from the left in black ink, the cores could be placed in a single container for histopathological processing.

SUMMARY

The biopsy protocol should be tailored to the individual patient. In a patient with a palpably normal prostate and an abnormal serum PSA level or other diagnostic parameter, a 10-core biopsy is appropriate, and local anaesthetic infiltration of the prostatic apex may be valuable in optimising tissue yield and improving patient comfort. If the sextant biopsy is negative, then repeat biopsy involving anterior TZ cores in addition to PZ systematic cores is appropriate and colour Doppler may be useful in highlighting core positions at the repeat biopsy session. In a patient with a clinically advanced cancer by PSA or palpation, fewer cores are normally sufficient for diagnosis.

REFERENCES

1 Jemal A, Murray T, Ward E et al. Cancer statistics, 2005. CA Cancer J Clin 2005; 51: 10–30.
2 Plawker MW, Fleisher JM, Vapnek EM et al. Current trends in prostate cancer diagnosis and staging among United States urologists. J Urol 1997; 158: 1853–8.
3 Obek C, Onal B, Ozkan B et al. Is periprostatic local anesthesia for transrectal ultrasound guided prostate biopsy associated with increased infectious or hemorrhagic complications? A prospective randomized trial. J Urol 2002; 168: 558–61.
4 American Urological Association Prostate-specific antigen (PSA) best practice policy. Oncology (Huntington) 2000; 14: 267–72.
5 Aron M, Rajeev TP, Gupta NP. Antibiotic prophylaxis for transrectal needle biopsy of the prostate: a randomized controlled study. BJU Int 2000; 85: 682–5.
6 Lindert KA, Kabalin JN, Terris MK. Bacteremia and bacteriuria after

transrectal ultrasound guided prostate biopsy. *J Urol* 2000; **164**: 76–80.

7 Carey JM, Korman HJ. Transrectal ultrasound guided biopsy of the prostate. Do enemas decrease clinically significant complications? *J Urol* 2001; **166**: 82–5.

8 Ihezue CU, Smart J, Dewbury KC *et al.* Biopsy of the prostate guided by transrectal ultrasound: relation between warfarin use and incidence of bleeding complications. *Clinical Radiology* 2005; **60**: 459–63.

9 Zhu J-P, Davidsen MB, Meyhoff HH. Aspirin, a silent risk factor in urology. *Scand. J. Urol. Nephrol* 1995; **29**: 369–74.

10 Rodriguez LV, Terris MK. Risks and complications of transrectal ultrasound.*Curr Opin Urol* 2000; **10**: 111–6.

11 Connor SEJ, Wingate JP. Management of patients treated with aspirin or warfarin and evaluation of haemostasis prior to prostatic biopsy; a survey of current practice amongst radiologists and urologists. *Clin Radiol* 1999; **54**: 598–603.

12 Herget EJ, Saliken JC, Donnelly BJ *et al.* Transrectal ultrasound-guided biopsy of the prostate: relation between ASA use and bleeding complications *Can Assoc Radiol J* 1999; **50**: 173–6.

13 Clements R, Aideyan OU, Griffiths GJ *et al.* Side effects and patient acceptability of transrectal biopsy of the prostate. *Clin Radiol* 1993; **47**: 125–6.

14 Desgrandchamps F, Meria P, Irani J *et al.* The rectal administration of lidocaine gel and tolerance of transrectal ultrasonography-guided biopsy of the prostate: a prospective randomized placebo-controlled study. *BJU Int* 1999; **83**: 1007–9.

15 Schostak M, Christoph F, Muller M *et al.* Optimizing local anesthesia during 10-core biopsy of the prostate. *Urology* 2002; **60**: 253–7.

16 Wu CL, Carter HB, Naqibuddin M *et al.* Effect of local anesthetics on patient recovery after transrectal biopsy. *Urology* 2001; **57**: 925–9.

17 Lee-Elliott CE, Dundas D, Patel U. Randomised trial of lidocaine vs. lidocaine/bupivacaine periprostatic injection on longitudinal pain scores after

prosate biopsy. *J Urol* 2004; **171**: 247–50.

18 Hodge KK, McNeal JE, Terris MK *et al.* Random systematic versus directed ultrasound guided transrectal core biopsies of the prostate. *J Urol* 1989; **142**: 71–5.

19 Bauer JJ, Zeng J, Weir J *et al.* 3-D computer simulated prostate models: lateral prostate biopsies increase the detection rate of prostate cancer. *Urology* 1999; **53**: 961–7.

20 Liu P, Terris M, McNeal JE. Indications for ultrasound guided transition zone biopsies in the detection of prostate cancer. *J Urol* 1995; **153**: 1000–3.

21 Salomon L, Colombel M, Patard JJ *et al.* Use of three additional mid biopsies to improve local assessment of prostate cancer in patients with one positive sextant biopsy. *Eur Urol* 1998; **34**: 313–7.

22 Presti JC, Jr., Chang JJ, Bhargava V *et al.* The optimal systematic prostate biopsy scheme should include 8 rather than 6 biopsies: results of a prospective clinical trial. *J Urol* 2000; **163**: 163–6.

23 Eskew LA, Bare RL, McCullogh DL. Systematic 5 region prostate biopsy is superior to sextant method for diagnosing carcinoma of the prostate. *J Urol* 1997; **157**: 199–203.

24 Stewart CS, Leibovich BC, Weaver AL *et al.* Prostate cancer diagnosis using a saturation needle biopsy technique after previous negative sextant biopsies. *J Urol* 2001; **166**: 86–92.

25 Brossner C, Madersbacher S, Klinger HC *et al.* A comparative study of a double-line versus a fan-shaped technique for obtaining transrectal ultrasound-guided biopsies of the prostate. *Eur Urol* 1998; **33**: 556–61.

26 Ghani K, Dundas D, Patel U. Bleeding after transrectal ultrasonography-guided prostate biopsy: a study of 7-day morbidity after a six-, eight- and 12-core biopsy protocol. *BJU Int* 2004; **94**: 1014–20.

27 McNeal JE, Redwine EA, Freiha FS *et al.* Zonal distribution of prostatic adenocarcinoma. *Am J Surg Pathol* 1988; **12**: 897–906.

28 Vanasupa B, Miller T, Schwartz B. Diagnosis of prostate adenocarcinoma using transurethral resection of the

prostate after multiple negative transrectal biopsies and persistently elevated prostate-specific antigen level. *Urology* 2000; **56**: 1056xi–xii.

29 Perrotti M, Han K-R, Epstein R *et al.* Prospective evaluation of endorectal magnetic resonance imaging to detect tumor foci in men with prior negative prostatic biopsy: a pilot study. *J Urol* 1999; **162**: 1314–17.

30 Vilanova JC, Comet J, Capdevila A *et al.* The value of endorectal MR imaging to predict positive biopsies in clinically intermediate-risk prostate cancer patients. *Eur Radiol* 2001; **11**: 229–35.

31 Griffiths GJ, Clements R, Jones DR *et al.* The ultrasound appearances of prostatic cancer with histologic correlation. *Clin Radiol* 1987; **38**: 219–27.

32 Lee F, Torp-Pedersen S, Littrup PJ *et al.* Hypoechoic lesions of the prostate: clinical relevance of tumor size, digital rectal examination, and prostate-specific antigen. *Radiology* 1989; **170**: 29–32.

33 Rifkin MD, Sudakoff GS, Alexander AA. Prostate: Techniques, results, and potential applications of color Doppler US scanning. *Radiology* 1993; **186**: 509–13.

34 Kelly IMG, Lees WR, Rickards D. Prostate cancer and the role of color Doppler US. *Radiology* 1993; **189**: 153–6.

35 Lavoipierre AM, Snow RM, Frydenberg M *et al.* Prostatic cancer: role of color Doppler imaging in transrectal sonography. *Am J Roentgenol* 1998; **171**: 205–10.

36 Rickards D, Gillams AR, Deng J *et al.* Do intravascular ultrasound Doppler contrast agents improve transrectal ultrasound diagnosis of prostate cancer? *Radiology* 1998; Supplement: (RSNA 98 meeting).

37 Halpern EJ, McCue PA, Aksnes AK *et al.* Contrast-enhanced US of the prostate with Sonazoid: Comparison with whole-mount prostatectomy specimens in 12 patients. *Radiology* 2002; **222**: 361–6.

38 Halpern EJ, Frauscher F, Rosenberg M *et al.* Directed biopsy during contrast-enhanced sonography of the prostate. *Am J Roentgenol* 2002; **178**: 915–9.

39 Frauscher F, Klauser A, Volgger H *et al.* Comparison of contrast-enhanced color Doppler targeted biopsy to conventional systematic biopsy: impact on Gleason score. In: L Derchi, ed. *European Radiology Annual Meeting of the European Society of Urogenital Radiology 2002.* Springer, Genova, 2002: D13.

40 Haggarth L, Ekman P, Egevad L. A new core-biopsy instrument with an end-cut technique provides prostate biopsies with increased tissue yield. *BJU Int* 2002; **90**: 51–5.

41 Rogatsch H, Mairinger T, Horninger W *et al.* Optimized preembedding method improves the histologic yield of prostatic core needle biopsies. *Prostate* 2000; **42**: 124–9.

42 Terris MK, McNeal JE. Application of tissue-marking ink to prostate biopsy specimens. *Prostate* 2002; **50**: 247–51.

9: Counselling Patients with Early Prostate Cancer

Gail Beese and Christopher Edmunds

SPOILT FOR CHOICE: THE DILEMMAS FACING MEN DIAGNOSED WITH EARLY PROSTATE CANCER

Early prostate cancer is taken to be a malignancy that is confined to the prostate gland. The diagnosis is made from the following tests and procedures:

- prostate-specific antigen (PSA) testing (specific assay title standardised test);
- a digital rectal examination (DRE); and
- transrectal ultrasound (TRUS) guided needle biopsy.

These can also be supported by ultrasound and radiological imaging, such as computerised tomography (CT) or magnetic resonance (MR) imaging. In the United Kingdom the definitive working diagnosis is to be reached following a discussion of all the established clinical information by a specialist multidisciplinary oncology team (MDT). This MDT includes all those health professionals who are involved in patient management. The team's role is to make collective and effective decisions regarding the diagnosis, treatment and care of individual patients.

Following the diagnosis of organ-confined prostate cancer, a range of treatments have to then be considered. A short list of these can then be drawn up to form the basis for counselling and discussion with patients (Box 9.1). Another issue to be addressed by the clinician at this stage of the counselling process is whether there are not only clinical, but also geographical and political influences that will affect the options available to each patient. Ethically, do we as clinicians inform patients of the full range of treatments whose clinical criteria they meet, or simply those that are

---

Box 9.1 *Treatment options for men with early prostate cancer.*

Treatment choices:

- Radical prostatectomy
    1 Open radical prostatectomy (+/− PLND[a])
    2 Perineal radical prostatectomy (+/− PLND[a])
    3 Lararoscopic radical prostatectomy (+/− PLND[a])

- Radical radiotherapy; different techniques:
    1 Standard external beam radiotherapy
    2 3D conformal radiotherapy

- Brachytherapy

- Watchful waiting/Active monitoring

- High intensity focused ultrasound (HIFU)

- Cryotherapy/cryoabolation.

[a]PLND = pelvic lymph node dissection

---

available locally. It may be that other treatments offer greater benefits to an individual but are only available in other parts of the United Kingdom, or further afield. This opens up a debate regarding just what constitutes patient choice; that is, what is available in theory, and what is available in practice.

The subject of prostate cancer is an emotive one. There is almost incessant media coverage of the disease, which on the one hand helps to raise public awareness, but on the other, helps fuel male anxiety about the chances and consequences of developing the disease. It is possible that prostate cancer is being used as a means to raise the profile of changing attitudes of men towards health generally, in much the same way that the breast cancer awareness campaign has done for women.

In terms of epidemiology and aetiology, there are similarities between breast and prostate cancer; however, in terms of the depth of knowledge, and certainly in terms of public profile, there is an ever-increasing gulf between the two diseases. The most striking contrast between prostate cancer and breast cancer care is with respect to the advice and support services that we, as health-care professionals, offer patients. Men who come to us seeking advice and reassurance, about a disease that kills approximately 10 000 per year in the United Kingdom alone, have recourse to very scant support networks, together with inconsistent and uncoordinated information materials. Men have every right to be anxious about prostate cancer, given the level of uncertainty and conjecture surrounding this disease amongst health professionals, and the need for counselling is paramount at every stage of the diagnostic and treatment process. Confusion reigns to such a degree that the opening sentence of the NHS 'Prostate Cancer Plan' [1] states that 'prostate cancer is the most mysterious of all cancers. It is often impossible to distinguish between slow growing tumours that cause no harm and fast growing tumours which kill'.

The dedicated pages on their website [2], which clearly illustrate the level of uncertainty surrounding the disease, list the following features of the disease:

- The cause or causes are not clearly understood.
- The natural history is unclear – it is not even clear whether there is a single entity called prostate cancer or a number of different types of cancer.
- The effectiveness of early detection as a means of reducing mortality remains contentious.
- The treatment of both early and advanced cancer remains a matter on which there is little clinical consensus.

PSA TESTING

In relation to its clinical significance, the issue of PSA testing has had a disproportionate degree of importance placed upon it, in terms of its contribution to the diagnosis and prognosis of prostate cancer. PSA is often taken out of context and highlighted as a panacea for all the difficulties we have in managing the disease. This is far from the truth.

When mountain climbers are asked why they risk their lives to climb Everest, they say, 'because it is there'. PSA was going to be discovered sooner or later, because it was there. There is no unmaking of science. Unfortunately, in medicine, some discoveries may lead to more harm than good.

It remains to be seen whether there will be a net benefit following the discovery of PSA. In the mean time, a large population of men who, 15 years ago, would have remained happily unaware of any problem, now have an impaired quality of life because they are consumed by anxiety about their PSA [3].

WHEN DOES THE COUNSELLING PROCESS BEGIN?

Clearly, the availability of counselling, albeit in a limited form, has to be introduced at the earliest possible stage of the diagnostic process. The PSA test request offers just such an opportunity. The uncertainties that pervade prostate cancer should not be unfamiliar to the patient by the time diagnosis is confirmed and discussions are centred on the choice of treatment. 'Patients, families and carers need access to support from the time that the cancer is suspected through death and into bereavement' [4].

The counselling process for early prostate cancer must start with the first approach to their family doctor, if not before. There needs to be a structured and consistent response to men asking for or being offered a PSA test. They need to understand and appreciate the consequences of the course of action that they are about to take. Men need to acknowledge that where early prostate cancer is concerned we are facing a conundrum that is unlikely to be solved in the near future.

The patient's journey has to be seen as a continuous process, not as separate stages, and therefore patient support has to be viewed in the same way. Every health-care professional with whom the patient comes into contact will have a counselling role to play and it is vital that the advice and support offered to patients is as accurate and consistent as possible. The clinical dilemmas that confront us should not be permitted to exacerbate the high degree of anxiety that the patient and his family would already be experiencing. Patients must at least have confidence in our ability to support them, despite our inability to give them the unambiguous answers they seek.

With the growing demand for screening, this would be the obvious starting point for the counselling process. However, screening is contentious in itself, particularly in the case of prostate cancer. The arguments for and against screening are as diverse as they are vociferous, but it must be accepted that it brings both harm and benefits: 'By offering screening to 250 000 we have helped a few, harmed thousands, disappointed many, used £1.5 m each year, and kept a few lawyers in work' [5]. The positive and negative aspects of screening for prostate cancer should form the basis of the initial aspect of the counselling process for those men who are concerned about prostate cancer. The counselling process can facilitate the required consent. Information for the patient, on which he can base his decisions, will also form the foundation of a successful relationship between the professional and the patient. The General Medical Council have addressed this specific topic, and their guidance on informed consent is as follows:

> Successful relationships between doctors and patients depend on
> trust. To establish that trust you must respect a patient's

autonomy – their right to decide whether or not to undergo any medical intervention. . .[They] must be given sufficient information, in a way they can understand, in order to enable them to make informed decisions about their care [6].

The purpose, then, of counselling men diagnosed with early prostate cancer is to enable them to decide which treatment is best suited to them. Some medical decisions are complex because evidence on outcomes is uncertain or the options have different risk-benefit profiles that patients value differently. Practice guidelines for these difficult decisions recommend that patients understand the probable outcomes of options, consider the personal value they place on benefits versus risk, and participate with their practitioners in deciding about treatment [7].

What form should this counselling take and what are the principles that are involved? The British Association for Counselling and Psychotherapy [8] suggests six ethical principles:

1 Fidelity: honouring the trust placed in the practitioner.
2 Autonomy: respect for the client's right to be self-governing.
3 Beneficence: a commitment to promoting the client's well being.
4 Non-malfeasance: a commitment to avoiding harm to the client.
5 Justice: the fair and impartial treatment of all clients and the provision of adequate services.
6 Self-respect: fostering the practitioner's self-knowledge and care for self.

Combining these elements will certainly help; however, it is the individualisation of the discussion that we see as of the greatest importance.

WHAT INFORMATION SHOULD BE GIVEN?

Counselling must have a clearly defined purpose. Does it aim to enable patients to assimilate information so that they can give informed consent to a planned investigation or treatment, or does it aim to enable patients to actively participate in the decision-making process? We must recognise that there is a distinction between these two objectives. As Fallowfield [9] points out:

Two fundamental issues should be determined when discussing treatment choices with patients – their own preferences about the amount and type of information that is needed and their actual rather than perceived desire for participation in decision making. A clear distinction needs to be made between a desire for information and a wish to assume responsibility for decision making [9].

Communication of Risk

Much of the discussion around treatment choices will be based upon effective communication of the comparative risks involved. One of the key issues surrounding cancer is the communication of such risks [10].

The individual patient will have a unique perception of, first, the risks involved in developing the disease; second, the risks of participating in a particular treatment modality; and, third, the risk of the treatment being unsuccessful and the potential cost to quality of life. Value judgements will have a major impact here; we cannot assume rational processes will be at work. Calman [10] goes on to say: 'How people perceive health issues and risk and how they make choices about their own behaviour do not always fall into a rational pattern'.

We need to make sure that patients are able to distinguish between absolute risk and relative risk. In the case of early prostate cancer, the patient is faced with an array of potential treatments. The temptation on the part of the clinician is to compare comparative risks of potential side-effects; for example, the relative risk of impotency between radical prostatectomy and radical radiotherapy is small, however, the absolute risk with either treatment is significant.

The language we use to describe different types of treatment and our knowledge of each treatment will influence the manner in which the information we offer is understood. One day, we may say to one patient that a particular risk is minimal, and then quantify the same risk to another as small. Different patients may perceive each term in entirely differing ways. We need to be conscious of the language we use and recognise when there is a need for explanation rather than simply a regurgitation of facts; one man's meat is very much another man's poison.

The ethos has to be one of information sharing, not just giving. That information should also state that as clinicians we are making the best use of the information we have and that we may not know all the answers. The patient needs to appreciate the degree of uncertainty that undermines much of what science has to offer. It is possible to argue that part of the counselling process should involve preparing the patient to participate in clinical trials and research, thereby taking the concept of partnership one step further. Evidence-based care should be founded on the analysis of data collected from those treated to date; each patient treated should offer something new to the next *ad infinitum*. We should all be engaged in the cyclical analysis of clinical practice as part of our professional routine.

We must not lose sight of the opportunity to use clinical practice to perform qualitative as well as quantitative research. There must be a drive towards improving not only what we do, but how we do it. A recent review [11] on the recording or summaries of consultations for people with cancer addressed the implications for both practice and research.

In terms of practice: 'Each cancer patient should be assessed carefully in terms of his or her needs, preferences, access to support and likely responses' [11]. The consultation should be viewed as an opportunity to discuss which types of information would best suit the individual patient's needs. The review identified the implications for research as wide reaching and illustrated the dearth of research into the impact of information giving to cancer patients.

Although it is clear that many people with cancer find consultation tapes and letters useful, further research is needed to assess the impact of these interventions on health status. Other outcomes which could usefully be explored include psychosocial adaptation and coping behaviour, and the quality of relationships between patients and their families and health-care providers.

The report goes on to highlight the lack of evidence relating to the information exchange processes within the oncology consultation, its quality and the manner of its delivery. Stage context of the consultation, that is, new diagnosis, treatment follow up or disease progression, and its impact on the exchange of information could also be the subject of research. Much needs to be done in relation to what we say, together with how and when we say it.

A major influence on the content and manner of consultation is the difference between the priorities and values of the clinician and those of the patient. There is clearly a wide variation in the risk–benefit analysis applied to different treatment modalities by individual clinicians. In the case of early prostate cancer, often a surgeon's interpretation of a particular set of diagnostic data will differ from that of the oncologist. In addition, a recent survey conducted by Donovan *et al.* [12] revealed that there is a wide variation between clinicians within the same speciality. When presented with a hypothetical patient, a total of 202 urologists who responded collectively recommended a total of seven different treatment modalities for the same patient. It could be argued that such a wide variation in the recommended treatment is a result of the poor evidence base that such recommendations are made on.

The ProtecT study [13], a randomised controlled trial comparing active monitoring, radical prostatectomy and radical radiotherapy in screened men with localised prostate cancer, which is currently running in the United Kingdom, is designed to address this issue. Rakow [14] attempts to address the reasons behind the variations in the preferences of doctors. It highlights one of the fundamental differences between doctors and patients, with doctors tending to look at long-term survival and patients looking at the impact on quality of life. The study found a clear association between belief about likely outcomes and option preference. The better informed a clinician is about a particular treatment, the more likely he or she is to recommend that treatment. Hence, a urologist specialising in radical prostatectomy will favour their modality, whereas the radiologist will advocate the benefits of radiotherapy.

In the case of patients, the preferences they demonstrate tend to be based upon their lack of knowledge rather than its depth. The decision-making process is not strictly rational but rather is subject to systematic biases. The evidence suggests that people use short cuts when making decisions in order to simplify the decision-making process, resulting in these biases [15]. This introduces the concept of heuristics, which is simply a method of problem solving by trial and error.

Familiarity tends to lead to an over-estimation of the risk. Slovic et al. [16] found that survey respondents over-estimated the frequency of rare causes of death (e.g. murder, car accidents, etc.) and under-estimated the frequency of more common causes (e.g. stroke and cancer).

Other factors that can affect perception of risk include immediacy of effect, controllability, novelty and catastrophe. Experimental studies have demonstrated that when assimilating information about risk, patients tend to just use the basic outline and base their decision on this. They simply perceive risk as big or small, not quantitatively valued in terms of percentages, as it is often presented [17].

This idea has been supported by Mazur et al. [18], who found that in discussions with doctors a large proportion of patients prefer qualitative terms, such as 'possible and probable', as opposed to an illustration of risk based on percentages. How the risk is presented, or how it is framed, affects the way it is received by the patient. A simple choice of providing information on survival, as opposed to mortality, will have a significant impact. A survival rate of 90% following major surgery will project the risk in a positive light, while the same information presented as a 10% death rate will achieve the opposite. It is vitally important for clinicians to be conscious of such factors when counselling patients about treatment choice.

Even more subtle differences, such as presenting risk as a rate rather than proportion, can influence a patient's decision. Indeed, studies have shown that even fundamental information, such as diagnosis, can be lost by a significant proportion of patients. Ellis *et al.* [19] reported that 38% of patients, who were counselled verbally by clinicians, could not remember their diagnosis when questioned later. Lloyd [15] defines risk as being made up of two parts: 'the product of the probability of an outcome and the severity of that outcome'. The first part constitutes the quantitative element of risk, and the second part, the more qualitative dimensions. It may be one thing for patients to be told a radical prostatectomy carries a 20% risk of permanent urinary incontinence, but quite another for the patient to have a clear understanding of what impact that incontinence will have on his quality of life, both in the short- and long-term.

Gattellari *et al.* [20] found that 80% of cancer patients, who had been told by their doctors that they had no chance of cure, reported that they had some chance of cure, and 15% reported their chance of cure as being 75%. Clearly, it is difficult to draw a direct comparison with such patients and those diagnosed with early prostate cancer; however, it clearly illustrates just what an emotive subject cancer is.

We cannot afford to under-estimate the negative psychological impact the word 'cancer' has. We have to also acknowledge that, especially in terms of a cancer diagnosis, the cognitive impact may make truly informed consent an impossible goal. The protective instinct of denial may prove to be a barrier that cannot be completely overcome. The ability to prove that the patient has actually given informed consent can be difficult.

Older patients' experiences of health-care, including many already undergoing treatment for prostate cancer, will have done little or nothing to suggest they should do anything other than comply with medicines' traditionally paternalistic approach of 'doctor knows best'. Recent demands to ensure that the patient is fully informed can leave many patients bombarded with a mass of information and choices to make regarding their treatment, which they feel unable or unwilling to make. This issue, in the case of prostate cancer, is further compounded by a lack of evidence proving any kind of benefit of one treatment over another. If clinicians provide information in equipoise, but no guidance on what to do, there may well be a feeling of abandonment. Clinicians often under-estimate a patient's need for information, but over-estimate their need to be involved in the decision-making process [21]. Providing information in a way that is appropriate for the patient to assimilate can result in benefits, such as a faster recovery and improved compliance with treatment. Patients also tend to demonstrate reduced levels of anxiety and increased levels of satisfaction in relation to their treatment [22].

The concept of shared decision-making can help to facilitate this. This process encourages patients to express their views and to participate in making clinical decisions. The following skills and steps have been identified [23], which may help to assist in this process:

- develop a partnership with the patient;
- establish or review the patient's preference for information, for example, amount and format;
- establish or review the patient's preferences for role in decision-making;
- ascertain and respond to patients' ideas, concerns and expectations;
- identify choices and evaluate the research evidence in relation to the individual patient;
- present (or direct to) evidence, taking into account the above steps, and help the patient reflect upon and assess the impact of alternative decisions with regard to their values and lifestyles;
- make or negotiate a decision in partnership, manage conflict; and
- agree upon an action plan and complete arrangements for follow up.

Informing and assisting the patient to choose the option most appropriate for them and providing the patient with a patient-centred approach to their care is time consuming. Therefore, it is vital that these aspects of care are co-ordinated in terms of how, when and by whom this information is to be delivered.

The use of specialist nurses to assist in the process of providing information is beneficial. This can also allow the patient faster access, allowing questions to be answered as they occur, and can often prove to be less intimidating to those who favour the more paternalistic approach. Patient support groups should also play a part in the decision-making process by providing first-hand accounts of the treatment in layman's terms. They can illustrate effects on quality-of-life of urinary incontinence or radiation proctitis, both of which will sound different from a personal experience perspective than when described as a percentage. The use of patient support groups for this purpose may vary with gender: Women are more likely to use support groups to access information on certain treatment aspect's 'feel' than men, who may seek out technical information and concentrate less on emotional issues [24]. This fact should be borne in mind when developing local support mechanisms.

Technology needs to be explored further as a method of assisting patients to reach their treatment of choice. Onel *et al.* [25] found that the use of a standardised video to explain treatment choice does not shorten the length of time the clinician spends with the patient. However, it does improve the quality of the consultation for both the patient and clinician. It allows the discussion to focus on critical risk–benefit tradeoffs rather than simply the description of treatment alternatives. The internet can also be a rich source of information.

Holmes-Rovner *et al.* [26] suggest that the producers of major patient websites, such as NHS Direct Online, National Electronic Library for Health, professional websites and voluntary organisations, could even include decision modules and complementary decision aids. Details of appropriate quality websites should be provided as an option for those patients and their families who wish to access this format for information.

A clinical pathway will facilitate the giving and reinforcement of information and offer a structured approach. A clinical pathway is defined as 'a documented sequence of clinical interventions, placed in an appropriate timeframe, written and agreed by a multidisciplinary team'. Its function is in turn described as: 'allowing a multidisciplinary team to co-ordinate care by setting out all the activities involved in the care of a patient with a defined condition. They lead each patient towards a set of desired outcomes and ensure that specified interventions are delivered at the appropriate time, in the right way and by the right professional' [27]. A clinical pathway facilitates information giving in a structured and co-ordinated way. This allows the patient time to assimilate all the information required, and to engage clinicians in discussion, thereby offering the partnership an opportunity to reach a consensual decision.

Initial discussions should be centred on the need for a PSA test and then move onto the subsequent results of the test. Box 9.2 provides an example of how decision-making may be assisted. In the first instance, emphasis should be given to what PSA and prostate cancer is. As the patient moves along the pathway, more in depth information is required and the emphasis should be shifted to allow larger involvement by health-care professionals and patient support groups. Such a pathway would have safeguards built in to ensure that information is given at key points, is relevant to each stage of the process and is allowed to accumulate in a sequential pattern. Each stage will allow patients and clinicians to revisit specific aspects of the planned treatment, building towards a comprehensive form of consent and partnership. To provide truly patient-centred care, information giving and the decision-making process need to be formalised, thus ensuring that all

Box 9.2 *Structured approach to information and decision aids for patients on the prostate cancer diagnosis pathway.*

Patients stage in pathway	Information required	Format/decision aids
Prior to PSA testing	What is PSA? What is prostate cancer? What are the treatments?	Leaflets Video Contacts for further information, that is, support groups, internet addresses
Raised PSA/ abnormal	How is prostate cancer diagnosed? How is prostate cancer treated?	Leaflets Video Specialist, that is, urologist, uro-oncology nurse
On diagnosis/ treatment decision	What are the different treatment options?	Specialist, that is, urological surgeon, oncologist, uro-oncology nurse, patient, support groups Leaflets, information should include complication rates (national & local) Videos Internet addresses Interactive CD ROM

patients can make an educated decision about the most appropriate treatment. The use of a template or pathway to assist in this process would bring structure to 'when, how and where' specific information should be given. This should not only include a description of the disease, what options are available (including their absolute and comparative advantages and disadvantages), but also strategies for communicating with the full range of health-care professionals, families and partners who are involved.

The complex nature of the diagnostic process for establishing whether a patient has or does not have prostate cancer will benefit from establishing a systematic approach. The use of a clinical pathway will facilitate this approach. The pathway can be constructed in such a way that it improves communication across the perceived barriers between primary and secondary care, while ensuring that the appropriate discussions with the patient takes place and that the discussions are supported by standard written materials. At each subsequent stage of the process each health professional who sees the patient will know what and how much the patient has been told. This will then provide the doctor or nurse with the opportunity to check the patient's understanding of the process thus far and to ensure that (s)he is ready to utilise the information necessary to move onto the next phase of the pathway. If the patient was adequately informed at each stage, then each subsequent consultation would have the potential to be more purposeful and focussed on the issues that concern both the patient and the clinician. Information and clinical procedures and their significance would be co-ordinated, which in turn would facilitate their consent. Standardised data collection leading to improved research opportunities and audit would be additional clinical benefits of a systematic approach to care.

It is our belief that the most effective way to ensure that patients are well informed about the investigations, diagnosis and treatment is to engage them in this structured and individualised programme of counselling. Information given verbally is then supported in a tactile format, such as written or video/audio material. Following a set pathway will regulate the rate and timing of information giving, providing co-ordination and consistency. Patients and clinicians will be offered protected time for clarification and validation of all aspects of both diagnosis and treatment of early prostate cancer.

The fundamental principle of any partnership is the ability of the parties involved to share. The introduction of consumerism into health-care has certainly contributed to the erosion of the paternalistic approach to medicine, but has done little to promote patient responsibilities. Partnership has to be seen as the middle way, with its emphasis on shared information, shared evaluation, shared decision-making and, most significantly, shared responsibility [28].

REFERENCES

1 Department of Health, *The NHS Prostate Cancer Plan*. 2000. Department of Health: London.

2 National Electronic Library for Health. Prostate Cancer Information. http://www.nelc.org.uk/risk/risk.htm.

3 Klotz LH. PSAdynia and other PSA-related syndromes: a new epidemic a – case history and taxonomy. *Urology* 1997; **50**: 831–2 (www.necl.org.uk/docs/risk/risk.htm).

4 Department of Health. *The NHS cancer plan. A plan for investment. A plan for reform.* 2000. Department of Health: London.

5 Austoker J. Gaining informed consent for screening. *BMJ* 1999; **319**: 722–3.

6 General Medical Council. *Seeking patient's consent: the ethical considerations.* 1998: General Medical Council: London.

7 O'Conner A, Rostom A, Fiset V, *et al.* Decision aids for patients facing health treatment or screening decisions: systematic review. *BMJ* 1999; **319**: 731–4.

8 British Association for Counselling and Psychotherapy. *Ethical Framework for Good Practice in Counselling and Psychotherapy.* 2002. British Association for Counselling and Psychotherapy: London.

9 Fallowfield L. Participation of patients in decisions about treatment for cancer. *BMJ* 2001; **323**: 1144.

10 Calman K. Cancer: science and society and the communication of risk. *BMJ* 1996; **313**: 799–802.

11 O'Conner A, Fiset V, Rosto A, *et al.* Decision aids for people facing health treatment or screening decisions. In: *Cochrane Collection.* Cochrane Library. Issue 1. Oxford: 1999.

12 Donovan J, Frankel S, Faulkener A, Selly S, Gillat D, Hamdy F. Dilemmas in treating early prostate cancer: the evidence and a questionnaire survey of consultant urologists in the United Kingdom. *BMJ* 1999; **318**: 299–300.

13 National Coordinating Centre for Health Technology Assessment. www.hta.nhsweb.nhs.uk/projectdata

14 Rakow T. Differences in belief about likely outcomes account for differences in doctor's treatment preferences: but what accounts for differences in belief? *Quality in Health Care* 2001; **10**: i44–9.

15 Lloyd A. the extent of patient's understanding of the risk of treatments. *Quality in Health Care* 2001; **10**: i14–18.

16 Slovic P, Fischhoff B, Lichtenstien S, Facts versus fears: understanding perceived risk. In: Khahneman D, Slovic P, Tversky A, eds. *Judgement under uncertainty: heuristics and biases.* Cambridge University Press, Cambridge, 1982: 463–89.

17 Reyna V, Brainerd C. Fuzzy – trace theory and framing effects in choice: gist extraction, truncation and conversion. *J Behav Decis Making* 1991; **4**: 249–62.

18 Mazur D, Hickam D, Mazur M. How patient's preferences for risk information influence treatment choice in a case of high risk and high therapeutic uncertainty: asymptomatic localised prostate cancer. *Med Decis Making* 1999; **19**: 394–8.

19 Ellis D, Hopkin J, Leitch A, *et al.* 'Doctor's orders': controlled trial of supplementary, written information for patients. *BMJ* 1979; **1**: 456.

20 Gattellari M, Butow P, Tattersall M, *et al.* Misunderstanding in cancer patients: why not shoot the messenger? *Ann Oncol* 1999; **10**: 39–46.

21 Wong F, Stewart D, Dancey J, *et al.* Men with prostate cancer: influence of psychological factors on informational needs and decision making. *J Psychosom Res* 2000; **49**: 13–9.

22 Bertakis K. the communication of information from physician to patient: a method for increasing patient retention and satisfaction. *J Fam Pract* 1997; **5**: 217–22.

23 Towle A. *Physician and patient communication skills: competencies for informed shared decision-making.*

Vancouver, Canada: University of British Columbia, 1997.

24 Volkers N. In coping with cancer, gender matters *Journal of the National Cancer Institute* 1999; **91**: 1712–14.

25 Onel E, Hamnd C, Wasson J.H, *et al.* Assessment of the feasibility and the impact of shared decision making in prostate cancer *Urology* 1998; **1**: 63–6.

26 Holmes-Rovner M, Llewellyn-Thomas H, Entwistle V, Coulter A, O'Conner A, Rovner D. Patient choice modules for summaries of clinical effectiveness: a proposal. *BMJ* 2001; **322**: 664–7.

27 NHS Cymru Wales. *Clinical Pathways*. 2000: National assembly for Wales: Cardiff.

28 Coulter A. Parternalism or partnership? *BMJ* 1999; **319**: 719–20.

10: The Role of Pelvic Node Dissection in Prostate Cancer

Owen Niall and Jamie Kearsley

INTRODUCTION

Prostate carcinoma is a major cause of cancer-related morbidity and mortality in the developed world. If detected, then localised, radical treatments, such as surgery or radiotherapy, may be offered in an attempt to cure. Once disseminated to local lymph nodes there is no strong evidence that radical surgery offers a survival advantage over conservative management in prostate carcinoma even if the microscopically involved nodes are resected. The goal of clinicians is to detect and treat those men with localized disease while avoiding costly and invasive treatments in those who will not benefit.

STAGING LYMPHADENECTOMY

Pelvic lymph node dissection has historically been an essential part of nodal staging of prostate carcinoma prior to or during curative treatment. It is not widely regarded as a therapeutic intervention as there is as yet no evidence of a survival advantage. It remains the gold standard for assessment of nodal metastases prior to or concomitant with therapy with curative intent. It can be undertaken through a lower mid-line incision during radical retropubic prostatectomy (RRP) or separately through either a minilaparotomy incision or laparoscopically prior to RRP, radical perineal prostatectomy (RPP), radiotherapy or brachytherapy.

However the absence of lymph node metastases may be predicted with a false negative rate of 2% or less using clinical criteria such as prostate-specific antigen (PSA), Gleason score and clinical stage in a logarithm. In the United States, up to 50% of patients fall into this low-risk category [1]. The remaining patients have a significant risk of greater than 20% [2].

Pelvic lymphadenectomy is a staging procedure without any therapeutic benefit except possibly in a very small subset of patients. There is no way to identify these patients, so there is no indication for pelvic lymphadenectomy on that basis alone. It is only necessary when a positive result will alter the proposed treatment such as aborting the radical prostatectomy, or introducing adjunctive treatment such as hormones, along with the primary curative therapy such as radiation.

Pelvic lymphadenectomy in conjunction with a RRP offers little extra in morbidity compared to prostatectomy alone as it is done via the same incision, whereas RPP or radical radiotherapy would require a separate procedure for the assessment of the pelvic nodes.

For radical radiotherapy, the treatment field with conformal therapy does not include the nodes so assessment of the nodal status would assist selection of appropriate patients.

In a study looking at laparoscopic lymphadenectomy in patients with locally advanced disease prior to possible treatment with radical radiotherapy, those in the high-risk group underwent laparoscopic lymphadenectomy [2]. 24% were found to have positive nodes and were treated with hormones. There was no significant differences in the PSA level, Gleason score or clinical stage between those with positive or negative nodes, so there was no way of selecting patients for the radiotherapy without lymph node sampling. The authors felt that a 20% risk of metastases justified pelvic lymphadenectomy.

However it is becoming a standard treatment to give adjuvant hormone therapy combined with radiotherapy for patients with locally advanced disease, often for several years, so that the presence of lymph node metastases may not matter.

Node dissection in conjunction with a retropubic prostatectomy is usually performed under the same anaesthetic, requiring the nodal tissue to be examined as a frozen section. The surgeon plans to abandon the prostatectomy if nodal metastases are present. Frozen section examination in this context has been shown to have a significant false negative rate of 7–33% [3–7] as well as a significant increase in theatre time. This can be avoided by performing the staging lymphadenectomy prior to prostatectomy but this requires a second admission and anaesthetic with subsequent increased cost and potential morbidity.

Other surgeons perform a node dissection for paraffin section only, unless the nodes are macroscopically involved, and use the presence of micrometastases to plan follow-up therapy. Even the accuracy of paraffin analysis has been questioned with Okegawa *et al.* showing that in 7 of 38 'node negative' patients, micrometastases could be detected using nested reverse transcriptase-polymerase chain reaction (RT-PCR) for prostate specific membrane antigen [8].

With the advent of serum PSA testing in the 1980s there has been a stage migration of newly diagnosed prostate adenocarcinoma with an increase in the number and percentage of men being diagnosed with localised disease [9].

This has been reflected in the low incidence (5–12%) of nodal disease in modern series [10–16]. Various groups have therefore questioned the need for routine node dissection in all patients during or prior to radical prostatectomy, and have attempted to predict those who are likely to harbour nodal metastases in apparently clinically localised prostate cancer [17–20].

IMAGING

There are no non-histological tests that can detect lymph node metastases with an adequate true-positive rate. CT and MR require enlargement of the nodes rather than actually detecting the metastatic deposits within the nodes. This may change with improvements in MR spectroscopy or contrast-enhanced MR.

Modern imaging techniques such as CT, MR and PET have not been shown to be adequately sensitive in the staging of pelvic 1ymph nodes [21–26]. It has been demonstrated however that at least in the United States, many urologists [27,28] continue to overuse imaging studies for patients who do not fall into the guidelines summarised by O'Dowd *et al.* [29]. After review of the current literature, they summarised that CT scans of the pelvis were only indicated in those men at high risk of nodal metastases; a PSA greater than 20 ng/mL. Gleason 8–10 carcinoma on biopsy, 5 or more (of 6) positive biopsies, clinically T3 or T4 disease or positive seminal vesicle biopsy.

Radioscintigraphy using radio-isotope labelled monoclonal antibody to prostate specific membrane antigen (111-In-capromab pendetide, Prostacint scan) has shown a 67% positive predictive value in patients at a high risk of nodal metastases (T2, T3) [30], there is yet no evidence for its use in low-risk patients.

Another alternative use of imaging reported is fine needle aspiration of suspicious lymph nodes under CT guidance. Oyen and Van Poppel [31] studied 285 patients with 43 patients (15%) showing suspicious nodes. The sensitivity, specificity and accuracy of needle aspiration was 77.8%, 100%, and 96.5% respectively, after correlating with lymph node dissection or the appearance of the node on follow-up CT after hormone therapy. The results were better than CT alone. However these are only reported on enlarged suspicious nodes and therefore not appropriate for the great majority of patients without evidence of node enlargement.

NOMOGRAMS

Nomograms that have been developed in an attempt to predict the chance of metastatic disease are numerous [32], but few have been validated outside their place of origin [33] and may not represent what occurs in community-based cohorts compared to academic centers [34].

The most widely known nomogram having been produced by Partin *et al.* [11] after logistic regression analysis of 4133 men, who had undergone RRP and node dissection in three major academic centres. Pre-operative PSA, Gleason score and clinical stage were used to predict final pathological outcomes such as organ confinement, capsular penetration, seminal vesicle and nodal involvement. It is most accurate in predicting nodal metastases (82.9%) over the other pathological findings and was used by Meng and Carroll in their study [35] that used formal decision analysis, using probability data from the available literature, to determine that pelvic lymphadenectomy was unnecessary in patients whose risk of nodal involvement was less than 18%.

Therefore a man with a PSA of 6 ng/mL, clinically T2a disease, Gleason 7 on biopsy would not benefit from a node dissection as his risk of nodal involvement is only 4%, while a man with a PSA of 12 ng/mL, clinically T2b disease and Gleason 8 has a risk of 29%.

Wolf identified low (2%), moderate (20%), and high-risk (40%) groups for pelvic lymph node metastases [36]. The low-risk group has stage T2c or less, Gleason <7 and PSA <10 ng/mL; moderate risk is Gleason 7 or greater or PSA >10; the high risk includes Gleason 7 or greater and PSA >20, Gleason 8 or greater and PSA >10, or PSA >50 ng/mL. To justify separate laparoscopic pelvic lymphadenectomy prior to RRP, the patient must be in the high-risk group. The low-risk group does not require lymphadenectomy, while the moderate group warrants lymphadenectomy prior to perineal prostatectomy or radiotherapy, or together with retropubic prostatectomy.

More recently, there has been work on neural networks in which many variables can be entered in the belief that they may be more accurate than regression analysis, this has not yet proven to be the case [37]. Other factors that have been suggested as having prognostic value are perineural invasion [38], positive seminal vesicle biopsy [39,40] and serum percent free PSA [41].

Crawford *et al.* [42] used artificial intelligence technology to predict lymph node spread in 4133 patients. They derived cut-off values of Gleason score 6 or less, PSA <10.6 ng/mL and clinical stage T2a or less to identify a low risk of lymph node metastasis with a false negative rate of <1%.

The surgeon and patient together must decide the level of 'risk' of missing nodal metastases they are willing to accept to avoid the potential morbidity of a node dissection. Bluestein *et al.* [16] studied retrospective data from 1632 patients who underwent pelvic lymphadenectomy at the Mayo Clinic. Using regression analysis of PSA, clinical stage and Gleason grade and an 'acceptable' false negative rate of 3%, they determined that 61% of men with T1a to T2b disease and 29% of men with T1a to T2c disease could be spared a lymphadenectomy. In 481 patients, Bishoff *et al.* [43] demonstrated that depending on what level of certainty (2–10%) was required, 20–63% of patients could forego their pelvic lymphadenectomy by simple assessment of their PSA, clinical stage and Gleason score.

OPERATIVE FIELDS

The operative fields of pelvic lymphadenectomy have developed over the years. Initially a wide excision of all lymphatic tissue between the external and internal iliac arteries from the bifurcation of the common iliac to the endopelvic fascia was recommended [44]. The pelvic lymph node dissection encompassed nodal tissue from the common, external and internal iliac arteries, obturator nerve and presacral area [45]. Brendler *et al.* modified the dissection to include only the obturator and hypogastric nodes [46]. Of 125 patients who underwent this procedure, only 7% had a complication and there were no lymphoceles, lymph fistulas or persistent lymphoedema. Modified or obturator node dissection became the lymphadenectomy of choice due to the lower morbidity compared to the extended lymphadenectomy.

Recently, however, the adequacy of this limited node dissection has been questioned. In the late 1980s up to 25% of men having radical prostatectomy were found to have positive lymph nodes but this is now reported in large series to be 2–3% [47]. Some authors question whether this is due to better patient selection with PSA or anatomically worse lymph node dissection. It has been suggested that up to a fifth of node-positive cases may be understaged without dissection of nodal tissue around the internal iliac vessels.

Studer [48] found that 19% of positive nodes are missed when the area around the internal iliac vessels is not dissected. However in this series, 70% of the patients with nodal metastases had seminal vesicle involvement or extracapsular spread of disease, both being poor prognostic factors associated with a high risk of biochemical failure even in the absence of nodal disease. There is no definite evidence that removing the affected nodes will improve survival.

Scheussler [49] suggested that modified node dissection may miss 30% of cases that may have lymph node metastasis outside the field of the modified dissection, as he reported a 23% rate of positive nodes. However, the apparently higher positivity rate for the extended dissection can be explained by the more tightly defined indications for this procedure that have become standard practice over the last 10 years. The extended dissection group had more high-risk patients, which explains the higher positive node rate.

Heindenreich *et al.* [50] compared 103 patients undergoing extended pelvic lymphadenectomy, with 26% showing metastatic deposits, to

100 patients having a standard lymphadenectomy with 12% found to have metastases, despite no significant differences in pre-op clinical criteria of PSA, Gleason score and clinical stage. 42% of all metastatic deposits were outside the field of a standard lymphadenectomy. In those with a pre-operative PSA <10.5 and a Gleason score of 6 or less, the risk of lymph node metastases was only 2.4%. There were no significant differences in regard to interoperative or post-operative complications in the two groups.

But in a recent randomised prospective evaluation of extended versus limited node dissection Clark *et al.* concluded that extended node dissection identified few patients with nodal metastases not found by a limited dissection and resulted in a three-fold increase in complications [51]. Brendler [42] also reported that the extranodal tissue removed via the standard pelvic node dissection did not significantly alter the overall results. However the majority of cases undergoing radical prostatectomy would not have require lymphadenectomy due to the low risk of lymph node metastases, so comparing two techniques in patients who are unlikely to have positive nodes will limit the power of the study [52].

Most urologists use PSA recurrence rather than pathological staging to determine the need for adjuvant therapy, such as hormones or radiotherapy. It is unclear whether removing all diseased nodes will prevent a PSA recurrence and therefore render any additional treatment unnecessary.

Sentinel node biopsy has become common place with breast cancer and melanoma but has yet to be clinically validated in prostate cancer although it has been shown to be technically feasible [53]. It relies on a predictable pattern of lymphatic spread and therefore is complicated by the variability of lymph drainage from the prostate including significant lymphatic drainage to sacral lymphatics [54] although the clinical significance of this is uncertain.

The modified dissection has been shown to yield similar node-positive results as the extended dissection, but the complication rates are much higher with the latter procedure. Stone [55] reported a 39% complication rate for the extended dissection versus 2% for the modified dissection, and Scheussler reported a 31% complication rate for the extended template [56]. Complications such as oedema and pelvic haematoma are a result of more extended node dissection and not the longer operative time nor the surgical approach.

OPERATIVE TECHNIQUE

Whether the operative field is the standard obturator dissection or the extended dissection, there are currently three main techniques of pelvic lymphadenectomy; the traditional open dissection, laparoscopic (either trans-peritoneal or extraperitoneal), or minilaparotomy.

Minimally invasive staging in men with clinically localised prostate cancer is well suited for patients treated with perineal prostatectomy, external beam or interstitial radiotherapy and before radical retropubic prostatectomy, if the risk of lymph node metastasis is high.

The advent of laparoscopic node dissection in the early 1990s [57] also encouraged a more limited dissection for technical ease. Its proponents believe it to be a viable alternative to an open procedure although with significant potential complications and learning curve [58].

The open procedure has traditionally used an extraperitoneal approach due to the lower risk of intra-abdominal complications, such as bowel adhesions or bowel injury. Most modern series put the complication rate at 20% using the modified template.

Minilaparotomy was introduced in 1993, as an alternative to open surgery, using only a 6 cm incision in the lower mid-line [59]. It allows for excellent surgical visualisation while reducing costs and morbidity, and has a minimal learning curve in comparison to laparoscopy.

Laparoscopic Technique

Under general anaesthesia, the patient is placed supine in the Trendelenberg position, a urethral catheter inserted, and compression stockings are used. Chest straps rather than shoulder braces are better to secure the patient in the Trendelenberg position as the latter have an increased risk of brachial plexus injuries.

Transperitoneal access is via the umbilicus. A 5 or 10 mm port can be used for the telescope, depending on the equipment. Three or four secondary ports are then inserted under direct vision after pneumoperitoneum is achieved. The ports can be either 5 or 10 mm in diameter, but one of the ports should be 10–12 mm to allow easier removal of the specimen.

In most patients, a diamond configuration is used, with ports placed at the umbilicus and just above the pubis, with lateral ports placed at the lateral edge of the rectus midway between the umbilicus and the anterior-superior iliac spine. Obese patients may require a different configuration to fit in another port.

First, the posterior peritoneum has to be incised in a line from a point between the medial umbilical ligament and the deep inguinal ring. The incision is extended along the medial aspect of the external iliac vessels. The boundaries of dissection are the external iliac vein laterally, the obturator nerve, the pubic symphysis and node of Cloquet distally, and the bifurcation of the common iliac vein proximally. The operative dissection is the same as for the open approach.

With the extended technique, the dissection takes in the lymph node tissue lateral to the genito-femoral nerve, around the external iliac artery and cephalad to the common iliac artery.

Dissection is begun medial to the external iliac vein, with the lymphatic tissue mobilised bluntly with a sucker, and bipolar cautery or clips used as necessary. The lymph packet is stripped proximally with identification of the obturator nerve. Gradually the packet tapers down to small lymphatic trunks at the bifurcation of the common iliac vein and these are clipped.

The nodal package can be removed either with a grasper or in a retrieval bag. The area is lavaged and inspected for bleeding. The ports sites are inspected visually, with the pressure reduced, for venous bleeding. The 10 mm ports are then closed in the fascial layer but 5 mm ports only need skin closure.

An extraperitoneal approach can also be made depending on the surgeon's preference. This may avoid potential intraperitoneal complications.

A 15 mm incision is made just below the umbilicus. Blunt dissection is carried down to the rectus sheath and the fascia secured with stay sutures. The anterior rectus fascia is then incised just off the midline. Blunt finger dissection is then carried out deep to the rectus muscle and superficial to the posterior rectus fascia and peritoneum toward the symphysis pubis. A balloon dilator can be used to develop this extraperitoneal space under visual observation, using a zero degree telescope placed into the trocar of the balloon dilator, and dissection performed with air insufflation. This can help to reduce the risk of injury to the epigastric vessels. The balloon is then deflated and removed and a normal Hassan port inserted into the space and secured.

The extraperitoneal approach has some theoretical advantages such as shortened operative time and reduced ileus, but no definite reduction in hospital stay. One study comparing transperitoneal and extraperitoneal approaches in a randomised fashion found that the extraperitoneal technique had a higher complication rate and similar hospital stay [60].

Raboy *et al.* [61] reported 125 patients who had the endoscopic extraperitoneal technique. Mean operative time was 104 min, length of stay 2.1 days and mean nodal yield was 10.2 nodes. 32.9% of patients who met at least two of three selection criteria (stage T2b-3a, PSA >20, Gleason score 7 or higher) had positive nodes. None of 52 patients who met one or none of the selection criteria had positive nodes.

The complication rate was low at 3.2%. Conversion to open surgery occurred in 2.4% due to pelvic adhesions but there were no conversions in the last 50 cases as experience improved. A lymphocele rate of 2.4% was similar to that seen in the trans-peritoneal approach [62].

Overall results of laparoscopic (whether trans- or extraperitoneal), and minilaparotomy pelvic node dissection are similar in experienced hands and the choice should be determined by surgeon experience. Data from centres that perform laparoscopic and minilaparotomy techniques for pelvic lymph-adenectomy report similar results in terms of the number of lymph nodes removed and node positivity.

A comparison of the three surgical techniques of transperitoneal laparoscopic, Minilap and open limited dissection found than laparoscopic and minilap techniques demonstrated similar staging efficacy with number of nodes sampled, decreased complications and hospital stay [63]. Minilaparotomy should be the procedure of choice where the learning curve and costs of laparoscopy cannot be overcome.

COMPLICATIONS

Aside from general post-operative complications, such as ileus, UTI, urinary retention, deep venour thrombosis, wound infection or cardiovascular events, there are complications specific to pelvic lymphadenectomy. These include vascular injury, lymphoceles, scrotal or penile oedema, leg oedema, obturator nerve palsy, pelvic haematoma, pelvic abscess and high inspiratory pressures. Also, as with any laparoscopic procedure there is risk of conversion to an open procedure or conversion from extraperitoneal to trans-peritoneal approach. The extended dissection results in increased risk of scrotal oedema or leg oedema.

There is a definite learning curve with laparoscopic surgery and complication rates decrease significantly with surgical experience. Lang *et al.* reported a 14% complication rate in their first 50 cases compared to 4% in the subsequent 50 cases. This learning curve is well documented and is the major reason preventing widespread use of laparoscopy in urology, together with a lack of an easy procedure to gain experience.

One study [64] reported 30% risk of lymphoceles on CT after transperitoneal node dissection, all asymptomatic and none requiring intervention. The risk of lymphoceles is lower in the transperitoneal technique than extraperitoneal method due to the opportunity of lymphatic drainage to escape into the peritoneal cavity.

Vascular injuries occur with port placement or during dissection. A careful technique and knowledge of the vascular anatomy will avoid most injuries, as will use of the open Hassan technique rather than the Veress needle.

Port-site-tumour recurrence is very rare with pelvic lymphadenectomy with one case reported. The patient had gross spillage of a large lymph node during dissection, soon developed bony metastases and 6 months later developed tumour in a port site. He died 2 months later.

A study of pelvic lymphadenectomy post-radiotherapy in patients considered for salvage treatment [65] found increased risk of complications due to more difficult dissection, less surgical planes, lymph node packages being smaller and more fibrotic and a longer operative time. Of 14 patients, 4 (28%) were positive and treated with hormone therapy, 10 were negative, with 1 receiving radical prostatectomy and 9 receiving salvage brachytherapy.

Treatment failure, post-initial definitive treatment, is a difficult management challenge. Accurate staging prior to any further definitive treatment is essential due to the increased risk of morbidity and distant disease resulting in failure. Laparoscopic lymphadenectomy post-radiotherapy is a feasible option for experienced surgeons but it is technically demanding.

CONCLUSIONS

Pelvic lymphadenectomy is currently the gold standard to stage lymph node involvement in patients with prostate cancer and a limited node dissection appears to have a low risk of complications, while demonstrating most positive cases. It should be omitted when the risk of lymph node metastasis is low and only high-risk patients need be selected to undergo pelvic lymphadenectomy prior to definitive local therapy. Either the laparoscopic or minilaparotomy techniques are appropriate, depending on surgeon expenence.

Nomograms using PSA, clinical stage and Gleason score allow urologists to stratify their patients into risk groups, with low risk being PSA <10 ng/mL, stage T2a or less, and Gleason 6 or less.

If it is shown that a complete node dissection improves the chance of cure of prostate cancer, then the role of pelvic node dissection will have to be reassessed, but at present the evidence is not definitely proven.

With improved use of PSA and clinical criteria the need for pelvic node dissection in men with prostate cancer is becoming uncommon. The future is moving away from a staging pelvic lymphadenectomy and will eventually incorporate imaging or systemic testing of molecular features of prostate cancer.

REFERENCES

1 Wolf J, Andriole G. The selection of patients for cross-sectional imaging and pelvic lymphadenectomy before radical prostatectomy. *AUA Update series* 1997; 15: 114–119.

2 Parkin J, Keeley F, Timoney A. Laparoscopic lymph node sampling in locally advanced prostate cancer. *BJU* 2002; 89: 14–18.

3 Epstein JI, Oesterling JE, Eggleston JC, Walsh PC. Frozen section detection of lymph node metastases in prostatic carcinoma: accuracy in grossly uninvolved pelvic lymphadenectomy specimens. *J Urol* 1986; 136: 1234.

4 Sadlowski RW, Donahue DJ, Richman AV, Sharpe JR, Finney RP. Accuracy of frozen section diagnosis in pelvic lymph

node biopsies for adenocarcinoma of the prostate. *J Urol* 1983; **129**: 324.

5 Catalona WJ, Stein AJ. Accuracy of frozen section detection of lymph node metastases in prostatic carcinoma. *J Urol* 1982; **127**: 460.

6 Beissner RS, Stricker JB, Coffield KS, Spiekerman AM, Riggs M. Frozen section diagnosis of metastatic prostate adenocarcinoma in pelvic lymphadenectomy compared with nomogram prediction of metastasis. *Urology* 2002; **59**: 721.

7 Kramolowsky EV, Narayana AS, Platz CE, Loening SA. The frozen section in lymphadenectomy for carcinoma of the prostate. *J Urol* 1984; **131**: 899.

8 Okegawa T, Nutahara K, Higashihara E. Detection of micrometastatic prostate cancer cells in the lymph nodes by reverse transcriptase polymerase chain reaction is predictive of biochemical recurrence in pathological stage T2 prostate cancer. *J Urol* 2000; **163**: 1183.

9 Catalona WJ, Smith DS, Ratcliff TL *et al.* Detection or organ-confined prostate cancer is increased through prostate-specific antigen-based screening. *JAMA* 1993; **270**: 948.

10 Danella JF, deKernion JB, Smith RB *et al.* The contemporary incidence of lymph node metastases in prostate cancer: implications for laparoscopic node dissection. *J Urol* 1993; **149**: 1488.

11 Partin AW, Kattan MW, Subong EN *et al.* Combination of prostate-specific antigen, clinical stage, and Gleason score to predict pathological stage of localized prostate cancer. A multi-institutional study. *JAMA* 1997; **277**: 1445.

12 Petros JA, Catalona WJ. Lower incidence of unsuspected lymph node metastases in 521 consecutive patients with clinically localized prostate cancer. *J Urol* 1992; **147**: 1574.

13 Zincke H, Oesterling JE, Blute ML *et al.* Long-term (15 years) results after radical prostatectomy for clinically localized (stage T2c or lower) prostate cancer. *J Urol* 1994; **152**: 1850.

14 Quinn DI, Henshall SM, Haynes A-M, Brenner PC *et al.* Prognostic significance of pathologic features in localized prostate cancer treated with radical prostatectomy: Implications for staging systems and predictive models. *J Clin Oncol* 2001; **19**: 3692.

15 Han MH, Partin AW, Pound ChR, Epstein JI, Walsh PC. Long-term biochemical disease-free and cancer-specific survival following anatomical radical retropubic prostatectomy: the 15-year Johns Hopkins experience. *Urol Clin North Am* 2001; **28**: 555.

16 Bluestein DL, Bostwick DG, Bergstralh EJ *et al.* Eliminating the need for bilateral pelvic lymphadenectomy in select patients with prostate cancer. *J Urol* 1994; **151**: 1315.

17 Campbell SC, Klein EA, Levin HS *et al.* Open pelvic lymph node dissection for prostate cancer: a reasessment. *Urology* 1995; **46**: 352.

18 Sullivan LD, Rabbani F. Should we reconsider the indications for ileo-obturator node dissection with localized prostate cancer? *Br J Urol* 1995; **75**: 33.

19 Bundrick WS, Culkin DJ, Mata JA *et al.* Evaluation of the current incidence of nodal metastasis from prostate cancer. *J Surg Oncol* 1993; **52**: 269.

20 Fournier GR Jr, Narayan P. Re-evaluation of the need for pelvic lymphadenectomy in low grade prostate cancer. *Br J Urol* 1993; **72**: 484.

21 Albertsen PC, Hanley JA, Harlan LC. *et al.* The positive yield of imaging studies in the evaluation of men with newly diagnosed prostate cancer: A population based analysis. *J Urol* 2000; **163**: 1138.

22 The Royal College of Radiologists' Clinical Oncology Information Network/British Association of Urological Surgeons: Guidelines on the management of prostate cancer. *BJU Int* 1999; **84**: 987.

23 Moul JW, Kane CJ, Malkowicz SB. The role of imaging studies and molecular markers for selecting candidates for radical prostatectomy. *Urol Clin North Am* 2001; **28**: 459.

24 Effert PJ, Bares R, Handt S, Wolff JM, Büll U, Jakse G. Metabolic imaging of untreated prostate cancer by positron emission tomography with 18-fluorine-labeled deoxyglucose. *J Urol* 1996; **155**: 994.

25 Hoh CK, Seltzer MA, Franklin J, DeKernion JB, Phelps ME, Belldegrun A.

Positron emission tomography in urological oncology. *J Urol* 1998; **159**: 347.

26 Sanz G, Robles JE, Arocena J *et al.* Positron emission tomography with 18-fluorine-labelled deoxyglucose: utility in localized and advanced prostate cancer. *BJU Int* 1999; **84**: 1028.

27 Cooperberg MR, Lubeck DP, Grossfield GD, Mehta SS, Carroll PR. Contemporary trends in imaging test utilization for prostate cancer staging: Data from the Cancer of the Prostate Strategic Urologic Research Endeavor. *J Urol* 2002; **168**: 491.

28 Plawker MW, Fleischer JM, Vapnek EM, Macchia RJ. Current trends in prostate cancer diagnosis and staging among United States urologists. *J Urol* 1997; **158**: 1853.

29 O'Dowd GJ, Veltri RW, Orozco R, Miller MC, Oesterling JE. Update on the appropriate staging evaluation for newly diagnosed prostate cancer. *J Urol* 1997; **158**: 687.

30 Polasicik TJ, Manyak MJ, Haseman MK *et al.* Comparison of clinical staging algorithms and 111-indium-capromab pendetide immunoscintigraphy in the prediction of lymph node involvement in high risk prostate carcinoma patients. *Cancer* 1999; **85**: 1586.

31 Oyen R, Van Poppel H, Ameye F *et al.* Lymph node staging of localised prostatic carcinoma with CT and CT guided fine needle aspiration. *Radiology* 1994; **190**: 315.

32 Ross PL, Scardino PT, Kattan MW. A catalog of prostate cancer nomograms. *J Urol* 2001; **165**: 1562.

33 Blute ML, Bergstralh EJ, Partin AW *et al.* Validation of Partin tables for predicting pathological stage of clinically localised prostate cancer. *J Urol* 2000; **164**: 1591.

34 Penson DF, Grossfield GD, Li Y-P, Henning JM, Lueck DP, Carroll PR. How well does the Partin nomogram predict pathological stage after radical prostatectomy in the community based population? Results of the cancer of the Prostate Strategic Urological Research Endeavor. *J Urol* 2002; **167**: 1653.

35 Meng MV, Carroll PR. When is pelvic lymph node dissection necessary before radical prostatectomy? A decision analysis. *J Urol* 2000; **164**: 1235.

36 Wolf JS. Indication, technique, and results of laparoscopic pelvic lymphadenectomy. *J Endourol* 2001; **15**: 427.

37 Borque A, Sanz G, Allepuz C, Plaza L, Gil P, Rioja LA. The use of neural networks and logistic regression analysis for predictmg pathological stage in men undergoing radical prostatectomy: A poopulation based study. *J Urol* 2001; **166**: 1672.

38 Stone NN, Stock RG, Parikh D, Yeghiayan P, Unger P. Perineural invasion and seminal vesicle involvement predict pelvic lymph node metastasis in men with localized carcinoma of the prostate. *J Urol* 1998; **160**: 1722.

39 Stone NN, Stock RG, Unger P. Indications for seminal vesicle biopsy and laparoscopic pelvic node dissection in men with localized carcinoma of the prostate. *J Urol* 1995; **154**: 1392.

40 Vallancien G, Bochereau G, Wetzel O, Bretheau D, Prapotnich D, Bougaran, J. Influence of positive seminal vesicle biopsy on the staging of prostatic carcinoma. *J Urol* 1994; **152**: 1152.

41 Southwick PC, Catalona WJ, Partin AW *et al.* Prediction of post-radical prostatectomy pathological outcome for stage T1c prostate cancer with percent free prostate specific antigen: A prospective multicenter clinical trial. *J Urol* 1999; **162**: 1346.

42 Crawford E, Batuello J, Snow P. The use of artificial intelligence technology to predict lymph node spread in men with clinically localised prostate cancer. *Cancer* 2000; **88**: 2105.

43 Bishoff JT, Reyes A, Thompson IM *et al.* Pelvic lymphadenectomy can be omitted in selected patients with carcinoma of the prostate: Development of a system of patient selection. *Urology* 1995; **45**: 270.

44 Weingärtner K, Ramaswamy A, Bittinger A, Gerharz EW, Vöge D, Riedmiller H. Anatomical basis for pelvic lymphadenectomy in prostate cancer. Result of an autopsy study and implications for the clinic. *J Urol* 1996; **156**: 1969.

45 Flocks R. Lymphatic spread from prostate cancer. *J Urol* 1959; **81**: 194.

46 Brendler C, Cleeve L, Anderson E, *et al.* Staging pelvic lymphadenectomy for

carcinoma of the prostate: risk versus benefit. *J Urol* 1980; **124**: 849.

47 Partin A. Editorial comment, *J Urol* 2003; **169**: 147.

48 Bader P, Burkhard FC, Markwalder R, Studer UE. Is a limited lymph node dissection an adequate staging procedure for prostate cancer? *J Urol* 2002; **168**: 514.

49 Scheussler W, Pharand D, Vancaille T. Laparoscopic standard pelvic lymph node dissection for carcinoma of the prostate: is it accurate? *J Urol* 1993; **150**: 898.

50 Heidenreich A, Varga Z, Von Knobloch R. Extended pelvic lymphadenectomy in patients undergoing radical prostatcetomy: high incidnec of lymph node mestasis. *J Urol* 2002; **167**: 1681.

51 Clark T, Parekh D, Smith J. Randomised prospective evaluation of extended versus limited lymph node dissection in patients with clinically localised prostate cancer. *J Urol* 2003; **169**: 145.

52 Studer U, Editorial comment. *J Urol* 2003; **169**: 148.

53 Wawroschek F, Vogt H, Weckermann D, Wagner T, Hamm M, Harzmann R. Radioisotope guided pelvic lymph node dissection for prostate cancer. *J Urol*, 2001; **166**: 1715.

54 Brössner C, Ringhofer H, Schatzl G, Madersbacher S, Powischer G, Kuber W. Sacral distribution of prostatic lymph nodes visualized on spiral computed tomography with three-dimensional reconstruction. *BJU Int* 2002; **89**: 44.

55 Stone N, Stock R, Unger P. Laparoscopic pelvic lymph node dissection for prostate cancer: comparison of the extended and modified techniques. *J Urol* 1997; **158**: 1891.

56 Scheussler W, Pharand D, Vancaille T. Laparoscopic standard pelvic lymph node dissection for carcinoma of the prostate: is it accurate? *J Urol* 1993; **150**: 898.

57 Schuessler WW, Vancille TG, Reich H *et al.* Transperitoneal endosurgical lymphadenectomy in patients with localised prostate cancer. *J Urol* 1991; **145**: 988.

58 Kavoussi LR, Sosa E, Chandhoke, P *et al.* Complications of laparoscopic lymph node dissection. *J Urol* 1993; **149**: 322.

59 Steiner M, Marshall F. Mini-laparotomy staging pelvic lymphadenectomy (MINILAP). *Urology* 1993; **41**: 201.

60 Persson D, Haggman M. Minimally invasive techniques for prostate cancer pelvic lymph node dissection: a randomised trial of trans and extraperitoneal methods. *J Urol* 1996; **155**: 658A.

61 Raboy A, Adler H, Albert P. Extraperitoneal endoscopic pelvic lymph node dissection. A review of 125 patients. *J Urol* 1997; **158**: 2202–2204.

62 Kavoussi L, Sosa E, Chodak G *et al.* Complications of laparoscopic pelvic lymph node dissection. *J Urol* 1993; **149**: 322.

63 Herrell D, Trachtenberg J, Theodorescu D. Staging pelvic lymphadenectomy for localised carcinoma of the prostate: a comparison of three surgical techniques. *J Urol* 1997; **157**: 1337–1339.

64 Freid J. in *J Endourol* 2001; **15**: 434.

65 Lund G, Winfield H, Donovan J *et al.* Laparoscopic pelvic lymph node dissection following definitive radiotherapy for carcinoma of the prostate. *J Urol* 1997; **152**: 548–551.

Part 3: Initial Treatment Policies

11: Laparoscopic Radical Prostatectomy

Mark Wright

INTRODUCTION

At the time of writing this chapter over 500 Laparoscopic Radical Prostatectomies (LRPP) have been performed in the United Kingdom. With the increasing numbers of surgeons performing the procedure this chapter looks to review the technique, and critique the published results and functional outcomes.

HISTORY

The first attempt to perform laparoscopic prostatectomy was presented by Schussler et al. at the American Urological Association meeting in 1992. In 1997, the same group published their experience of nine cases [1]. They concluded that initial operations appeared to have little advantage over open surgery primarily due to the long operation times (mean 9.4 h).

In 1998, Vallancien and Guilloneau refined and standardised the procedure using a transperitoneal approach to the seminal vesicles and ampullae and intra-corporeal suturing [2]. In the same year the first extra peritoneal LRPP was described by Ralboy et al. [3]. Over 3000 cases have been subsequently recorded in the world literature.

INDICATIONS

Patients with clinically organ confined prostate cancer in males with a greater than 10 year life expectancy. As in open surgery, coagulopathies are a contraindication, however, there are no other absolute contraindications to a LRPP. Patients who have previously undergone trans-urethral prostate surgery, or laparoscopic hernia (mesh) repair, or who are on anti-androgen medication should be approached with caution.

Reuseable	Singleuse
	Laparoscopic pledgets
Johann forceps×2	
Needle holders×2	
Laparoscopic J hook	
Maryland forceps	
Suction irrigation device	
Bipolar forceps	
Weck clip applicator	
Urethral sound	
Laparoscopic scissors	

Table 11.1 Laparoscopic equipment

EQUIPMENT

Table 11.1 lists the equipments recommended as a basic armamentarium for pelvic laparoscopic surgery.

PATIENT PREPARATION

Patients are anaesthetised with a general anaesthesia and muscle relaxant (Figure 11.1). Intravenous cephalosporin is administered on induction and an arterial line is placed to monitor blood pH [4]. The patient is placed in a supine position on the operating table with 10–20° of Trendelenberg. The abdominal wall is shaved from the costal margins to the symphysis pubis and the skin is prepped with an iodine-based disinfectant. Once draped, a 20 Foley catheter is inserted per urethra and 20 cc of water inserted into the catheter balloon. The catheter is placed on free drainage.

Operative Steps

Extra-peritoneal laparoscopic radical prostatectomy

Introduction of primary port. A 10 mm incision is made just inferior to the umbilicus and the anterior rectus sheath is incised using MacIndoe scissors. The anterior sheath is then retracted vertically using a 5 mm retractor.

Creation of cave of Retzius. A 10 mm diameter inflatable balloon port (Tyco XB2 Endoview) is inserted through the incision in the anterior rectus sheath and passed caudally until the symphysis pubis can be palpated. A 0° laparoscope is then passed into the port and the balloon is inflated with a hand pump. Approximately 400 cc of air is insufflated until the following

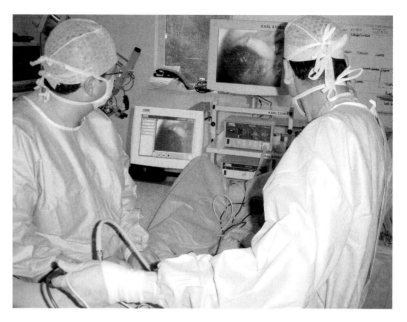

Fig. 11.1 Patient set-up for LRPP.

landmarks can be identified:
(a)   left and right inferior epigastric arteries;
(b)   pubic arch and symphysis;
(c)   external iliac vessel pulsation.
The internal inguinal rings are checked for any signs of herniation. The balloon is then deflated and the preperitoneal space is checked for haemorrhage.

   Port placement. The placements of ports are very much operator dependent, however, the following points need to be considered:
(a)   with one assistant only three ports are required – two for the surgeon and one for the free hand of the assistant for traction and suction;
(b)   if an additional assistant is used or robotic camera holder employed, four ports can be utilised;
(c)   a minimum of one 10 mm port is required to allow introduction of sutures for intra-corporeal stitching. Two 10 mm ports allow more flexibility;
(d)   if the surgeon's operating ports are placed on either side of the primary camera port, this allows easier triangulation, but is less ergonomic. The alternative is to have the two operating ports to the left of the camera.
All ports should be inserted under endoscopic vision, angled down towards the prostate. Structures to be avoided during placement include the inferior epigastric arteries, iliac veins, bladder and peritoneum.

   Pelvic lymphadenectomy. A bilateral lymphadenectomy is conducted, removing lymphatic tissue in the area bounded by the pubic bone, external iliac vein and obturator nerve. The lymphatic channels are sealed using 5 mm titanium ligaclips to prevent a postoperative lymphocele.

Endopelvic fascia incision. The prostate is retracted medially using a laparoscopic pledget, thus placing the endopelvic fascia under tension. A 1 mm puncture is made in the fascia using a monopolar hook and then a linear incision is made in the endopelvic fascia from the vesico-prostatic junction to the edge of the pubo-prostatic ligaments using cold scissors. The lateral edge of the dorsal venous complex is then defined using a lap pledget. This process is repeated on the contralateral side (Plate 6).

Dorsal venous complex ligation. The prostate is retracted inferiorly and a 1 Polysorb suture cut to 20 cm is mounted in a needle holder in a plane parallel to the pubic arch. The needle is then rotated between the dorsal venous complex (DVC) and urethral wall and withdrawn at the contralateral side of the apex. A surgeon's knot tied intracorporeally is then used to secure the DVC and pubo-prostatic ligaments. A helpful technique to facilitate this manoeuvre includes replacing the catheter with the urethral sound so that the prostate can be moved from side to side to facilitate the entry point of the needle and pick-up. A further suture is then placed at the level of the anterior bladder neck to prevent back-bleeding from the superficial vesical veins (Plate 7).

Anterior bladder neck dissection. The preprostatic veins are divided between the sutures with cold scissors and a lateral release performed bilaterally to allow the neuro-vascular bundles (NVBs) to fall posteriorly. The anterior neck is then identified by gentle to-and-fro traction on the urethral catheter. A combination of sharp and blunt dissection is then used to delineate the anterior and lateral walls of the bladder neck. Extra care on the lateral aspect of the anterior bladder neck will help prevent ureteric damage at the next step of the procedure. The bladder neck and urethra is then incised anteriorly, the catheter balloon deflated and the catheter is grasped with a Johann forceps and used to retract the prostate superiorly by the assistant.

Posterior bladder neck dissection. The posterior bladder neck is easily visualised with the prostate retracted and is then assessed for the presence of a median lobe and the exact location of the ureteric orifices. A horizontal incision is then made at the proposed line of transection. As this incision is developed, the posterior edge of the bladder neck is grasped in the midline with a Johann forceps and retracted anteriorly. The posterior bladder wall is then peeled off the prostate with a combination of sharp and blunt dissection. Care must be taken not to button-hole the posterior wall of the bladder. The anterior layer of Denonvillier's fascia is then identified as a midline raphe and incised horizontally (Plate 8).

Dissection of ampullae. Incision of the midline raphe allows access to the paired ampullae, which are grasped and retracted cranially. The vasa deferentia are dissected free of their investing tissue and ligated with locking nylon clips. These are then divided with cold scissors.

Dissection of seminal vesicles. The freed ampullae are then grasped and retracted anteriorly. This allows lateral access to the seminal vesicles. While it is safe to perform the circumferential dissection with bipolar diathermy, the tips of the vesicles lie very close to the NVBs and it is important not to use any thermal or electrical energy in this region. The artery is therefore ligated with locking nylon clips (Plate 9).

Lateral pedicles. Both seminal vesicles are then grasped and retracted anteriorly. The urethral sound is re-inserted and the prostate angled laterally. This places the lateral pedicle under tension and allows accurate vision of the NVB. If a nerve-sparing procedure is to be carried out, then each feeding vessel to the prostate is individually clipped and divided and all forms of thermal energy are avoided. This process is repeated on the contralateral side (Plate 10).

Apical dissection. The prostate is then retracted posteriorly placing it under tension. Cold scissors are then used to dissect the apex of the free prostate taking care to preserve the external-urethral sphincter mechanism and the NVBs that pass just lateral to the sphincter complex.

Transection of urethra. The anterior urethra is transsected just distal to the apex of the prostate and the urethral sound advanced. The urethra is then elevated anteriorly and the posterior wall and recto-urethralis divided. The specimen is then placed in an entrapment bag.

Vesico-urethral anastomosis. Two 3/0 laparoscopic sutures (EV-23 17 mm needle) are then tied together and introduced via one of the 10 mm ports. Van Velthoven described a technique of a continuous vesico-urethral anastomosis that, once mastered results in a tension-free, water-tight anastomosis that takes 30 min to complete [5]. This technique is endorsed by the author (Plate 11).

Specimen removal. An 18 F silicon catheter is inserted and the anastomosis is checked for integrity by filling the bladder with 250 cc of warm saline. The specimen is delivered via the camera (sub umbilical) port.

Transperitoneal laparoscopic radical prostatectomy

The steps for this procedure are almost identical, except for the initial dissection that involves a peritoneal incision over the seminal vesicles and a further incision through the median umbilical ligament to gain entry into the Cave of Retzius.

COMPLICATIONS

No intra-operative mortalities have been reported in the literature till date (July 2005). Conversion rates to open surgery vary between 0.3–2.4% but

	Mean (%)
Urinary retention	4.6
Anastomotic stricture	2.5
Postoperative ileus	2.3
Rectal injury	1.9
Bladder injury	1.4
Deep vein thrombosis	1.3
Conversion to open surgery	1.3
Rectal injury	0.9
Iliac vein injury	0.8
Epigastric artery damage	0.5

Table 11.2 LRPP postoperative complications

are higher in the first 50 cases [6–9]. The most common cause for conversion is uncontrollable haemorrhage. Rectal injury, as in open radical prostatectomy (ORPP), is rare (1.4–2.4%) in LRPP and usually occurs at the apex of the prostate in non-nerve sparing procedures [6]. The important management point is to recognise the injury at the time of surgery and repair the defect with two layers of interrupted sutures [10]. Prolonged catheterisation (14 days) is recommended.

Ureteric injury (0.8%) most commonly occurs during posterior bladder neck dissection when a median lobe is present. Injury, in this scenario, can be avoided by careful lateral dissection of the bladder neck and making a sharp horizontal incision in the posterior urethral urothelium overlying the median lobe. The posterior wall is then retracted anteriorly using a Johann forceps and the bladder is peeled off the prostate until the posterior median raphe is identified. The ureteric orifices should then be checked with the laparoscope.

Other complications include inferior epigastric artery and iliac vein damage, Anastomotic stricture and deep vein thrombosis [11] (see Table 11.2)

Blood loss and transfusion rates.   In a review of 1228 LRPP at six European centres, the mean blood loss was 448 mL with an overall transfusion rate of 3.5% [11]. Farouk from the Cleveland clinic reported a mean blood loss of 332 cc and a similar transfusion rate of 2% in 100 consecutive LRPPs [12].

CONTINENCE

Urinary incontinence is a serious concern for patients undergoing radical prostate surgery. Continence rates from published studies range from 82–92% [6–9], which compare favourably with open RPP (61–95%) [13,14] (see Table 11.3).

Table 11.3 Continence rates following LRPP

Author	Centre	N	Urinary continence (%)	Follow-up (months)
Guillonneau	Paris	550	82.3	12
Rassweiller	Heidelberg	438	90.3	12
Salomon	Creteil	235	90	12
Turk	Berlin	125	92.1	12
Eden	Basingstoke	100	90	12

In a prospective comparison – non-randomised – between two cohorts of patients undergoing RPP ($n = 70$) and LRPP ($n = 230$) there was no significant difference in continence rates at 1 year, however the LRPP group had an earlier return to continence resulting in a significant benefit to quality of life [15].

ERECTILE DYSFUNCTION

The preservation of the neurovascular bundles in order to preserve erectile function is a well known challenge to open prostatectomists. A laparo-scopic approach should give a magnified, well illuminated view of the NVBs, however, long-term data is not yet available.

The three largest studies (see Table 11.4) report potency rates of 58.8–82.3% [6–9]. In these cohorts there was at least 6 months follow-up, however the definitions of erectile function varied from 'spontaneous' erections to others including sildenafil use.

Longer follow-up is required as it is well known from ORPP studies that erectile function can return up to 15 months post procedure.

A new technique in the refinement of nerve sparing procedure has been described by Gill and co-workers [14]. A trans-rectal ultrasound and colour Doppler probe is used to monitor the NVBs during resection of the lateral pedicles. Functional results are awaited.

Oncologic Outcome

Surgical margins

One of the potential concerns about LRPP has been positive margin rates due to the lack of tactile feedback that is possible in open surgery. Results from open series for positive margins range from 19.9–37% [16]. Data from larger laparoscopic series range from 13.8–26.4%, which compare favourably but

Centre	N	Potency with nerve sparing procedure in previously potent Patients (%)
Creteil	235	58.8
Montsouris	550	82.3
Basingstoke	100	62

Table 11.4 Potency rates following LRPP

no firm comparison can be drawn as prospective nor randomised data are yet available.

A comparative study from Paris analysed a cohort of 139 ORPP and 139 LRPP performed by senior surgeons between 1994 and 1997. There was no statistical difference in tumour grade or volume, however the rate of positive surgical margins was statistically lower in the LRPP group compared to open (13.7% versus 25.9% $p < 0.02$) [17].

PSA recurrence

As yet, the long-term efficacy of LRPP is unproven. Guilloneau and co-workers reported on 1000 LRPP patients with a minimum follow-up of 3 years [6]. Of this 91.8% patients with pT2a tumours exhibited no PSA progression, 88% for pT2b and 77% for pT3a. They also noted that 94% of patients with negative surgical margins had progression free survival. Eden reported a 100% disease free progression with a mean follow-up of 9.8 months [9].

COST

In other areas of surgical intervention, laparoscopic surgery has benefited the patient by reducing length of hospital stay, operation related morbidity and a speedier recovery. In Bristol, the average length of stay for LRPP is 2 days with even shorter length of stay elsewhere (Cleveland). A quality of life study on 50 consecutive LRPP patients reported that 68% of patients could return to work 2 weeks after the procedure [18].

To date, there is a paucity of data on cost analysis between the two approaches. The Montsouris group evaluated the differences between LPPP and ORPP and found that average costs were lower for LRPP ($5058 versus $6295) [2]. An American study, however, showed that LRPP was theoretically 1.2 times more expensive than an open procedure [19].

CONCLUSION

LRPP has been shown to be an effective treatment for localised prostate cancer. The advantages of magnification and better visualisation afforded by the laparoscopic approach herald the possibility of improving the procedure of radical prostatectomy rather than replacing it. While the procedure has a steep learning curve, the complication rates and functional outcomes of LRPP compare favourably to open prostatectomy. Long-term survival results are awaited, but disease progression data obtained thus far are encouraging.

REFERENCES

1 Schuessler WW, Schulam PG, Clayman RV, Kavoussi LR. Laparoscopic radical prostatectomy: initial short term experience. *Urology* 1997; **50**: 854–57.

2 Guillonneau B, Vallancien G. Laparoscopic radical prostatectomy: the Montsouris technique. *J Urol* 2000; **163**: 1643–49.

3 Raboy A, Ferzli G, Albert P. Initial experience with extraperitoneal endoscopic radical retropubic prostatectomy. *Urology* 1997; 859–62.

4 Meininger D, Byhahn C, Bueck M *et al*. Effects of prolonged pneumoperitoneum on hemodynamics and acid-base balance during totally endoscopic robot-assisted radical prostatectomies. *World J Surg* 2002; **26**: 1423–27.

5 Van Velthoven RF, Ahlering TE, Peltier A, Skarecky DW, Clayman RV. Technique for laparoscopic running urethrovesical anastomosis: the single knot method. *Urology* 2003; **61**: 699–702.

6 Guillonneau B, el-Fettouh H, Baumert H *et al*. Laparoscopic radical prostatectomy: oncological evaluation after 1,000 cases a Montsouris Institute. *J Urol* 2003; **169**: 1261–66.

7 Rassweiler J, Schulze M, Teber D *et al*. Laparoscopic radical prostatectomy with the Heilbronn technique: oncological results in the first 500 patients. *J Urol* 2005; **173**: 761–64.

8 Turk I, Deger S, Winkelmann B, Schonberger B, Loening SA. Laparoscopic radical prostatectomy. Terchnical aspects and experience with 125 cases. *Eur Urol* 2002; **40**: 46–50.

9 Eden CG, Cahill D, Vass JA, Adams TH, Dauleh MI. Laparoscopic radical prostatectomy: the initial UK series. *BJU Int* 2002; **90**: 876–82.

10 Guillonneau B, Gupta R, El Fettouh H, Cathelineau X, Baumert H, Vallancien G. Laparoscopic management of rectal injury during laparoscopic radical prostatectomy. *J Urol* 2003; **169**: 1694.

11 Susler T, Guillonneau B, Vallancien G, Gaston R, Piecchaud T, Turk I. Complications and initial experience with 1228 laparoscopic prostatectomies at 6 European centres. *J Urol* 2001; **165**: 615A.

12 Farouk A, Gill I, Kaouk J *et al*. 100 laparoscopic radical prostatectomy (LRP): learning curve in the United States. *J Endourol* 2002; **16**: 33A.

13 Walshe PC, Marschke P, Ricker D. Patient reported urinary continence and sexual function after anatomic radical prostatectomy. *Urology* 2000; **55**: 58–61.

14 Gill IS, Ukimura O, Rubinstein M *et al*. Lateral pedicle control during laparoscopic radical prostatectomy: refined technique. *Urology* 2005; **65**: 23–7.

15 Rassweiler J, Seemann O, Schulze M, Teber D, Hatzinger M, Frede T. Laparoscopic versus open radical prostatectomy: a comparative study at a single institution. *J Urol* 2003; **169**: 1689.

16 Pound CR, Partin AW, Epsein JI, Walshe PC. Prostate-specific antigen after anatomic radical prostatectomy. Patterns of recurrence and cancer control. *Urol Clin North Am* 1997; **24**: 1821–29.

17 Salomon L, Levrel O, de la Taille A, Antiphon P, Abbou CC. Radical prostatectomy by the retropubic, perineal and laparoscopic approach: 12 years experience.

18 Zippe CD, Meraney AM, Sung GT, Gill IS. Laparoscopic radical prostatectomy in the USA. Cleveland clinic series of 50 patients. *J Urol* 2001; **165**: 135A.

19 Link RE, Su LM, Bhayani SB, Pavlovich CP. Making ends meet: a cost comparison of laparoscopic and open radical retropubic prostatectomy. *J Urol* 2004; **172**: 6–7.

12: Endocrine Therapy for Prostate Cancer: the Latest

A. Goyal and W. Bowsher

INTRODUCTION

Since the first documented use of hormonal therapy in prostate cancer by Nobel laureate Huggins and colleague Hodges [1] in the early 1940s, a significant amount of progress has been made in this particular treatment modality of the disease. Akin to the treatment of other hormone dependent disorders, improvements in the side effect profile of existing drugs, new methods of delivery, research into novel agents, intermittent therapy and combination therapy has brought great promise and occasional dilemmas to this subject. Despite ever-increasing focus on gene therapy, chemoprevention and the role of diet in prostate cancer, hormonal manipulation remains the mainstay of treatment thus far, in the large majority of prostate cancer presenting to the medical profession. Furthermore, although traditionally it has only played a part in the treatment of locally advanced and metastatic disease, it is now finding an ever-expanding role as adjuvant, concomitant or neo-adjuvant therapy (or a combination of the above) in both early and advanced prostatic adenocarcinoma.

In this chapter, we attempt to summarise the current practice employing endocrine manipulation in prostate cancer and its future direction based on evidence from established studies and ongoing research.

SURGICAL CASTRATION

This remains the gold standard against which all hormonal manipulation in prostate cancer has to be weighed. Its popularity has waned as evidenced both by patient and clinician surveys alike, mainly due to it being deemed a permanent and irreversible physical and psychological insult to manhood. Although other androgen ablative methods have been developed and refined,

137

it still remains a viable and sometimes the best option in certain situations, for example,

• Where there may be concerns with regards to poor compliance or non-compliance with pharmacological treatment, for example, debilitated or demented elderly patients forgetting to attend for their depot injections.

• When rapidity of reduction in serum testosterone is necessary, for example, in impending spinal cord compression, renal impairment from locally advanced disease or ureteric obstruction secondary to lymphadenopathy. Castrate testosterone levels are achieved within 3 to 12 h, with a mean of 8.6 h post-orchidectomy (Testosterone mean half-life 45 min) [2].

Although clearly the more cost effective option (see below), it has now been superseded by medical castration in the large majority.

OESTROGENS

Use of oestrogenic agents such as diethylstilbestrol as first-line androgen deprivation has dwindled, due to their unacceptable cardiovascular side effects [3], which often compound the pre-existing cardiovascular co-morbidity in the elderly population being treated.

However, recently some renewed interest has been seen in this area, as the oestrogenic effects of diethylstilbestrol protects against bone resorption and subsequent osteoporosis when compared to patients treated with other forms of androgen deprivation therapy [4].

Diethylstilbestrol continues to play an important role as second-line hormone manipulative therapy in androgen independent prostate cancer.

GnRH ANALOGUES

Since their first commercial use in the 1980s (based on the original work of another Nobel Laureate Schally and group [5]) gonadotrophin-releasing hormone (GnRH) analogues have stood the test of time and remain the mainstay of endocrine manipulation in current practice. Various trials comparing it against surgical castration and oestrogens confirm no significant difference in various efficacy end-points including response to treatment, time to progression and overall survival or tolerability [6,7].

However, GnRH analogues have two main shortcomings. First, unique to this form of castration is the initial tumour flare, which can result in devastating consequences when treating advanced disease states. Second, the cumulative financial cost burden with continued treatment on GnRH analogues needs to be carefully considered when comparing them with the cheaper option of surgical orchidectomy. It was concluded by Bonzani *et al.* [8] that GnRH analogues have a financial advantage only if the life expectancy of the patient being treated is less than 9 months. This is roughly the point at which the cost of GnRH analogues equals the one-off price of surgical castration.

Leuprorelin acetate (Wyeth Pharmaceuticals) holds the biggest market share worldwide. The main competitor to this product is Goserelin (AstraZeneca). Both can be administered as subcutaneous depot preparations in various settings, ranging from specialised urology clinics to General Practice, with recent attempts also having been made at patient self-administration schemes. A small scale study [9] showed that it was feasible for a selected group of patients to be taught self-injection of depot leuteinising hormone-releasing hormone (LHRH) analogues, and that some of these patients preferred this mode of drug administration.

Furthermore, with continual progress in drug development, more robust preparations of a sustained release formulation of GnRH analogues are now available. We return to this at the end of the chapter.

MAXIMUM ANDROGEN BLOCKADE

The biggest and most comprehensive collaborative meta-analysis to date on the effect of the addition of anti-androgen therapy to androgen suppression was published by the Prostate Cancer Trialists' Collaborative Group in the year 2000 [10]. This incorporated 27 randomised controlled trials conducted before 1991, on a combined total of 8275 patients. The final conclusion drawn from this large body of work was that in advanced prostate cancer, the addition of an antiandrogen improves the absolute 5-year survival by about 2% or 3%, with a range of uncertainty that runs from 0–5%. This variation correlates with whether a non-steroidal or steroidal antiandrogen is used as part of the maximum androgen blockade (MAB). The benefits of combination therapy were restricted to the use of non-steroidal antiandrogens, as cyprotrone acetate resulted in increased non-prostate cancer deaths. Furthermore, the survival advantage was only seen in patients with metastatic disease, and not in those with locally advanced disease, although it may be argued that the cohort of patient with locally advanced disease (12%; $n = 1000$) was too small for any meaningful data analysis.

This meta-analysis however, only looked at one endpoint, that is, survival, and did not address other issues such as medical outcomes, quality of life, or treatment costs, which may make the modest improvement in survival less valuable when the aims of treatment are viewed from a more holistic perspective.

A more recent meta-analysis [11] declared a statistically significant difference in survival at 5 years in favour of combined androgen blockade (10 trials; hazard ratio = 0.871; 95% confidence interval, 0.805–0.942). However, adverse events leading to withdrawal of therapy occurred with greater frequency in the combined hormone therapy arms of the various trials analysed. Although little is known with regards to the effects of combined androgen blockade (CAB) versus monotherapy on quality of life parameters, the one trial within this meta-analysis that addressed quality of life outcomes, reported a clear advantage for monotherapy, over CAB [12]. Once again, the authors concluded that derivation of any benefit in terms of increased survival must be balanced against the increased risk of adverse effects and the potential for affecting the patient's overall quality of life.

Neither of the afore-mentioned meta-analyses [10,11] included trials where Bicalutamide had been used as the additive anti-androgen to the androgen suppressive therapy. This was addressed in a study by Schell-hammer et al. [13], which demonstrated a trend favouring MAB (using Bicalutamide plus LHRH agonist), showing it to be well tolerated and resulting in equivalent time to progression (hazard ratio 0.93, 95% confidence interval 0.79–1.10; $p = 0.41$) and survival (hazard ratio 0.87, 95% confidence interval 0.72 to 1.05; $p = 0.15$) when compared to treatment with Flutamide plus LHRH agonist, at a median follow-up of 160 weeks.

INTERMITTENT VERSUS CONTINUOUS HORMONAL THERAPY

Several experimental, pre-clinical and phase II clinical studies have shown clear benefits of intermittent androgen therapy over continuous androgen ablative therapy. These have been carefully summarised in a review article by Wolff [14]. Eventual and inevitable progression to a hormone refractory state remains a major obstacle in the treatment of advanced prostate cancer. As the burden of prostate cancer increases, with demographic trends towards detection of early disease in younger men, it is inevitable that overall time on treatment will increase. Intermittent androgen blockade (IAB) therefore provides an avenue whereby time on active treatment, (along with the treatment related side effects and expense) is kept to a minimum without any compromise on survival end points.

The benefits derived from this are reversal of treatment induced side-effects such as impotence, loss of libido, hot flushes and nocturia during periods off treatment, leading to a significant improvement in the quality of life, in addition to delaying the onset of hormone refractory disease.

Re-commencement and cessation of hormone suppression therapy resulting in cyclical hormonal influences is usually guided by serum PSA, using various cut-offs to indicate reactivation and quiescence of the cancer. Several cycles can be achieved in this manner before an androgen independent state is reached.

A recent small-scale study [15] where patients with advanced hormone-naive prostate cancer were randomised to intermittent androgen deprivation ($n = 35$) or to a continuous regimen, showed that the estimated 3-year progression rate was significantly lower in the intermittent androgen deprivation group ($7\% \pm 4.8\%$) than in the continuous androgen deprivation group ($38.9\% \pm 11.2\%$; $p = 0.0052$).

However, it remains unclear as to which patient groups would be best suited to this form of androgen deprivation. Therefore, at present, this approach remains experimental and current treatment protocols continue to adopt continuous therapy with clear consensus on IAB eagerly awaited, based on more conclusive data from prospective larger-scale randomised trials with longer follow-up times. A number of these are ongoing as outlined below:

• An intercontinental study (SWOG 9346; CAN–NCIC–JPR8; CLB-9594; INT-0612; CAN–NCIC–PR). A phase III randomised study to compare intermittent versus continual combined androgen deprivation using Bicalutamide and Goserelin in stage IV prostate cancer, with survival as the main endpoint. Study coordinator is M Hussain.

• A SEUG phase III international study of IAB versus continuous MAB. Study coordinator is C Da Silva.

ADJUVANT AND NEO-ADJUVANT HORMONAL THERAPY IN LOCALLY ADVANCED DISEASE

Endocrine therapy has taken on an important role in complementing the local treatment modalities for prostate cancer. This increasingly popular multi-modal approach offers a survival advantage.

Within this setting, complementary androgen suppression using GnRH analogues with external radiotherapy for locally advanced disease has been best studied and found to be of clear and unquestionable benefit in preventing relapse from disease, and thereby improving disease free survival. This is therefore now widely adopted in everyday standard clinical practice. There is a large body of trial evidence to support this and it has been concisely summarised in a recent review article by Pisansky [16].

In particular, two large-scale prospective randomised trials [17–19 – see Table 12.1] have clearly shown better results with this approach, for many endpoints including overall survival, disease free survival and freedom from loco-regional or metastatic progression.

The optimal overall duration of supplemental hormonal therapy in this setting remains to be clearly established, based on the final results of two recent prospective randomised phase III trials – the RTOG (Radiation

Table 12.1 Survival data from studies combining adjuvant hormonal therapy with radiotherapy in the treatment of prostate cancer

Study	n	Eligibility	Treatment arms	Follow-up (years)	Outcome
RTOG 8531 [17,18]	945	T3 ± N+ or T1–T2, + N+	EBRT alone versus EBRT + Goserelin (continued indefinitely)	10 (live patients)	Improved 10-year absolute survival with adjuvant Goserelin (53% versus 38%; $p < 0.0043$) [18]
EORTC 22863 [19]	415	T1–T2, (WHO grade 3) or T3–T4 (any grade)	EBRT alone versus EBRT + Goserelin (for 3 years)	5.5	Improved 5-year prostate cancer-specific survival with adjuvant Goserelin (94% versus 79%; $p < 0.0001$)

EBRT = external beam radiotherapy
N+ = node positive

Therapy Oncology Group) 92-02 and the EORTC (European Organisation for Research and Treatment of Cancer) 22961.

Preliminary data from the RTOG 92-02 [20] showed patients receiving long-term (an additional 2 years of Goserelin) androgen suppression following external beam radiotherapy, had a significant improvement in several efficacy endpoints including local progression, freedom from distant metastasis and disease free survival, when compared to the short-term androgen suppression (only 2 months of Goserelin and Flutamide before and 2 months during the radiotherapy) arm, at 5-year follow-up. More mature data is awaited, but this current analysis supports the use of adjuvant long-term androgen suppression with radiotherapy in prostate cancer.

The EORTC 22961 recruited 966 patients with T1C – T2B; N 1–2 or T2C – T4; N 0–2, between 1997 and 2002. All patients initially receive an LHRH agonist plus a non-steroidal antiandrogen for 6 months during and after radiotherapy, and are then randomised to a further 30 months of LHRH agonist therapy or no further hormonal therapy [21].

Although the most conclusive trials have been with the use of GnRH analogues, adjuvant/ neoadjuvant therapy can take any form. The early prostate cancer programme, which is discussed below seeks to elucidate the additive benefit of antiandrogens to standard care for prostate cancer.

Neo-adjuvant Hormonal Treatment with Radiotherapy for Locally Advanced Disease

Neo-adjuvant therapy is best described as a treatment method administered before radiotherapy to enhance, primarily, its efficacy by reducing the likelihood for tumour recurrence at the primary site [16].

In the prospective randomised phase III RTOG 86-10 trial the benefits of neo-adjuvant hormonal therapy were investigated in patients with bulky T2–T4 disease ± nodal involvement undergoing radiotherapy. Randomisation was either to 4 weekly maximum androgen blockade (Goserelin plus Flutamide) for 2 months before and concurrently with external radiotherapy ($n = 226$) or to radiotherapy alone ($n = 230$). The most recent analysis of this study [22] showed that receipt of neo-adjuvant hormonal therapy resulted in significant prevention of local progression (30% versus 43%; $p = 0.016$), metastatic progression (34% versus 45%; $p = 0.040$), disease-free survival (33% versus 21%; $p = 0.004$) and disease specific mortality (23% versus 31%; $p = 0.05$), over an 8-year period. However, an overall survival benefit (70% versus 52% alive at 8 years; $p = 0.015$) was only seen in the sub-group of the patients with a Gleason score ≤6.

As in the case of adjuvant hormonal therapy, there are further ongoing trials in an attempt to elucidate what would be the optimal duration of neo-adjuvant androgen suppression prior to radiotherapy. These include the multi-centre phase III Canadian trial that randomises to maximal androgen blockade (Goserelin plus Flutamide) for 3 months or 8 months prior to radiotherapy. The larger ongoing phase III study (RTOG 9910) is of a similar design, randomising to maximal androgen blockade for an 8-week or 28-week period before and concomitantly with radiotherapy [16].

ANTI-ANDROGEN MONOTHERAPY

Quite clearly, the shortcoming of GnRH analogues is the development of other androgen deprivation induced disorders such as osteoporosis [23,24], hot flushes, loss of libido, impotence, and fatigue. Quality of life considerations continue to become more important as we see trends towards identifying earlier stage disease in younger patients. These patients are therefore likely to be treated for longer periods often at a point in their lives when they remain sexually and physically active.

Cross-sectional surveys of patients with prostate cancer have shown their desires to trade-off life years for preservation of sexual function [25]. Within this survey significantly more patients ($p < 0.01$) were willing to accept a treatment associated with a higher mortality to avoid a 100% chance of becoming impotent.

This is where anti-androgens (which help maintain testosterone levels) appear to provide an attractive alternative in helping overcome the unwanted side effects of castration. Surveys on quality of life parameters such as sexual desire and physical capacity, have clearly demonstrated improved satisfaction when non-steroidal anti-androgen monotherapy (Bicalutamide) is used to treat locally advanced disease, when compared to castration [26]. Trends in favour of Bicalutamide were also identified in six other quality of life domains, although these did not reach statistical significance. The main side effects seen with the use of Bicalutamide were gynaecomastia and mastalgia, although withdrawal from the study as a result of intolerability of these specific drug-related events remained low (1.3%).

Furthermore, it is important to note that the above gains were not at the expense of other efficacy end points. Bicalutamide monotherapy matched castration (no statistically significant difference demonstrated) in terms of overall survival ($p = 0.70$) and time to progression ($p = 0.11$), at median follow-up of 6.3 years [26].

A recent prospective open label study revealed that bone mineral density (BMD – measured in the lumbar spine and the hip) was maintained during Bicalutamide 150 mg/ once daily monotherapy, while castration was associated with a significant loss in BMD, after 96 weeks of treatment [27]. Concerns over minimisation of osteoporotic losses secondary to long-term androgen deprivation therapy are of critical importance, as it is now established that patients with advanced prostate cancer often have underlying osteoporosis even prior to being subject to castration [28].

THE EARLY PROSTATE CANCER PROGRAMME

The Early Prostate Cancer Programme (EPC) is the largest ongoing multi-centre randomised double blind, placebo-controlled prospective study in prostate cancer. It comprises of three similar designed, but geographically separated trials, grouped as follows:

- IL0023 – North America – 3292 patients
- IL0024 – Europe, Australia, South Africa and Mexico – 3603 patients
- IL0025 – Scandinavia – 1218 patients

The EPC programme seeks to address as to whether the addition of the non-steroidal anti-androgen Bicalutamide 150 mg to standard care (either as adjunctive to radiotherapy, or radical prostatectomy, or as mono-therapy in patients unfit for radical treatment), can reduce the risk of objective disease progression and improve survival in patients with organ-confined and locally advanced prostate cancer.

The secondary endpoints the programme hopes to examine are time to treatment failure, time to PSA progression and tolerability [29].

The early prostate cancer study design randomised patients ($n = 4052$) to 150 mg/ once daily Bicalutamide or ($n = 4061$) to placebo, in addition to standard care.

The first combined analysis, at a median of 3 years of this EPC study showed that treatment with Bicalutamide provided a highly significant reduction of 42% (hazards ratio 0.58; 95% confidence interval 0.51, 0.66; $p \ll 0.0001$) in the risk of objective progression compared to standard care alone [29]. This result was only seen in trials IL0024 and IL0025, with trial IL0023 not reporting any significant difference at this stage. Objective clinical progression was defined on the basis of evidence from radionucleotide bone scan, MRI or CT. Changes in PSA levels or physical examination findings were not considered evidence of objective progression.

PSA progression is often considered to be the earliest evidence of persistent or recurrent disease after primary therapy of curative intent. In a separate analysis by the same group [30] it was found that addition of Bicalutamide 150 mg to standard care significantly reduced the risk of PSA progression-free interval by 59% when compared to standard care alone (hazards ratio 0.41; 95% confidence interval 0.38, 0.45; $p \ll 0.0001$) at a median follow-up of 3 years. This benefit was observed irrespective of whether patients had undergone radical prostatectomy or radiotherapy as standard care. Time to PSA progression was defined as the time from randomisation to the earliest occurrence of PSA doubling from the baseline, objective progression or death from any cause.

Gynaecomastia and mastodynia remained the most frequently reported side effects of Bicalutamide therapy, as has been noted in previous studies with this anti-androgen [26].

Mature data on survival is awaited following longer follow-up periods from the EPC programme in order to establish whether the afore-mentioned benefits will translate into a long-term survival advantage with this treatment approach.

Casodex License Withdrawal for Treatment of Organ-Confined Prostate Cancer

Following a review of trial data [31] by the committee on the safety of medicines in the United Kingdom, the product license for the use of Bicalutamide (Casodex 150 mg) in localised prostate cancer was withdrawn in November 2003. This was in light of data results from the planned second per protocol analysis of the EPC programme carried out in 2003, after a median follow-up period of 5.4 years. This revealed, Casodex use in the sub-group of patients with localised disease who would otherwise have been managed by watchful waiting only, had resulted in increased mortality when compared to patients on placebo (25.2% deaths versus 20.5% deaths; hazards ratio = 1.23; 95% confidence interval, 1.00, 1.50). This trend towards reduced overall survival was attributed to an increase in non-prostate cancer deaths, as relatively few patients had died from prostate cancer in the Casodex arm of the trial in this sub-group.

However, in patients with locally advanced disease, who would otherwise have been managed by watchful waiting, overall survival tends to favour Casodex treated patients (hazards ratio 0.81).

AstraZeneca sources reported, having conducted an extensive review of their safety databases, that they were unable to find any evidence of a direct causal link between the increase in mortality and use of Casodex in patients with localised disease.

However, it is felt there may be a case for its use in patients with more aggressive localised disease. The confirmatory trials on this are eagerly awaited. This came as a surprise to many prostate cancer specialists who remain optimistic about the beneficial use of Bicalutamide in localised disease, claiming that this has been an over-reaction on part of the medicines regulatory authorities.

Data from the third planned analysis is awaited; expected to be published in 2005.

EARLY VERSUS DEFERRED TREATMENT FOR METASTATIC DISEASE

A large MRC study was commenced in 1984 to assess whether immediate hormonal therapy in advanced or asymptomatic metastatic prostate cancer conferred any benefits over therapy that was deferred until clinically significant progression occurred.

Although the study was heavily criticised on several accounts [32], the one useful conclusion drawn from analysis of the patients with metastasis was that early introduction of hormonal therapy can prevent the onset of serious complications of metastatic prostate cancer, while not necessarily prolonging the life of most patients.

Several other studies, as listed in a review article by Newling [32], also aimed to look at the benefits of instituting hormonal therapy at the time of diagnosis in patients with asymptomatic or symptomatic metastatic disease. The results once again showed a reduction in serious complications, thereby ensuring a reasonable quality of life in patients with metastatic prostate carcinoma. No studies have however demonstrated a clear overall survival advantage.

SIDE EFFECTS OF ENDOCRINE THERAPY AND ITS TREATMENT

Over 50% of prostate cancer patients treated with androgen deprivation therapy experience hot flushes within a few months of having commenced their treatment. The incidence of hot flushes tends to be even higher in the medical castrated patients. These hot flushes can be very annoying and severely disruptive to the patient's quality of life [33].

Treatment is often individualised to the patient's needs. Both oral and transdermal oestrogens have been shown to be effective in reducing the incidence of hot flushes, however their high risk of thromboembolic side effects often makes them unfavourable choices.

Progesterogenic agents such as megesterol acetate [34–36] and cyproterone acetate [37] have been shown to be efficacious in several clinical studies. Their slightly more favourable side-effect profile over exogenous oestrogen replacement therapy often makes them the first-line choice in the treatment of hot flushes secondary to androgen deprivation therapy in prostate cancer.

Skeletal complications secondary to osteoporotic bone loss following androgen deprivation therapy [38] are a common cause of morbidity and mortality in prostate cancer patients. One study showed that approximately 14% of orchidectomised men experienced at least one osteoporotic fracture compared with only 1% of men without a history of androgen deprivation therapy ($p = 0.001$) [39]. Long-term follow up revealed osteoporotic fractures to be more common than traumatic or pathological types, with approximately 38% of the men surviving for more than 5 years after bilateral orchidectomy experiencing one or more osteoporotic fracture.

Furthermore, skeletal fractures in prostate cancer patients on chronic androgen deprivation therapy have been shown to be an independent and adverse predictor of survival [40]. Preventative measures to curb the accelerated bone loss during androgen deprivation therapy should therefore be encouraged by lifestyle modifications, stopping smoking, moderation of alcohol consumption and regular weight-bearing exercises. Vitamin D and calcium supplementation may also be of some benefit. The role of anti-androgen monotherapy (Bicalutamide) in minimising osteoporotic bone loss has already been alluded to above.

Finally, bisphosphonates such as Pamidronate [41,42] and the new third-generation Zoledronic Acid [43] (Novartis Pharmaceuticals, United Kingdom) have been shown to not only prevent bone loss, but also increase the bone mineral density in the hip and the spine during androgen deprivation therapy in non-metastatic prostate cancer.

NOVEL AGENTS

The Implantable Leuprolide Delivery System

This is a subcutaneous implant (Viadur – Bayer Corporation) that releases leuprolide acetate at a constant rate of 120 μg/day over a year [44]. The implant can be removed and replaced with another implant after 12 months for continuous therapy. The implant is considered safe and is well tolerated. All reported adverse events with this device have been mild and most were attributable to testosterone suppression as opposed to the physical properties of the implant itself. Where reactions did occur at the insertion site they tended to be mild and transient, and resolved within 2 weeks of insertion or removal of the implants. The most common local reaction noted was bruising. Efficacy data from 4 years of clinical experience indicates uniform testosterone suppression into the castrate range and a high degree of patient satisfaction [44].

GnRH Antagonists

Unlike the GnRH analogues, GnRH antagonists do not result in an initial stimulation of gonadotrophin release, but cause an immediate, rapid and reversible suppression of gondatrophin secretion. This in turn results in the avoidance of an initial testosterone surge. The principal mechanism of their action is competitive receptor occupancy of the GnRH receptor [45]. An additional benefit seen with GnRH antagonists is the long-term suppression of follicle-stimulating hormone (FSH), as FSH has been implicated as a potential independent growth factor in prostate cancer [46].

Studies on normal volunteers demonstrate that GnRH agonists appear to only suppress FSH levels to a nadir of 30% of pre-treatment values, but even this escapes from suppression shortly after reaching the nadir [47]. A similar escape pattern in FSH suppression is observed in patients with prostate cancer treated with GnRH agonists [48].

The new GnRH antagonist Abarelix (Plenaxis® – marketed by Praecis Pharmaceuticals) has recently been approved by the Food and Drug Administration (FDA) for use in prostate cancer patients with advanced symptomatic disease when treatment with conventional GnRH analogues is contraindicated [49]. The approval was based on an open label clinical study (81 men from 17 centres) where the drug was shown to be effective in lowering testosterone levels to a castrate state [50]. The authors concluded that the major clinical benefit was avoidance of surgical castration (in 97% of the subjects, by undergoing therapy for at least 12 weeks), likely to have been required had Aberelix not been available. Benefits were observed in other biochemical and clinical endpoints too. These include a reduction in PSA levels, a decrease in pain intensity from skeletal metastases, a decrease in analgesic requirements and the resolution of obstructive uropathy.

Abarelix is administered as an intra-muscular injection every 2 weeks during the first month of therapy, followed by a 4-weekly depot injections thereafter. Although approved, in view of an allergic-type reaction experienced by two patients, the FDA and the manufacturer have limited its use only under a risk management programme, whereby clinicians need to enrol onto the Plenaxis user safety programme in order to be able to prescribe Abarelix.

CONCLUSIONS

At present GnRH analogues, with or without an anti-androgen, remain the most common form of hormonal manipulation in prostate cancer patients.

Although we continue to witness significant advances in understanding the aetiological basis of prostate cancer and its treatment, many unanswered questions and challenges remain within the remit of hormonal management of this disease.

Quality-of-life considerations are of paramount importance and impact on the patients' and clinicians' choice of treatment, especially when efficacy outcomes may be similar with differing therapeutic options.

REFERENCES

1 Huggins C, Hodges CV. Studies on prostate cancer I: the effects of castration on oestrogen and of androgen injection on serum phosphatases in metastatic carcinoma of the prostate gland. *Cancer Res* 1941; **1**: 293.

2 Khoury S. Testicular androgen ablation. In: Kaisary AV, Murphy GP, Denis L, Griffiths K, eds. *Textbook of prostate cancer: Pathology, Diagnosis and Treatment,* Martin Dunitz Ltd, London, 1999; 291.

3 Byar DP, Corle DK. Hormone therapy for prostate cancer: results of the VACURG studies. *NCI Monogr* 1988; (7): 165–70.

4 Scherr D, Pitts WR Jr, Vaughn ED Jr. Diethylstilbesterol revisited: androgen deprivation, osteoporosis and prostate cancer. *J Urol* 2002; **167**: 535–8.

5 Schally AV, Arimura A, Baba Y *et al.* Isolation and properties of the FSH and LHRH. *Biochem Biophys Res Commun* 1971; **43**: 393–9.

6 Turkes AO, Puelling WB, Griffith H. Treatment of patients with advanced cancer of the prostate: phase III trial. Zolazex against castration: a study of the British Prostate Group. *J Steroid Biochem* 1987; **27**: 543–9.

7 Volgelzang NY, Chodak GW, Soloway MS *et al.* Goserelin versus orchidectomy in the treatment of advanced prostate cancer: final results of a randomised trial. Zolazex Prostate Study Group. *Urology* 1995; **46**: 220–6.

8 Bonzani RA, Stricker HJ, Peabody JO, Menon M. Cost comparison of orchidectomy and leuprolide in metastatic prostate cancer. *J Urology* 1998; **160**: 2446–9.

9 Hamm R, Patel B, Whittlestone T, Persad R. Patient self-injection: a new approach to administering luteinizing hormone-releasing hormone analogues. *BJU International* 2000; **86**: 840–2.

10 Prostate Cancer Trialists' Collaborative Group. Maximum androgen blockade in advanced prostate cancer: an overview of randomised trials. *Lancet* 2000; **355**: 1491–8.

11 Samson DJ, Seidenfeld J, Schmitt B *et al.* Systematic review and meta-analysis of monotherapy compared with combined androgen blockade for patients with advanced prostate carcinoma. *Cancer* 2002; **95**: 361–76.

12 Moinpour CM, Savage MJ, Troxel A *et al.* Quality of life in advanced prostate cancer: results of a randomised therapeutic trial. *J Natl Cancer Inst* 1998; **90**: 1537–44.

13 Schellhammer P, Sharifi R, Block N *et al.* for the Casodex Combination Study Group. Clinical benefits of Bicalutamide compared with Flutamide in combined androgen blockade for patients with advanced prostatic carcinoma: final report of a double-blind, randomised multicenter trial. *Urology* 1997; **50**: 330–6.

14 Wolff JM, Tunn UW. Intermittent androgen blockade in Prostate Cancer: rationale and clinical experience. *Eur Urol* 2000; **38**: 365–71.

15 De Leval J, Boca P, Yousef E *et al.* Intermittent versus continuous total androgen blockade in the treatment of patients with advanced hormone-naïve prostate cancer: results of a prospective randomised multicenter trial. *Clin Prostate Cancer* 2002; **1**: 163–71.

16 Pisansky TM. Use of neoadjuvant and adjuvant therapy to prevent or delay recurrence of prostate cancer in patients undergoing radiation treatment for prostate cancer. *Urology* 2003; **62**: 36–45.

17 Pilepich MV, Caplan R, Byhardt RW *et al.* Phase III trial of antiandrogen suppression using goserelin in unfavourable-prognosis carcinoma of the prostate treated with definite radiotherapy: report of Radiation Therapy Oncology Group Protocol 85-31. *J Clin Oncol* 1997; **15**: 1013–21.

18 Pilepich MV, Winter K, Lawton C, Krisch RE, Wolkov H, Movsas B, *et al.* Androgen suppression adjuvant to radiotherapy in carcinoma of the prostate. Long-term results of phase III RTOG study 85-31. *Int J Radiat Oncol Biol Phys* 2003; **57**: S172–3.

19 Bolla M, Gonzalez D, Warde P *et al.* Improved survival in patients with locally advanced prostate cancer treated with radiotherapy and Goserelin [EORTC

22863]. *N Engl J Med* 1997; **337**: 295–300.

20 Hanks GE, Pajak TF, Porter A *et al.* Phase III trial of long-term adjuvant androgen deprivation after neoadjuvant hormonal cytoreduction and radiotherapy in locally advanced carcinoma of the prostate: the Radiation Therapy Oncology Group Protocol 92-02. *J Clin Oncol* 2003; **21**: 3972–8.

21 Bolla M, de Reijke T. Long term adjuvant hormonal treatment with LHRH analogue versus no further treatment in locally advanced prostatic carcinoma treated by external irradiation and six months combined androgen blockade – a phase III study. EORTC trial 22961 – a joint trial of the EORTC Radiotherapy and EORTC Genito-urinary Tract Co-operative Group. EORTC Data Center, Brussels, 1997.

22 Pilepich MV, Winter K, John MJ *et al.* Phase III Radiation Therapy Oncology Group (RTOG) Trial 86-10 of androgen deprivation adjuvant to definitive radiotherapy in locally advanced carcinoma of the prostate. *Int J Radiat Oncol Biol Phys* 2001; **50**: 1243–52.

23 Ross RW, Small EJ. Osteoporosis in men treated with androgen deprivation therapy for prostate cancer. *J Urol* 2002; **167**: 1952–6.

24 Daniell HW, Dunn SR, Ferguson DW, Lomas G, Niazi Z, Stratte PT. Progressive osteoporosis during androgen deprivation therapy for prostate cancer. *J Urol* 2000; **163**: 181–6.

25 Mazur DJ, Hickman DH. Patient preferences: survival versus quality-of-life considerations. *J Gen Intern Med.* 1993; **8**: 374–7.

26 Iversen P, Tyrell CJ, Kaisary AV *et al.* Bicalutamide monotherapy compared with castration in patients with non-metastatic locally advanced prostate cancer: 6.3 years of follow-up. *J Urol* 2000; **164**: 1579–82.

27 Sieber PR, Keiller DL, Khanoski RJ, Gallo J, McFadden S. Bicalutamide 150 mg maintains bone mineral density during monotherapy for localised or locally advanced prostate cancer. *J Urol* 2004; **171**: 2272–6.

28 Hussain SA, Weston R, Stephenson RN, George E, Parr NJ. Immediate dual energy X-ray absorptiometry reveals a high incidence of osteoporosis in patients with advanced prostate cancer before hormone manipulation. *BJU International* 2003; **92**: 690–4.

29 See WA, Wirth MP, Wirth DG *et al.* on behalf of the Casodex Early Prostate Cancer Trialist Group. Bicalutamide as immediate therapy either alone or as adjunct to standard care of patients with localised or locally advanced prostate cancer: first analysis of the early prostate cancer program. *J Urol* 2002; **168**: 429–35.

30 See W, Iversen P, Wirth M, McLeod D, Garside L, Morris T. Immediate treatment with Bicalutamide 150 mg as adjunct therapy significantly reduces the risk of progression in early prostate cancer. *European Urology* 2003; **44**: 512–8.

31 Professor Gordon Duff. Casodex 150 mg (Bicaltumide): no longer indicated for treatment of localised prostate cancer. Safety message issued by the Committee on the Safety of Medicines, 2003.

32 Newling D. Early versus late androgen deprivation therapy in metastatic disease. *Urology* 2001; **58**: 50–5.

33 Kouriefs C, Georgiou M, Ravi R. Hot flushes and prostate cancer: pathogenesis and treatment. *BJU International* 2002; **89**: 379–83.

34 Loprinzi CL, Michalak JC, Quella SK *et al.* Megestrol acetate for the prevention of hot flashes. *N Engl J Med* 1994; **331**: 347–52.

35 Quella SK, Loprinzi CL, Sloan JA *et al.* Long term use of megesterol acetate by cancer survivors for the treatment of hot flashes. *Cancer* 1998; **82**: 1784–8.

36 Smith JA Jr. A prospective comparison of treatments for symptomatic hot flushes following endocrine therapy for carcinoma of the prostate. *J Urol* 1994; **152**: 132–4.

37 Eaton AC, McGuire N. Cyproterone acetate in the treatment of post-orchidectomy hot flushes. Double-blind cross-over trial. *Lancet* 1983; **2**: 1336–7.

38 Smith MR. Diagnosis and management of treatment-related osteoporosis in men with prostate carcinoma. *Cancer* 2003; **97**: 789–95.

39 Daniell HW. Osteoporosis after orchidectomy for prostate cancer. *J Urol* 1997; **157**: 439–44.

40 Oefelein MG, Ricchiuti V, Conrad W, Resnick MI. Skeletal fractures negatively correlate with overall survival in men with prostate cancer. *J Urol* 2002; **168**: 1005–7.

41 Smith MR, McGovern FJ, Zietman AL *et al.* Pamidronate to prevent bone loss in men receiving gonadotrophin releasing hormone agonist therapy for prostate cancer. *N Engl J Med* 2001; **345**: 948–55.

42 Diamond TH, Winters J, Smith A *et al.* The antiosteoporotic efficacy of intravenous pamidronate in men with prostate carcinoma receiving combined androgen blockade: a double blind, randomised, placebo-controlled crossover study. *Cancer* 2001; **92**: 1444–50.

43 Smith MR, Eastham J, Gleason DM, Shasha D, Tchekmedyian S, Zinner N. Randomised controlled trial of zoledronic acid to prevent bone loss in men receiving androgen deprivation therapy for nonmetastatic prostate cancer. *J Urol* 2003; **169**: 2008–12.

44 Marks LS. Leuteinizing Hormone-Releasing Hormone Agonists in the management of men with prostate cancer: timing, alternatives, and the 1-year implant. *Urology*, 2003; **62**: 36–42.

45 Huirne J, Lambalk CB. Gonadotropin-releasing-hormone-receptor antagonists. *Lancet* 2001; **358**: 1793–803.

46 Ben-Josef E, Yang SY, Ji TH *et al.* Hormone refractory prostate cancer cells express functional FSH receptor. *J Urol* 1999; **161**: 970–6.

47 Bhasin S, Berman N, Swerdloff RS. Follicle-stimulating hormone (FSH) escape during chronic gonadotrophin-releasing hormone (GnRH) agonist and testosterone treatment. *J Androl* 1994; **15**: 386–91.

48 Mahler C, Verhelst J, Chaban M, Dennis L. Prolactin and pituitary gonadotrophin values and responses to acute LHRH challenge in patients having long-term treatment with a depot LHRH analogue. *Cancer* 1991; **67**: 557–9.

49 FDA Talk Paper. FDA approves new drug for advanced prostate cancer. Nov 2003. Information retrieved from website http://www.fda.gov/bbs/topics/ANSWERS/2003/ANS01268.html on the 7th May 2004.

50 Koch M, Steidle C, Brosman S, Centeno A, Gaylis F, Campion M, Garnick M for the Abarelix Study Group. An open-label study of abarelix in men with symptomatic prostate cancer at risk of treatment with LHRH agonists. *Urology* 2003; **62**: 877–82.

13: The Role of Conservative Policies in the Treatment of Prostate Cancer

Stijn de Vries, Christopher Bangma and Fritz Schröder

INTRODUCTION

Males diagnosed with organ-confined adenocarcinoma of the prostate (PCa) have four treatment options: surgery, radiation therapy, endocrine treatment or an expectant regimen. Most patients, like the majority of urologists, will prefer radical treatment in order to eliminate all cancer tissue. This train of thought is a logical consequence of the impressive long-term disease-specific survival results of organ-confined prostate cancer. With time, these survival prospects have only increased due to improved skill and more sophisticated treatment techniques, but this is mainly accredited to the introduction of prostate-specific antigen (PSA) as a screening tool for the detection of prostate cancer. PSA driven screening allows earlier diagnosis and it is possible that prostate cancer is diagnosed in males who would not develop symptoms of this disease during their normal life span. These males could be candidates for a more conservative policy, which could protect selected patients from treatment related side effects and diminish the burden imposed on the health care systems by the increasing incidence of PCa in the current PSA era. This chapter gives a review of the role for conservative management policies in prostate cancer patients.

DEFINITIONS OF EXPECTANT MANAGEMENT

The literature suggests different protocols for monitoring PCa patients on a conservative treatment policy [1–5]. Conservative policies can be divided into two entities. The first regimen provides delayed palliative treatment in previously untreated males and in this chapter will be called expectant management (EM), because there is no intention to cure. If however both the patient and his tumour characteristics are closely monitored and treatment with curative intent is provided at a later time, this will be called watchful waiting with deferred treatment, or in brief deferred treatment (DT).

WINDOW OF OPPORTUNITY

It is estimated that a 50-year-old male has a 42% lifetime risk of developing histological evidence of prostate cancer, a 9.2% risk of developing clinical disease and a 2.9% risk of dying of Pca [6]. Though these are estimated risks, they reflect the relatively slow progression of this disease in most cases and the observation that many men will not die of their PCa. This can be visualised with the Albertsen tables in Fig. 13.1 [7]. The graphs show the disease specific and overall survival of the males stratified per age group and

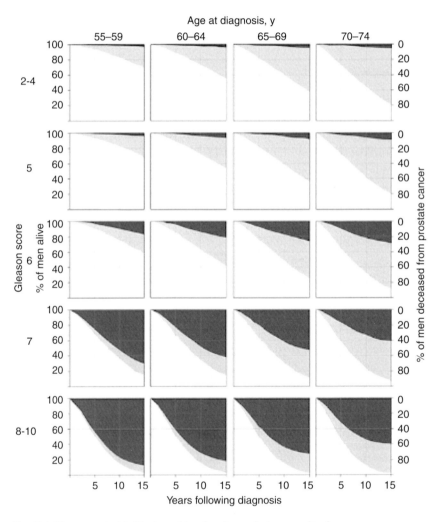

Fig. 13.1 Shows survival (white lower) band and cumulative mortality from prostate cancer (dark grey upper band) and other causes (light grey middle band) up to 15 years after diagnosis stratified by age at diagnosis and Gleason score. Percentage of men alive can be read from the left-hand scale, and percentage of men who have died from prostate cancer or other causes from the right hand scale. (Ref Albertsen et al JAMA 1998).

Gleason score, determined by biopsy over time. The Gleason score is currently the gold standard to describe PCa differentiation grade. The Gleason score is based on the two most prevalent architectural acinar and glandular patterns. The Gleason pattern can range from 1 (highly differentiated) to 5 (poorly differentiated). The Gleason score is the sum of both patterns and can thus range from 2 to 10. Earlier studies use the MD Anderson grading system, which has three grades. Grade 1 disease can roughly be compared with a Gleason score of 6, grade 2 with a Gleason score of 7 and grade 3 PCa with a Gleason score of 8 or higher. The 767 men in the study of Albertsen *et al.* all had clinically localised disease and received palliative treatment when developing symptoms. More interesting is that all these males were diagnosed without the use of PSA testing, thus in males with symptomatic disease. The white lower band represents survival, the black upper band depicts the cumulative disease-specific mortality, and the grey middle band shows the cumulative mortality from other causes. When looking at the patients with well-differentiated PCa, indicated by a Gleason score of 2–5, 2–10% died of PCa after 15 years, while 30–80% did die of other causes. In the patients with a moderate to poorly differentiated PCa, that is, a Gleason score of 7 and higher, the percentage of males dying from PCa increases, though in the older age groups 40–50% will die of other causes. On this basis it does not seem appropriate to select younger patients with a Gleason score 7 or higher for watchful waiting (WW) with deferred treatment (DT), but males with lower Gleason scores have a low chance of dying of PCa so may be more suitable. Comparing different treatment modalities Lu-Yao *et al.* report similar disease specific survival percentages for treatment with curative intent, 90–94%, and conservative management policies, 93%, in patients with grade 1 PCa on the basis of an intention to treat analysis [8]. Moreover 10 year overall survival was equal to slightly better for grade one patients compared to an age-matched cohort. Other studies from the pre-PSA era found comparable 5 to 10 years prostate cancer-specific survival outcomes for the patients with low-grade cancers treated with radical prostatectomy, external beam radiation or conservative management. Conservative policies however were less effective with increasing grade [9,10].

The introduction of PSA has drastically increased the incidence of prostate cancer. Recent studies provide growing evidence for a PSA-induced risk migration towards more favourable PCa characteristics at diagnosis [11]. This risk migration can be explained by lead-time and length-time bias. Lead-time bias can be defined as the advancement in time of diagnosis by PSA. Length time reflects the effect wherein slow growing cancers are more likely to be detected in a screening program as they remain longer in the pre-clinical detectable phase. Preliminary results of estimates for lead time in both hypothetical cohorts and prospective randomised screening studies for

(a)

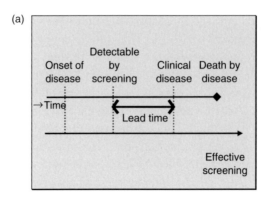

(b)

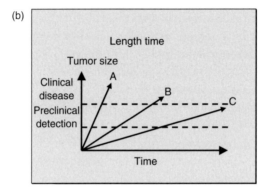

Fig. 13.2 (a) With an effective screening test diagnosis can be forwarded in time, ideally before the disease becomes clinically apparent. Screening is only effective if outcome prospects for these patients increases due to this earlier diagnosis, which is represented by arrow 'C'. A lead time bias occurs when the apparent gained period of life due to the earlier diagnosis is described a positive result of screening, while the patients still die at the same time due to their disease. (b) If time is plotted against tumor size fast growing PCa (arrow A) will be in the preclinical detectable phase for a shorter interval than slower growing PCa (arrow B and C). The longer a tumor is in the preclinical phase the higher is the chance that it will be detected during screening. Thus screening will preferably detect PCa with a long preclinical phase.

the detection of PCa have shown that the calculated lead time for prostate cancers ranges from 5–12 years, depending on the definition used [12,13]. Lead time is presumably shorter for aggressive cancers and older males while it is longer for latent cancers and younger patients. Figure 13.2(a) and (b) schematically explain lead- and length-time bias. Assuming that PSA-driven screening advances the diagnosis in time, prostate cancer can be diagnosed at an earlier pre-clinical asymptomatic stage. This earlier diagnosis explains the documented shift to lower tumour stage and grade in patients with newly diagnosed PCa in the PSA era [14].

Some of the slowly growing cancers will never enter the symptomatic phase and will not be detected if PSA is not used as a screening test. These cancers could be categorised as over-detected or clinically insignificant. The shift to lower stage and grade can also be explained using length-time bias, as most of these patients with low-stage, low-grade cancer are diagnosed due to the length time generated by PSA-driven screening. The definition of over-detection used in most studies is the amount of cancers that would not have been diagnosed, during lifetime, in the absence of screening. Calculations of over-detection range from 24–93%, depending on age and the definition used [12,15]. Males with 'over-detected' or clinically insignificant cancers could favourably bias the disease-specific survival after radical treatment, as over-treatment by definition has a 100% cure rate.

The rationale of watchful waiting with DT is to avoid unnecessary treatment, with its inherent side effects and costs in patients with PCa, who are not likely to progress to clinical disease during their lifetime, while offering these selected patients a possible cure at a later time. If as an experiment, a lead time of 7.5 years is added to Fig. 13.1, the middle of the black upper band would represent the disease-specific mortality after 15 years. Most probably, the overall mortality does not change, but the relative chance of dying of prostate cancer has now significantly diminished, especially for the older males and patients with Gleason score 6 and lower. The questions that follow are: who are the males that are likely to die before ever experiencing Pca-related symptoms, how can they be selected and how should they be monitored?

EXPECTANT MANAGEMENT – REVIEW OF LITERATURE

Most of the EM studies published, concern males diagnosed in the pre-PSA era. In the landmark study of the Scandinavian Prostate Group (SPG 4), a total 695 men were randomised either to a radical prostatectomy (RP) arm or an EM arm [1]. They found a statistically significant decrease after 8 years in Pca-specific mortality in the RP arm (7.1%) compared to the EM group (13.6%). The overall mortality did not differ between the two arms, the rate of developing metastases, however, was again significantly higher after 8 years, in the EM group (27.3%) compared to the RP group (13.4%). The results of this study therefore suggest that RP is the better treatment modality for clinically detected localised PCa. However, 60.7% of the patients in this study had a Gleason score of six or lower and half of the patients of this study had a WHO grade 2. Because in this study no data are available on disease-specific survival results stratified by differentiation grade, it remains unclear whether the survival benefit is present in all differentiation grades or only for patients with less differentiated PCa. Though in a pooled data analysis of six non-randomised studies of patients treated with expectant management no significant difference was noted in prostate cancer-specific survival for grade 1 and grade 2 cancers after 10 years [10], the rate of developing metastases increased from 19% to 42% and 74% for patients with grade 1, 2 and 3 prostate cancer respectively. However, using data from almost 60 000 patients from the SEER database (Surveillance, Epidemiology and End Results program) 'an intention to treat' analysis showed a deteriorating 10 year Pca-specific survival of 93%, 77% and 45% for patients with grade 1, 2 and 3 PCa respectively, managed on a conservative policy [8]. The corresponding survival figures for RP were 94%, 87% and 67%, supporting the proposition that patients with poorly differentiated organ-confined disease and a long-life expectancy should not be followed in a conservative way.

All these non-randomised studies concern PCa patients diagnosed in the pre-PSA era and comparisons between current patients diagnosed in the PSA era may not be justifiable. Most authors, however, agree that only patients with a well-differentiated organ-confined PCa or a limited life expectancy should be considered for EM.

WATCHFUL WAITING WITH DEFERRED TREATMENT – REVIEW OF LITERATURE

Though long-term results of patients, diagnosed in the PSA era are not yet available, several prospective studies have started evaluating the role of DT in organ-confined PCa diagnosed in the current PSA era. The prospective study of Choo *et al.* included 206 patients with a PSA level under 15 ng/mL, clinical stage T1b–2BN0M0 and a Gleason score 2–7, and confirmed review of the original low to moderate grade pathology. During follow-up, subsequent treatment was provided if either clinical, histological or biochemical evidence of progression was noted. Clinical progression was defined by worsening digital rectal examination (DRE) findings, symptoms requiring trans-urethral resection of the prostate or clinical evidence of metastases. Histological progression was assumed with a Gleason score of 8 or higher on a repeat biopsy 12 to 18 months after study enrollment. Patients with a calculated PSA doubling time (PSADT) <2 years were defined as having biochemical progression. The probability of remaining on the protocol, without signs of progression, after 4 years was 48%. Of the 69 patients, 33 discontinued the protocol without having signs of progression and were not included in this analysis, but they highlight the anxiety of patients monitored on a watchful waiting policy, who at follow-up prefer a definite treatment. The fact that the trial is still running shows that DT is a possible option in selected patients [2]. Though initial PSA, T-stage and Gleason score were not predictive of rapid progression in the preliminary analyses, this remains to be validated with a longer follow-up.

In another prospective study [16], 81 males with small volume PCa were identified using the Epstein criteria: stage T1C PCa, a PSA-density (PSAD)

<0.15 ng/mL/cc, absence of any Gleason pattern of 4 or 5 in the prostatic biopsies, less than three biopsy cores with cancerous invasion and under 50% invasion of any core [17]. Disease progression was noted in 25 of the included males after a median follow-up of 14 months and was exclusively based on adverse repeat biopsy findings, defined as a Gleason score of 7 or more or more than 2 cores with cancerous invasion. Of the 13 patients, 12 subsequently had a RP and had a calculated probability of over 70% 10 year disease-free progression after surgery, based on pathological stage and Gleason score, and were considered to still have had curable cancers. In this study, PSAD was significantly (p = 0.01) lower and percent free PSA was significantly (p = 0.04) higher in patients without progression. PSA at diagnosis, prostatic volume and age at diagnosis did not statistically differ between the two groups. The authors, recognising the limitations of identifying men with small volume disease concluded that DT may be a safe alternative for older men complying with the criteria for small volume disease, but that these patients have to be aware of the risk of loosing the opportunity of cure. Yet another group used the same biopsy-derived criteria together with a PSA cut-off of 20 ng/mL and a clinical stage ≤T2 at diagnosis to evaluate watchful waiting with DT in patients under 70 years of age [18]. After 2 and 4 years, 57.3% and 73.2% of the 313 patients respectively had chosen treatment. Of the 215 patients, 6 with DT received androgen deprivation. Using a univariate analysis age, clinical stage and PSADT were the strongest predictors of secondary treatment. In the multivariate analyses a shorter PSADT, that is, <2 years and higher clinical T-stage at diagnosis remained statistically significant predictors of secondary treatment. Though no information was available for the outcome of the treated patients to evaluate whether DT is an acceptable regimen in younger males, this analysis is currently being done.

De Vries et al. showed that of the 191 patients from the European Randomized Study of Screening for Prostate Cancer monitored with a DT policy, 161 (84%) had a PSA under 10 ng/mL, a maximum Gleason score of $3 + 3$ and a clinical T2A stage or lower [19]. In this study, 30 patients changed therapy, they had a mean follow-up of 27 months after treatment and one patient had signs of biochemical recurrence of disease after an RP. The reason to start active treatment ranged from the patient's wish to biochemical progression, whether or not combined with progression based on DRE. In this study, PSADT again was significantly lower for patients who crossed over to active treatment compared to men who stayed on the watchful waiting regimen. Like Choo et al. the authors noted that a considerable percentage of the males had a PSADT over 10 years suggesting indolent disease. Though this was not a prospective study designed to evaluate a DT regimen and males detected with PCa were free to choose any form of treatment, all patients had signed informed consent before being randomised into the intervention arm.

Taking these different studies into consideration it clearly emerges that (1) only patients with favourable tumour characteristics at diagnosis are selected, (2) different strategies to monitor disease progression are used ranging from gathering histological evidence to interpreting repeated PSA values, and assessing signs of clinical progression and (3) a significant number of patients request treatment without having signs of progression.

SELECTION OF PATIENTS

To minimise the chance of the doom scenario of a patient with apparently curable disease at diagnosis, who progresses beyond cure or even dies of prostate cancer, males with PCa opting for a conservative policy should be carefully selected and followed. Though at present no foolproof parameters are available, clinical stage, Gleason score and PSA at diagnosis are used to stratify patients into risk groups [20]. Favourable disease is usually defined as clinical stages T1A, T1C and T2A, combined with a PSA at diagnosis under 10 ng/mL and a Gleason score of 6 or less. There should not be a Gleason pattern 4 present in the pathological specimen. Patients with these favourable tumour characteristics, have similar 5-year biochemical relapse-free survival rates irrespective of treatment modality, which have increased in the PSA era to upto and even over 90% [21]. Supportive of these limits are the facts that less than 1% of the PCa patients have a nucleotide bone scan positive for skeletal metastases if the PSA value is less than 10, 50% of the males above this level have disease beyond the prostate [22], and that PSA levels under 4 ng/mL identified organ-confined disease in 80% of the patients [23]. The cut-off of the Gleason score of $3 + 3$ is not only explained by the Albertsen tables, but higher Gleason grades are correlated with worse pathological outcome and reduced survival in various nomograms [24,25]. These nomograms although predicting outcome for different radical treatment modalities can also be of use in selecting patients for a DT policy. When comparing the biopsy Gleason score with the gold standard pathological Gleason score both under- and over-grading are common [26]. Therefore the biopsy Gleason score should be interpreted with caution. However multiple studies have shown the statistically significant predictive value of biopsy derived Gleason score or its use as a predictive parameter [24,27,28].

Initial PSA, biopsy Gleason score and clinical T-stage are widely available and could be used as a basis for selecting males for a conservative policy. Meanwhile, researchers have continuously been exploiting known predictors and exploring new parameters that may enhance reproducibility, sensitivity and specificity of the different markers used in selecting patients with favourable characteristics at diagnosis. PSA derivatives as percent free PSA and PSAD could be valuable in this context [29,30]. Likewise, further evaluation of biopsy cores showed that the absolute length, the presence of perineural invasion and the amount of cores with cancerous invasion were all related to biochemical outcome after treatment [17,28,31]. All these studies showed the correlation of tumour load with (biochemical) recurrence of disease. Epstein *et al.* proposed an algorithm that could identify 16% of cases with insignificant prostate cancer out of 660 males treated for PCa. Insignificant PCa was defined as pathological organ-confined disease with no Gleason score over 6 and less that 0.2 cm^3 tumour. Their model was based on a PSAD less than 0.1 ng/mL/g and a Gleason score of 6 or less, less than 3 cores with PCa invasion and no more than 50% of invasion of any core, or a PSAD of 0.1 to 0.15 ng/mL/g, with a low- to intermediate-grade cancer smaller than 3 mm, found in only one needle biopsy core specimen [17]. The positive predictive value of this model was 95%, with a negative predictive value of 66%.

FOLLOW-UP OF PATIENTS

After the identification of apparent clinically insignificant PCa, only DT remains as a viable option if tumour dynamics can be monitored. PCa is by definition a progressive disease and progression can arise on three levels: biochemical, histological and clinical. Based on the assumption that PSA is correlated with PCa volume [32] and that the prostate cancer continues to produce PSA, sequential PSA measurements over time reflect tumour growth. Consequently, PSA velocity was introduced [33] for the detection of PCa and PSA DT for monitoring patients on a conservative policy [34]. Individual PSA and thus also PSADT values for patients with PCa are extremely variable, reflecting the natural and biochemical variation [35]. Although this feeds the controversy in the use of PSADT in monitoring patients with PCa, growing evidence in the contemporary literature is shifting the balance in favour of using PSADT as a more objective clinical parameter in conservative policies [5]. Carter estimated a normal baseline PSADT of 54 ± 30 years for patients without PCa in men aged 40 years [33]. Though an evidence based cut-off value cannot yet be determined, most authors using PSADT in PCa patients suggest that a PSADT over 10 years suggest minimal active disease [2,36,37]. This is supported by another report where 48% of 104 males with PCa had a PSADT <10 years, which correlated with histological and clinical progression [3]. A PSADT under 2 years should trigger treatment as it reflects an active growing PCa [38]. Formulas to calculate PSADT use natural, or two base logarithms [2,39], and are therefore not usable in daily practice.

However easy to use programs incorporating different nomograms are freely available to use and download on the internet like the nomograms developed by the Memorial Sloan-Kettering Cancer Center [40].

The only way to monitor histological progression is to perform repeat biopsies. The interval between biopsies and the biopsy regimen used may vary, taking into account initial PCa and patient characteristics. If a Gleason pattern 4 is encountered or the tumour load has dramatically increased, though most likely attributable to a sample error in the first biopsy [41], treatment should follow. Clinical disease as in developing symptoms, though unlikely in these patients, should not be neglected. Advancing clinical stage as estimated on DRE should trigger treatment especially if a previously impalpable disease transforms into a palpable lesion. This lesion however might also be the result of a previously performed biopsy procedure. Though these different progression criteria can be useful from a clinical point of view, the anxiety of the patient or his relatives could also result in a request for treatment. This reflects the psychological stress inherent to living with an identified cancer and uncertainties about the slow but steady rise in PSA level.

Table 13.1 summarises options for patient selection, follow-up and trigger points for treatment [42] and accurately reflects the data reviewed in their paper. Most criteria have been adapted, while some have been modified to further minimise the chance of including patients with extraprostatic disease. The authors recommend a 3-monthly evaluation for the first 2 years and semi-annually thereafter. The remark in Table 13.1 concerning an optional repeat biopsy should be interpreted as an extra precaution. Depending of the initial biopsy strategy and the prostatic volume measured, performing an early repeat biopsy, could further minimise the chance of a sample or grade error [43].

CONCLUDING REMARKS

Preliminary data on the natural history of screen-detected Prostate Cancer suggests there is a long interval in which curative treatment is possible, broadening the horizon for conservative policies, including younger patients with a long-life expectancy. Conservative policies should be divided into EM, and watchful waiting with DT with curative intent. Though selection criteria are obviously more stringent for patients with possible DT, both physician and patient should comprehend and accept both advantages and disadvantages of either conservative policy chosen. Further understanding of the aetiology of PCa provided by the ongoing randomised screening studies combined with longer follow-up of the prospective DT studies will mould DT into a mature and possibly equally effective treatment option in the future.

Table 13.1 Policy proposals for WW.

Proposal	Criteria
I Selection	Patients aged <75 years, life expectancy >10 years
	Good general health (ASA score ≤2, Charlson score ≤1) T1a, T1c or T2a
	PSA < 5–8 ng/mL (and/or PSAD < 0.1 and/or f/tPSA ≥ 19%?)
	Gleason score ≤6, no Gleason pattern 4
	Patient request (quality of life considerations), applicable to higher risk after proper information
	≤ one core positive for cancer with <30% cancer involvement
II Follow-up recommendations	
Timing	3–6 months, 3 monthly during year 1 and 2
Physical	DRE — exclude T progression
Laboratory	PSA and PSA-DT, creatinine
Imaging	TRUS yearly and upon indication, possibly together with biopsy (support for DRE, volume)
Biopsy	Every 12–18 months (grade progression?)
	Option: biopsy after 3 months
III Trigger points for treatment	
1	Patient request
2	Local T progression (DRE or TRUS)
3	PSA-DT < 2 years
4	Grade progression on biopsy (≥ two Gleason scores, or Gleason pattern 4)
5	Any combination of items 2–4

PSAV, PSA velocity; PSAD, PSA density; DRE, digital rectal examination; PSA-DT, PSA doubling time; TRUS, transrectal ultrasound.

REFERENCES

1 Holmberg L, Bill-Axelson A, Helgesen F et al. A randomized trial comparing radical prostatectomy with watchful waiting in early prostate cancer. *N Engl J Med* 2002; **347**: 781–9.

2 Choo R, Klotz L, Danjoux C et al. Feasibility study: watchful waiting for localized low to intermediate grade prostate carcinoma with selective delayed intervention based on prostate specific antigen, histological and/or clinical progression. *J Urol* 2002; **167**: 1664–9.

3 Stephenson AJ, Aprikian AG, Souhami L et al. Utility of PSA doubling time in follow-up of untreated patients with localized prostate cancer. *Urology* 2002; **59**: 652–6.

4 Koppie TM, Grossfeld GD, Miller D et al. Patterns of treatment of patients with prostate cancer initially managed with surveillance: results from The CaPSURE database. Cancer of the Prostate Strategic Urological Research Endeavor. *J Urol* 2000; **164**: 81–8.

5 Klotz LH, Choo R, Morton G et al. Expectant management with selective delayed intervention for favorable- risk prostate cancer. *Can J Urol* 2002; **9 Suppl 1**: 2–7.

6 Scardino PT, Weaver R, and Hudson MA. Early detection of prostate cancer. *Hum Pathol* 1992; **23**: 211–22.

7 Albertsen PC, Hanley JA, Gleason DF et al. Competing risk analysis of men aged 55 to 74 years at diagnosis managed conservatively for clinically localized prostate cancer. *JAMA* 1998; **280**: 975–80.

8 Lu-Yao GL, and Yao SL. Population-based study of long-term survival in patients with clinically localised prostate cancer. *Lancet* 1997; **349**: 906–10.

9 Barry MJ, Albertsen PC, Bagshaw MA *et al*. Outcomes for men with clinically nonmetastatic prostate carcinoma managed with radical prostatectomy, external beam radiotherapy, or expectant management: a retrospective analysis. *Cancer* 2001; **91**: 2302–14.

10 Johansson JE. Expectant management of early stage prostatic cancer: Swedish experience. *J Urol* 1994; **152**: 1753–6.

11 Chodak GW, Thisted RA, Gerber GS *et al*. Results of conservative management of clinically localized prostate cancer. *N Engl J Med* 1994; **330**: 242–8.

12 Aus G, Hugosson J, Norlen L. Long-term survival and mortality in prostate cancer treated with noncurative intent. *J Urol* 1995; **154**: 460–5.

13 Jani AB, Vaida F, Hanks G *et al*. Changing face and different countenances of prostate cancer: racial and geographic differences in prostate-specific antigen (PSA), stage, and grade trends in the PSA era. *Int J Cancer* 2001; **96**: 363–71.

14 Cooperberg MR, Lubeck DP, Mehta SS *et al*. Time trends in clinical risk stratification for prostate cancer: implications for outcomes (data from CaPSURE). *J Urol* 2003; **170**: S21–5; discussion S26–7.

15 Moul JW, Wu H, Sun L *et al*. Epidemiology of radical prostatectomy for localized prostate cancer in the era of prostate-specific antigen: an overview of the Department of Defense Center for Prostate Disease Research national database. *Surgery* 2002; **132**: 213–9.

16 Hoedemaeker RF, van der Kwast TH, Boer R *et al*. Pathologic features of prostate cancer found at population-based screening with a four-year interval. *J Natl Cancer Inst* 2001; **93**: 1153–8.

17 Etzioni R, Penson DF, Legler JM *et al*. Overdiagnosis due to prostate-specific antigen screening: lessons from U.S. prostate cancer incidence trends. *J Natl Cancer Inst* 2002; **94**: 981–90.

18 Hugosson J, Aus G, Becker C *et al*. Would prostate cancer detected by screening with prostate-specific antigen develop into clinical cancer if left undiagnosed? A comparison of two population-based studies in Sweden. *BJU Int* 2000; **85**: 1078–84.

19 Draisma G, Boer R, Otto SJ *et al*. Lead times and overdetection due to prostate-specific antigen screening: estimates from the European Randomized Study of Screening for Prostate Cancer. *J Natl Cancer Inst* 2003; **95**: 868–78.

20 Pearson JD, Carter HB. Natural history of changes in prostate specific antigen in early stage prostate cancer. *J Urol* 1994; **152**: 1743–8.

21 Gann PH, Hennekens CH, Stampfer MJ. A prospective evaluation of plasma prostate-specific antigen for detection of prostatic cancer. *Jama* 1995; **273**: 289–94.

22 Clegg LX, Li FP, Hankey BF, Chu K, Edwards BK. Cancer survival among US whites and minorities: a SEER (Surveillance, Epidemiology, and End Results) Program population-based study. *Arch Intern Med* 2002; **162**: 1985–93.

23 Han M, Partin AW, Chan DY, Walsh PC. An evaluation of the decreasing incidence of positive surgical margins in a large retropubic prostatectomy series. *J Urol* 2004; **171**: 23–6.

24 Zappa M, Ciatto S, Bonardi R, Mazzotta A. Overdiagnosis of prostate carcinoma by screening: an estimate based on the results of the Florence Screening Pilot Study. *Ann Oncol* 1998; **9**: 1297–300.

25 McGregor M, Hanley JA, Boivin JF, McLean RG. Screening for prostate cancer: estimating the magnitude of overdetection. *Cmaj* 1998; **159**: 1368–72.

26 Peschel RE, Colberg JW. Surgery, brachy therapy, and external-beam radiotherapy for early prostate cancer. *Lancet Oncol* 2003; **4**: 233–41.

27 Carter HB, Walsh PC, Landis P, Epstein JI. Expectant management of nonpalpable prostate cancer with curative intent: preliminary results. *J Urol* 2002; **167**: 1231–4.

28 Epstein JI, Walsh PC, Carmichael M, Brendler CB. Pathologic and clinical findings to predict tumor extent of nonpalpable (stage T1c) prostate cancer. *Jama* 1994; **271**: 368–74.

29 Carter CA, Donahue T, Sun L *et al.* Temporarily deferred therapy (watchful waiting) for men younger than 70 years and with low-risk localized prostate cancer in the prostate-specific antigen era. *J Clin Oncol* 2003; **21**: 4001–8.

30 de Vries SH, Raaijmakers R, Kranse R, Blijenberg BG, Schröder FH. Prostate cancer characteristics and prostate specific antigen changes in screening detected patients initially treated with a watchful waiting policy. *J Urol* 2004; **172**: 2193–6.

31 D'Amico AV, Whittington R, Malkowicz SB *et al.* Biochemical outcome after radical prostatectomy or external beam radiation therapy for patients with clinically localized prostate carcinoma in the prostate specific antigen era. *Cancer* 2002; **95**: 281–6.

32 Pound CR, Partin AW, Epstein JI, Walsh PC. Prostate-specific antigen after anatomic radical retropubic prostatectomy. Patterns of recurrence and cancer control. *Urol Clin North Am* 1997; **24**: 395–406.

33 Kupelian PA, Elshaikh M, Reddy CA, Zippe C, Klein EA. Comparison of the efficacy of local therapies for localized prostate cancer in the prostate-specific antigen era: a large single-institution experience with radical prostatectomy and external-beam radiotherapy. *J Clin Oncol* 2002; **20**: 3376–85.

34 Campbell. Diagnosis and staging of Prostate Cancer. *Campbell's Urology.* Walsh PC, Retik AB, Vaughan ED *et al.* Philadelphia, Saunders. 2003; **4**: 3055–3079.

35 Rietbergen JB, Hoedemaeker RF, Kruger AE, Kirkels WJ, Schroder FH. The changing pattern of prostate cancer at the time of diagnosis: characteristics of screen detected prostate cancer in a population based screening study. *J Urol* 1999; **161**: 1192–8.

36 Partin AW, Mangold LA, Lamm DM, Walsh PC, Epstein JI, Pearson JD. Contemporary update of prostate cancer staging nomograms (Partin Tables) for the new millennium. *Urology* 2001; **58**: 843–8.

37 Kattan MW, Eastham JA, Stapleton AM, Wheeler TM, Scardino PT. A preoperative nomogram for disease recurrence following radical prostatectomy for prostate cancer. *J Natl Cancer Inst* 1998; **90**: 766–71.

38 Narain V, Bianco FJ, Jr., Grignon DJ, Sakr WA, Pontes JE, Wood DP, Jr. How accurately does prostate biopsy Gleason score predict pathologic findings and disease free survival? *Prostate* 2001; **49**: 185–90.

39 Lattouf JB, Saad F. Gleason score on biopsy: is it reliable for predicting the final grade on pathology? *BJU Int* 2002; **90**: 694–8; discussion 698–9.

40 D'Amico AV, Whittington R, Malkowicz SB, Wu YH, Chen M, Art M *et al.* Combination of the preoperative PSA level, biopsy Gleason score, percentage of positive biopsies, and MRI T-stage to predict early PSA failure in men with clinically localized prostate cancer. *Urology* 2000; **55**: 572–7.

41 Haese A, Chaudhari M, Miller MC, Epstein JI, Huland H, Palisaar J *et al.* Quantitative biopsy pathology for the prediction of pathologically organ-confined prostate carcinoma: a multiinstitutional validation study. *Cancer* 2003; **97**: 969–78.

42 Badalament RA, Miller MC, Peller PA, Young DC, Bahn DK, Kochie P *et al.* An algorithm for predicting nonorgan confined prostate cancer using the results obtained from sextant core biopsies with prostate specific antigen level. *J Urol* 1996; **156**: 1375–80.

43 Benson MC, Whang IS, Olsson CA, McMahon DJ, Cooner WH. The use of prostate specific antigen density to enhance the predictive value of intermediate levels of serum prostate specific antigen. *J Urol* 1992; **147**: 817–21.

44 Stenman UH, Leinonen J, Alfthan H, Rannikko S, Tuhkanen K, Alfthan O. A scomplex between prostate-specific antigen and alpha 1-antichymotrypsin is the major form of prostate-specific antigen in serum of patients with prostatic cancer: assay of the complex improves clinical sensitivity for

cancer. *Cancer Res* 1991; **51**: 222–6.

45 Karazanashvili G, Abrahamsson PA. Prostate specific antigen and human glandular kallikrein 2 in early detection of prostate cancer. *J Urol* 2003; **169**: 445–57.

46 Polascik TJ, Oesterling JE, Partin AW. Prostate specific antigen: a decade of discovery – what we have learned and where we are going. *J Urol* 1999; **162**: 293–306.

47 Bonin SR, Hanlon AL, Lee WR, Movsas B, al-Saleem TI, Hanks GE. Evidence of increased failure in the treatment of prostate carcinoma patients who have perineural invasion treated with three-dimensional conformal radiation therapy. *Cancer* 1997; **79**: 75–80.

48 Nelson CP RM, Strawderman M, Montie JE, Sanda MG. Preoperative parameters for predicting early prostate cancer recurrence after radical prostatectomy. *Urology* 2002; **59**: 740–5; discussion 745–6.

49 Bastacky SI, Walsh PC, Epstein JI. Relationship between perineural tumor invasion on needle biopsy and radical prostatectomy capsular penetration in clinical stage B adenocarcinoma of the prostate. *Am J Surg Pathol* 1993; **17**: 336–41.

50 Schmid HP, McNeal JE, Stamey TA. Observations on the doubling time of prostate cancer. The use of serial prostate-specific antigen in patients with untreated disease as a measure of increasing cancer volume. *Cancer* 1993; **71**: 2031–40.

51 Carter HB, Morrell CH, Pearson JD, Brant LJ, Plato CC, Metter EJ. Estimation of prostatic growth using serial prostate-specific antigen measurements in men with and without prostate disease. *Cancer Res* 1992; **52**: 3323–8.

52 Stamey TA, Kabalin JN, Ferrari M, Yang N. Prostate specific antigen in the

diagnosis and treatment of adenocarcinoma of the prostate. IV. Anti-androgen treated patients. *J Urol* 1989; **141**: 1088–90.

53 Prestigiacomo AF, Stamey TA. Physiological variation of serum prostate specific antigen in the 4.0 to 10.0 ng./ml. range in male volunteers. *J Urol* 1996; **155**: 1977–80.

54 Egawa S, Matsumoto K, Suyama K, Iwamura M, Kuwao S, Baba S. Observations of prostate specific antigen doubling time in Japanese patients with nonmetastatic prostate carcinoma. *Cancer* 1999; **86**: 463–9.

55 McLaren DB, McKenzie M, Duncan G, Pickles T. Watchful waiting or watchful progression?: Prostate specific antigen doubling times and clinical behavior in patients with early untreated prostate carcinoma. *Cancer* 1998; **82**: 342–8.

56 Vollmer RT, Egawa S, Kuwao S, Baba S. The dynamics of prostate specific antigen during watchful waiting of prostate carcinoma: a study of 94 Japanese men. *Cancer* 2002; **94**: 1692–8.

57 Schroder FH, Kranse R, Barbet N, Hop WC, Kandra A, Lassus M. Prostate-specific antigen: A surrogate endpoint for screening new agents against prostate cancer? *Prostate* 2000; **42**: 107–15.

58 http://www.mskcc.org/mskcc/html/10088.cfm.

59 Epstein JI, Walsh PC, Carter HB. Dedifferentiation of prostate cancer grade with time in men followed expectantly for stage T1c disease. *J Urol* 2001; **166**: 1688–91.

60 Schroder FH, de Vries SH, Bangma CH. Watchful waiting in prostate cancer: review and policy proposals. *BJU Int* 2003; **92**: 851–9.

61 Vashi AR, Wojno KJ, Gillespie B, Oesterling JE. A model for the number of cores per prostate biopsy based on patient age and prostate gland volume. *J Urol* 1998; **159**: 920–4.

14: Complementary and Alternative Therapies for Prostate Cancer

Gary Deng and Barrie Cassileth

OVERVIEW

The terminology associated with therapies not commonly taught in modern western medical schools has evolved from a very negative 'quackery' to 'unorthodox', 'unconventional', 'questionable', 'unproved', and 'alternative.' Current, but still evolving terminology favours 'complementary' and 'alternative' medicine, or the acronym of both: CAM. The shifting language is exemplified by the creation in the United States, over a decade ago, of the National Institutes of Health 'Office of Alternative Medicine', which in 1999 was renamed the 'National Center for Complementary and Alternative Medicine' (NCCAM). CAM therapies may be categorised in a variety of ways. NCCAM currently classifies CAM therapies into five categories: alternative medical systems, mind-body interventions, biologically based therapies, manipulative and body-based methods and energy therapies.

There is a necessary distinction between 'complementary' and 'alternative' methods. Complementary therapies are promoted and used as adjuncts to mainstream cancer care. They are supportive measures that control symptoms, enhance well being, and contribute to overall patient care. Alternative therapies typically are promoted for use instead of mainstream treatment. This is especially problematic in oncology, when delayed treatment can diminish the possibility of remission and cure [1]. Over time, some complementary therapies are proven safe and effective. These become integrated into mainstream care, producing Integrative Oncology, a synthesis of the best of mainstream cancer treatment and rational, databased, adjunctive complementary therapies.

A growing number of patients with prostate cancer use CAM. This is in part due to publicity about saw palmetto to treat benign prostate hypertrophy (BPH), the use of PC-SPES (the trade name of a herbal preparation) for prostate cancer, and the clinical trials on cancer prevention with selenium [2], vitamin E and β-carotene [3]. Several surveys assessed the prevalence of use CAM of in prostate cancer [4]. Results vary depending on the definition of CAM [5–7]. When spiritual practices such as prayer were included, 43% of those surveyed were found to use CAM [8]. Patients use CAM remedies to suppress cancer progression, manage side effects and prevent cancer recurrence. The clinical effectiveness of most CAM therapies remains to be definitively demonstrated, but some relevant to prostate cancer have been subjected to scientific study. These therapies are discussed in the following sections.

LOW FAT, HIGH VEGETABLE AND FRUIT DIET

Epidemiologic studies suggest a role for low-fat diets in prostate cancer. Studies of Japanese and Chinese immigrants in the United States show an increase in incidence compared with men in their native countries [9–11]. In animal studies, low-fat diets decrease tumour growth [12–14]. Data from case-control and prospective studies are mixed. Some demonstrate a direct association between increased saturated and monounsaturated fat and increased risk of prostate cancer [15–19], while others find no relationship [20–21]. In a cohort study of more than 58 000 men, prostate cancer risk was not associated with the intake of total fat, total saturated fatty acids or total trans-unsaturated fatty acids in general, although lower risk was weakly associated with increased intake of linolenic acid [22].

Although the role of low-fat, high vegetable and fruit diets in prostate cancer prevention is not fully established, such diets reduce cardiovascular risk and offer other health benefits [23,24]. There is no evidence supporting the role of diet as prostate cancer treatment.

Soy

Soy contains isoflavones, including phytoestrogens genistein and daidzein [25]. Genistein and daidzein are Selective Estrogen-Receptor Modulators (SERMs). *In vitro* studies indicate that genistein inhibits the growth of prostate cancer cells, apparently independent of genistein's oestrogenic effects [26,27]. Soy intake and serum phytoestrogen levels are higher in Asia, where lower mortality rates from prostate cancer are seen.

Much research has been conducted on the relationship between phytoestrogen consumption and prostate cancer [28,29]. Current trials include a randomised, double blinded, placebo controlled post-radical prostatectomy study of men at high risk for recurrence. Started on soy protein powder, they are now being followed for PSA failure rate and time-to-PSA failure [30]. Another randomised, prospective trial enrolled men with clinically localised prostate cancer who had selected 'watchful waiting' as primary therapy.

A low-fat, soy-supplemented vegan diet along with other lifestyle changes was initiated and PSA and endorectal MRI data collected [31]. Results are pending.

Soy products attenuate bone loss in peri-menopausal women [32], and prevent post-menopausal osteoporosis [33]. They have beneficial effects on cardiovascular health [34,35]. Although preventive or therapeutic value in prostate cancer is not yet documented, consumption of a moderate amount of soy protein can be beneficial, especially to the cardiovascular system [36].

Vitamin D

Vitamin D is a fat-soluble secosteroid involved in the regulation of serum calcium and phosphorus levels. Calcitriol (1,25-dihydroxycholecalciferol) is responsible for most, if not all, of its biological activities. The possibility that vitamin D deficiency may be a risk factor for prostate cancer was first based on epidemiologic studies [36].

Vitamin D receptors have been found in prostate cancer cell lines [37], and treatment with vitamin D suppresses their proliferation [38] although the mechanism is not clearly defined. Some studies suggest that calcitriol alters cell cycle progression and may also initiate apoptosis [39,40]. Vitamin D analogues reduce tumour size and the number of lung metastases in an *in vivo* model of androgen-insensitive metastatic prostate cancer [41,42].

A pilot study of seven patients showed that calcitriol slows the rate of PSA rise in early recurrent prostate cancer [43]. In a phase I trial of a vitamin D analogue in 25 patients with advanced hormone-refractory prostate, two patients showed evidence of a partial response, and five others achieved disease stabilisation for more than 6 months [44]. Hypercalcaemia with associated renal insufficiency was the main toxicity reported in both of these studies.

Vitamin D, lowered the incidence of hip fractures in post-menopausal women in a large prospective study [45]. A small phase II study found some improvement in metastatic prostate cancer bone pain with vitamin D supplementation [45]. The use of vitamin D in prostate cancer remains an area of active research. There are as yet no conclusive data to warrant its use in non-deficient patients.

Vitamin E

Vitamin E includes tocopherols and tocotrienols, each having four subtypes, alpha, beta, gamma and delta [46]. They are potent free-radical scavengers and anti-oxidants [47]. Recent research revealed other functions unrelated to its anti-oxidant activity, such as inhibition of protein kinase C, 5-lipoxygenase, cell proliferation, platelet aggregation and monocyte adhesion [48].

Vitamin E inhibits the growth of prostate cancer cells *in vitro* at a concentration that may be achieved with oral supplementation [49,50], and enhances the cytotoxic effects of Adriamycin in human prostate cancer cell lines [51]. However, it had no effect on hyperplasia or carcinoma in a prostate cancer model in rats [52]. Several large clinical trials investigated the role of vitamin E in cardiovascular disease and cancer [3,53]. In the Finnish 'ATBC Trial' originally designed to study lung cancer, daily intake of α-tocopherol was associated with a 32% reduction in incidence and a 41% decrease in mortality of prostate cancer.

A randomised, placebo-controlled, double-blind, phase III prostate cancer prevention trial of 32 400 men [the Selenium and Vitamin E Cancer Prevention Trial (SELECT)] is underway to test the preventive efficacy of selenium and vitamin E [54,55]. Final results are anticipated in 2013.

Oral vitamin E appears very safe [56]. Double-blind studies involving large numbers of subjects demonstrated that oral doses up to 3200 USP – Units/day produced no consistent adverse effects [57]. In patients with vitamin K deficiency caused by malabsorption or anticoagulant therapy, however, oral intake of high levels of vitamin E exacerbated the blood coagulation defect [58].

Selenium

Dietary selenium intake and serum selenium level correlate inversely with cancer risk [59,60]. Selenium is a trace element required for the activity of the anti-oxidant enzyme glutathione peroxidase, which protects cell membranes from damage caused by the peroxidation of lipids [61,62]. How selenium exercises its biological activity remains unclear. Proposed mechanisms include interaction with redox pathways [63], inhibition of cell growth [64], induction of apoptosis [65,66], interference with cell cycle [67] and alteration of carcinogen metabolism [68,69].

In a multi-centre, randomised, placebo-controlled study of 1312 patients with history of non-melanoma skin cancer (the Nutritional Prevention of Skin Cancer Trial), daily intake of 200 μg of selenium lowered the incidence of prostate cancer by two-thirds [70]. The incidence of lung and colorectal cancers also was reduced. There was no significant effect on other cancers. In the 'Health Professionals Follow-Up Study', higher selenium levels were associated with reduced risk of advanced prostate cancer [71]. The association became stronger with additional controls for family history of prostate cancer, body mass index, calcium intake, lycopene and saturated fat intake, vasectomy and geographical region. The large-scale prostate cancer prevention trial noted above, the SELECT trial, is ongoing [54].

At the tested dose of 200 μg per day, selenium was found to be safe [72]. At more than 1000 μg per day, chronic ingestion of selenium can cause selenosis [73]. The Institute of Medicine set a tolerable upper intake at 400 μg of selenium per day.

Plants that grow in selenium-rich soil or animals that eat such plants are good sources of dietary selenium. One ounce of Brazil nuts contains 40 μg of selenium, while 3 ounces of canned Tuna contain about 70 μg of selenium [74,75]. In summary, there is evidence supporting the potential of selenium in prostate cancer prevention. A definitive trial is ongoing.

Saw Palmetto

An extract of the dwarf American palm, saw palmetto (*Serenoa repens*) is best known for its use in treating BPH [76,77]. Although popular and effective in relieving urinary frequency and nocturia [78], there is no evidence of benefit against prostate cancer when it is used alone. Laboratory studies show that Saw Palmetto extract inhibits human α-1-adrenoreceptors [79] and displays non-competitive 5-α-reductase inhibition activity directly [80]. No clinical trial of Saw Palmetto to treat prostate cancer has been reported, and no significant change of serum PSA level was found in patients taking Saw Palmetto [78].

Adverse effects are mild and infrequent [81,82]. The content of commercially available Saw Palmetto supplements varies widely, with some samples containing virtually none of the active ingredient [83].

PC-SPES

PC for 'prostate cancer and' SPES, Latin for 'hope', PC-SPES was a popular herbal compound containing 8 herbs: chrysanthemum, isatis, liquorice, lucid ganoderma, pseudo-ginseng, rubescens, saw palmetto and scute. Although its mechanism of action is unclear, patients with androgen-dependent or -independent prostate cancer had lower PSA levels following PC-SPES treatment [84–86]. Patients previously treated with chemotherapy or ketoconazole treatment still responded to PC-SPES [84,86]. Toxicities in those trials were similar to those expected from oestrogen treatment, including gynecomastia, loss of libido and venous thrombosis [84,86–88].

The California Department of Health Services found that PC-SPES was contaminated with undeclared prescription drugs, including indomethacin and diethylstilbestrol (DES) [89]. In 2002, the FDA warned consumers to stop using PC-SPES, and the manufacturer (BotanicLab, Brea, CA) recalled the product. Despite promising clinical activity against prostate cancer, contamination with undeclared synthetic drugs rendered this product unavailable to patients.

Acupuncture

Acupuncture is the stimulation of certain points on the body by very thin, filiform needles. Modern research suggests that the effect of acupuncture may be mediated by the release of neurotransmitters [90–92]. An NIH consensus statement in 1997, supported the efficacy of acupuncture for adult postoperative and chemotherapy nausea and vomiting, and for post-operative dental pain [93]. Acupuncture is used for various symptoms associated with cancers, most commonly nausea, pain, anxiety and fatigue [94–102]. It relieves hot flashes in post-menopausal patients [103] and those on tamoxifen, an oestrogen antagonist [104]. In a small study of seven patients, acupuncture was reported to lower the frequency of vasomotor symptoms ('hot flashes') resulting from androgen ablation therapy [105].

Serious adverse events were rare and any such event reported was found to be associated with inadequately trained acupuncturists in several large studies [106,107]. Only 94 minor adverse events were reported across 65 000 treatments in a Japanese survey [106]. Acupuncture is safe when performed by qualified practitioners using disposable needles. It helps to control some symptoms associated with prostate cancer. Acupuncture for the control of yet additional symptoms remains an area of active research.

SUMMARY

The use of complementary and alternative therapies is prevalent among patients with prostate cancer, who seek them for many reasons, including desperation, dissatisfaction with conventional medicine, relief of symptoms and desire to participate actively in their own care. Internet vendors aggressively market many useless and possibly harmful products and approaches. Physicians should help patients in identifying false claims and to take advantage of helpful complementary modalities such as acupuncture and massage therapy [1]. Vigorous research is now devoted to botanicals and other complementary therapies for prostate cancer. The field is constantly evolving, with new information expected in the near future.

It is important for physicians and other health care practitioners to be knowledgeable about common CAM remedies used by their patients. Physicians should encourage open discussion about CAM and educate themselves so that they can offer informed advice or direct patients to reliable sources of information. A few helpful sources containing reliable information are listed in the reference section [108–115].

REFERENCES

1 Cassileth B. The Alternative Medicine Handbook. New York: W.W. Norton and Company, Inc, 1998.

2 Clark LC, Dalkin B, Krongrad A *et al.* Decreased incidence of prostate cancer with selenium supplementation: results of a double-blind cancer prevention trial. *Br J Urol* 1998; **81**: 730–4.

3 Heinonen OP, Albanes D, Virtamo J *et al.* Prostate cancer and supplementation with alpha-tocopherol and beta-carotene: incidence and mortality in a controlled trial. *J Natl Cancer Inst* 1998; **90**: 440–6.

4 Zimmerman RA, Thompson IM, Jr. Prevalence of complementary medicine in urologic practice. A review of recent studies with emphasis on use among prostate cancer patients. *Urol Clin North Am* 2002; **29**: 1–9, vii.

5 Nam RK, Fleshner N, Rakovitch E *et al.* Prevalence and patterns of the use of complementary therapies among prostate cancer patients: an epidemiological analysis. *J Urol* 1999; **161**: 1521–4.

6 Kao GD, Devine P. Use of complementary health practices by prostate carcinoma patients undergoing radiation therapy. *Cancer* 2000; **88**: 615–9.

7 Lerner IJ, Kennedy BJ. The prevalence of questionable methods of cancer treatment in the United States. *CA Cancer J Clin* 1992; **42**: 181–91.

8 Lippert MC, McClain R, Boyd JC, Theodorescu D. Alternative medicine use in patients with localized prostate carcinoma treated with curative intent. *Cancer* 1999; **86**: 2642–8.

9 Wynder EL, Mabuchi K, Whitmore WF, Jr. Epidemiology of cancer of the prostate. *Cancer* 1971; **28**: 344–60.

10 Haenszel W, Kurihara M. Studies of Japanese migrants. I. Mortality from cancer and other diseases among Japanese in the United States. *J Natl Cancer Inst* 1968; **40**: 43–68.

11 Shimizu H, Ross RK, Bernstein L, Yatani R, Henderson BE, Mack TM. Cancers of the prostate and breast among Japanese and white immigrants in Los Angeles County. *Br J Cancer* 1991; **63**: 963–6.

12 Connolly JM, Coleman M, Rose DP. Effects of dietary fatty acids on DU145 human prostate cancer cell growth in athymic nude mice. *Nutr Cancer* 1997; **29**: 114–9.

13 Wang Y, Corr JG, Thaler HT, Tao Y, Fair WR, Heston WD. Decreased growth of established human prostate LNCaP tumors in nude mice fed a low-fat diet. *J Natl Cancer Inst* 1995; **87**: 1456–62.

14 Pollard M, Luckert PH. Promotional effects of testosterone and high fat diet on the development of autochthonous prostate cancer in rats. *Cancer Lett* 1986; **32**: 223–7.

15 Ross RK, Shimizu H, Paganini-Hill A, Honda G, Henderson BE. Case-control studies of prostate cancer in blacks and whites in southern California. *J Natl Cancer Inst* 1987; **78**: 869–74.

16 Kolonel LN, Yoshizawa CN, Hankin JH. Diet and prostatic cancer: a case-control study in Hawaii. *Am J Epidemiol* 1988; **127**: 999–1012.

17 Whittemore AS, Kolonel LN, Wu AH *et al.* Prostate cancer in relation to diet, physical activity, and body size in blacks, whites, and Asians in the United States and Canada. *J Natl Cancer Inst* 1995; **87**: 652–61.

18 Le Marchand L, Kolonel LN, Wilkens LR, Myers BC, Hirohata T. Animal fat consumption and prostate cancer: a prospective study in Hawaii. *Epidemiology* 1994; **5**: 276–82.

19 Bairati I, Meyer F, Fradet Y, Moore L. Dietary fat and advanced prostate cancer. *J Urol* 1998; **159**: 1271–5.

20 Severson RK, Nomura AM, Grove JS, Stemmermann GN. A prospective study of demographics, diet, and prostate cancer among men of Japanese ancestry

in Hawaii. *Cancer Res* 1989; **49**: 1857–60.

21 Mills PK, Beeson WL, Phillips RL, Fraser GE. Cohort study of diet, lifestyle, and prostate cancer in Adventist men. *Cancer* 1989; **64**: 598–604.

22 Schuurman AG, van den Brandt PA, Dorant E, Brants HA, Goldbohm RA. Association of energy and fat intake with prostate carcinoma risk: results from The Netherlands Cohort Study. *Cancer* 1999; **86**: 1019–27.

23 Bosland MC, Oakley-Girvan I, Whittemore AS. Dietary fat, calories, and prostate cancer risk. *J Natl Cancer Inst* 1999; **91**: 489–91.

24 Moyad MA. Dietary fat reduction to reduce prostate cancer risk: controlled enthusiasm, learning a lesson from breast or other cancers, and the big picture. *Urology* 2002; **59**: 51–62.

25 Kris-Etherton PM, Hecker KD, Bonanome A, Coval SM, Binkoski AE, Hilpert KF, *et al.* Bioactive compounds in foods: their role in the prevention of cardiovascular disease and cancer. *Am J Med* 2002; **113**: 71S–88S.

26 Hempstock J, Kavanagh JP, George NJ. Growth inhibition of prostate cell lines in vitro by phyto-oestrogens. *Br J Urol* 1998; **82**: 560–3.

27 Peterson G, Barnes S. Genistein and biochanin A inhibit the growth of human prostate cancer cells but not epidermal growth factor receptor tyrosine autophosphorylation. *Prostate* 1993; **22**: 335–45.

28 Castle EP, Thrasher JB. The role of soy phytoestrogens in prostate cancer. *Urol Clin North Am* 2002; **29**: 71–81, viii–ix.

29 Messina MJ, Persky V, Setchell KD, Barnes S. Soy intake and cancer risk: a review of the *in vitro* and *in vivo* data. *Nutr Cancer* 1994; **21**: 113–31.

30 Bosland MC, Kato I, Melamed J *et al.* Chemoprevention trials in men with prostate-specific antigen failure or at high risk for recurrence after radical prostatectomy: Application to efficacy assessment of soy protein. *Urology* 2001; **57**: 202–4.

31 Ornish DM, Lee KL, Fair WR, Pettengill EB, Carroll PR. Dietary trial in prostate cancer: Early experience and implications for clinical trial design. *Urology* 2001; **57**: 200–1.

32 Alekel DL, Germain AS, Peterson CT, Hanson KB, Stewart JW, Toda T. Isoflavone-rich soy protein isolate attenuates bone loss in the lumbar spine of perimenopausal women. *Am J Clin Nutr* 2000; **72**: 844–52.

33 Chiechi LM, Secreto G, D'Amore M *et al.* Efficacy of a soy rich diet in preventing postmenopausal osteoporosis: the Menfis randomized trial. *Maturitas* 2002; **42**: 295–300.

34 Clarkson TB. Soy, soy phytoestrogens and cardiovascular disease. *J Nutr* 2002; **132**: 566S–569S.

35 Costa RL, Summa MA. Soy protein in the management of hyperlipidemia. *Ann Pharmacother* 2000; **34**: 931–5.

36 Schwartz GG, Hulka BS. Is vitamin D deficiency a risk factor for prostate cancer? (Hypothesis). *Anticancer Res* 1990; **10**: 1307–11.

37 Miller GJ, Stapleton GE, Hedlund TE, Moffat KA. Vitamin D receptor expression, 24-hydroxylase activity, and inhibition of growth by 1alpha, 25-dihydroxyvitamin D3 in seven human prostatic carcinoma cell lines. *Clin Cancer Res* 1995; **1**: 997–1003.

38 Blutt SE, Weigel NL. Vitamin D and prostate cancer. *Proc Soc Exp Biol Med* 1999; **221**: 89–98.

39 Zhuang SH, Burnstein KL. Antiproliferative effect of 1alpha, 25-dihydroxyvitamin D3 in human prostate cancer cell line LNCaP involves reduction of cyclin-dependent kinase 2 activity and persistent G1 accumulation. *Endocrinology* 1998; **139**: 1197–207.

40 Krishnan AV, Peehl DM, Feldman D. Inhibition of prostate cancer growth by vitamin D: Regulation of target gene expression. *J Cell Biochem* 2003; **88**: 363–71.

41 Lokeshwar BL, Schwartz GG, Selzer MG *et al.* Inhibition of prostate cancer metastasis *in vivo*: a comparison of 1,23-dihydroxyvitamin D (calcitriol) and EB1089. *Cancer Epidemiol Biomarkers Prev* 1999; **8**: 241–8.

42 Getzenberg RH, Light BW, Lapco PE *et al.* Vitamin D inhibition of prostate adenocarcinoma growth and metastasis in the Dunning rat prostate model system. *Urology* 1997; **50**: 999–1006.

43 Gross C, Stamey T, Hancock S, Feldman D. Treatment of early recurrent prostate cancer with 1,25-dihydroxyvitamin D3 (calcitriol). *J Urol* 1998; **159**: 2035–9; discussion 2039–40.

44 Liu G, Oettel K, Ripple G *et al.* Phase I trial of 1alpha-hydroxyvitamin d(2) in patients with hormone refractory prostate cancer. *Clin Cancer Res* 2002; **8**: 2820–7.

45 Feskanich D, Willett WC, Colditz GA. Calcium, vitamin D, milk consumption, and hip fractures: a prospective study among postmenopausal women. *Am J Clin Nutr* 2003; **77**: 504–11.

46 Brigelius-Flohe R, Traber MG. Vitamin E: function and metabolism. *Faseb J* 1999; **13**: 1145–55.

47 Herrera E, Barbas C. Vitamin E: action, metabolism and perspectives. *J Physiol Biochem* 2001; **57**: 43–56.

48 Ricciarelli R, Zingg JM, Azzi A. The 80th anniversary of vitamin E: beyond its antioxidant properties. *Biol Chem* 2002; **383**: 457–65.

49 Israel K, Yu W, Sanders BG, Kline K. Vitamin E succinate induces apoptosis in human prostate cancer cells: role for Fas in vitamin E succinate-triggered apoptosis. *Nutr Cancer* 2000; **36**: 90–100.

50 Sigounas G, Anagnostou A, Steiner M. dl-alpha-tocopherol induces apoptosis in erythroleukemia, prostate, and breast cancer cells. *Nutr Cancer* 1997; **28**: 30–5.

51 Ripoll EA, Rama BN, Webber MM. Vitamin E enhances the chemotherapeutic effects of adriamycin on human prostatic carcinoma cells *in vitro*. *J Urol* 1986; **136**: 529–31.

52 Nakamura A, Shirai T, Takahashi S, Ogawa K, Hirose M, Ito N. Lack of modification by naturally occurring antioxidants of 3,2′-dimethyl-4-aminobiphenyl-initiated rat prostate carcinogenesis. *Cancer Lett* 1991; **58**: 241–6.

53 The effect of vitamin E and beta carotene on the incidence of lung cancer and other cancers in male smokers. The Alpha-Tocopherol, Beta Carotene Cancer Prevention Study Group. *N Engl J Med* 1994; **330**: 1029–35.

54 Hoque A, Albanes D, Lippman SM *et al.* Molecular epidemiologic studies within the Selenium and Vitamin E Cancer Prevention Trial (SELECT). *Cancer Causes Control* 2001; **12**: 627–33.

55 Klein EA, Thompson IM, Lippman SM, *et al.* SELECT: the next prostate cancer prevention trial. Selenum and Vitamin E Cancer Prevention Trial. *J Urol* 2001; **166**: 1311–5.

56 Meydani SN, Meydani M, Rall LC, Morrow F, Blumberg JB. Assessment of the safety of high-dose, short-term supplementation with vitamin E in healthy older adults. *Am J Clin Nutr* 1994; **60**: 704–9.

57 Kappus H, Diplock AT. Tolerance and safety of vitamin E: a toxicological position report. *Free Radic Biol Med* 1992; **13**: 55–74.

58 Meyers DG, Maloley PA, Weeks D. Safety of antioxidant vitamins. *Arch Intern Med* 1996; **156**: 925–35.

59 Shamberger RJ, Tytko SA, Willis CE. Antioxidants and cancer. Part VI. Selenium and age-adjusted human cancer mortality. *Arch Environ Health* 1976; **31**: 231–5.

60 Willett WC, Polk BF, Morris JS *et al.* Prediagnostic serum selenium and risk of cancer. *Lancet* 1983; **2**: 130–4.

61 Young VR. Selenium: a case for its essentiality in man. *N Engl J Med* 1981; **304**: 1228–30.

62 Gronberg H. Prostate cancer epidemiology. *Lancet* 2003; **361**: 859–64.

63 Lu YP, Lou YR, Yen P *et al.* Enhanced skin carcinogenesis in transgenic mice with high expression of glutathione peroxidase or both glutathione peroxidase and superoxide dismutase. *Cancer Res* 1997; **57**: 1468–74.

64 Harrison PR, Lanfear J, Wu L, Fleming J, McGarry L, Blower L. Chemopreventive and growth inhibitory effects of selenium. *Biomed Environ Sci* 1997; **10**: 235–45.

65 Lanfear J, Fleming J, Wu L, Webster G, Harrison PR. The selenium metabolite selenodiglutathione induces p53 and apoptosis: relevance to the chemopreventive effects of selenium? *Carcinogenesis* 1994; **15**: 1387–92.

66 Lu J, Kaeck M, Jiang C, Wilson AC, Thompson HJ. Selenite induction of

DNA strand breaks and apoptosis in mouse leukemic L1210 cells. *Biochem Pharmacol* 1994; **47**: 1531–5.

67 Nelson MA, Porterfield BW, Jacobs ET, Clark LC. Selenium and prostate cancer prevention. *Semin Urol Oncol* 1999; **17**: 91–6.

68 Griffin AC. Role of selenium in the chemoprevention of cancer. *Adv Cancer Res* 1979; **29**: 419–42.

69 Marshall MV, Arnott MS, Jacobs MM, Griffin AC. Selenium effects on the carcinogenicity and metabolism of 2-acetylaminofluorene. *Cancer Lett* 1979; **7**: 331–8.

70 Clark LC, Combs GF, Jr., Turnbull BW *et al*. Effects of selenium supplementation for cancer prevention in patients with carcinoma of the skin. A randomized controlled trial. Nutritional Prevention of Cancer Study Group. *JAMA* 1996; **276**: 1957–63.

71 Yoshizawa K, Willett WC, Morris SJ *et al*. Study of prediagnostic selenium level in toenails and the risk of advanced prostate cancer. *J Natl Cancer Inst* 1998; **90**: 1219–24.

72 Schrauzer GN. Nutritional selenium supplements: product types, quality, and safety. *J Am Coll Nutr* 2001; **20**: 1–4.

73 Fan AM, Kizer KW. Selenium. Nutritional, toxicologic, and clinical aspects. *West J Med* 1990; **153**: 160–7.

74 Pennington JA, Young BE, Wilson DB, Johnson RD, Vanderveen JE. Mineral content of foods and total diets: the Selected Minerals in Foods Survey, 1982 to 1984. *J Am Diet Assoc* 1986; **86**: 876–91.

75 US Department of Agriculture ARS. Nutrient Database for Standard Reference, Release 17: Nutrient Data Lab Home Page. URL http://www.nal.usda.gov/fnic/foodcomp/Data/SR17/wtrank/sr17w317.pdf.

76 Wilt TJ, Ishani A, Stark G, MacDonald R, Lau J, Mulrow C. Saw palmetto extracts for treatment of benign prostatic hyperplasia: a systematic review. *JAMA* 1998; **280**: 1604–9.

77 Boyle P, Robertson C, Lowe F, Roehrborn C. Meta-analysis of clinical trials of permixon in the treatment of symptomatic benign prostatic hyperplasia. *Urology* 2000; **55**: 533–9.

78 Gerber GS, Zagaja GP, Bales GT, Chodak GW, Contreras BA. Saw palmetto (Serenoa repens) in men with lower urinary tract symptoms: effects on urodynamic parameters and voiding symptoms. *Urology* 1998; **51**: 1003–7.

79 Goepel M, Hecker U, Krege S, Rubben H, Michel MC. Saw palmetto extracts potently and noncompetitively inhibit human alpha1-adrenoceptors *in vitro*. *Prostate* 1999; **38**: 208–15.

80 Iehle C, Delos S, Guirou O, Tate R, Raynaud JP, Martin PM. Human prostatic steroid 5 alpha-reductase isoforms – a comparative study of selective inhibitors. *J Steroid Biochem Mol Biol* 1995; **54**: 273–9.

81 Wilt T, Ishani A, Mac Donald R. Serenoa repens for benign prostatic hyperplasia. *Cochrane Database Syst Rev* 2002: CD001423.

82 Cheema P, El-Mefty O, Jazieh AR. Intraoperative haemorrhage associated with the use of extract of Saw Palmetto herb: a case report and review of literature. *J Intern Med* 2001; **250**: 167–9.

83 Feifer AH, Fleshner NE, Klotz L. Analytical accuracy and reliability of commonly used nutritional supplements in prostate disease. *J Urol* 2002; **168**: 150–4; discussion 154.

84 Small EJ, Frohlich MW, Bok R *et al*. Prospective trial of the herbal supplement PC-SPES in patients with progressive prostate cancer. *J Clin Oncol* 2000; **18**: 3595–603.

85 Pfeifer BL, Pirani JF, Hamann SR, Klippel KF. PC-SPES, a dietary supplement for the treatment of hormone-refractory prostate cancer. *BJU Int* 2000; **85**: 481–5.

86 Oh WK, George DJ, Hackmann K, Manola J, Kantoff PW. Activity of the herbal combination, PC-SPES, in the treatment of patients with androgen-independent prostate cancer. *Urology* 2001; **57**: 122–6.

87 DiPaola RS, Zhang H, Lambert GH *et al*. Clinical and biologic activity of an estrogenic herbal combination (PC-SPES) in prostate cancer. *N Engl J Med* 1998; **339**: 785–91.

88 de la Taille A, Buttyan R, Hayek O *et al*. Herbal therapy PC-SPES: *in vitro* effects and evaluation of its efficacy in

69 patients with prostate cancer. *J Urol* 2000; **164**: 1229–34.

89 Sovak M, Seligson AL, Konas M *et al.* Herbal composition PC-SPES for management of prostate cancer: identification of active principles. *J Natl Cancer Inst* 2002; **94**: 1275–81.

90 Han JS. Acupuncture: neuropeptide release produced by electrical stimulation of different frequencies. *Trends Neurosci* 2003; **26**: 17–22.

91 Shen J. Research on the neurophysiological mechanisms of acupuncture: review of selected studies and methodological issues. *J Altern Complement Med* 2001; **7**: S121–7.

92 Foster JM, Sweeney BP. The mechanisms of acupuncture analgesia. *Br J Hosp Med* 1987; **38**: 308–12.

93 Acupuncture. *NIH Consens Statement* 1997; **15**: 1–34.

94 Shen J, Wenger N, Glaspy J *et al.* Electroacupuncture for control of myeloablative chemotherapy-induced emesis: A randomized controlled trial. *JAMA* 2000; **284**: 2755–61.

95 Lee A, Done ML. The use of nonpharmacologic techniques to prevent postoperative nausea and vomiting: a meta-analysis. *Anesth Analg* 1999; **88**: 1362–9.

96 Vickers AJ. Can acupuncture have specific effects on health? A systematic review of acupuncture antiemesis trials. *J R Soc Med* 1996; **89**: 303–11.

97 Alimi D, Rubino C, Leandri EP, Brule SF. Analgesic effects of auricular acupuncture for cancer pain. *J Pain Symptom Manage* 2000; **19**: 81–2.

98 Ernst E, Pittler MH. The effectiveness of acupuncture in treating acute dental pain: a systematic review. *Br Dent J* 1998; **184**: 443–7.

99 Melchart D, Linde K, Fischer P *et al.* Acupuncture for idiopathic headache. *Cochrane Database Syst Rev* 2001: CD001218.

100 Filshie J, Redman D. Acupuncture and malignant pain problems. *Eur J Surg Oncol* 1985; **11**: 389–94.

101 Leng G. A year of acupuncture in palliative care. *Palliat Med* 1999; **13**: 163–4.

102 Dillon M, Lucas C. Auricular stud acupuncture in palliative care patients. *Palliat Med* 1999; **13**: 253–4.

103 Wyon Y, Lindgren R, Hammar M, Lundeberg T. [Acupuncture against climacteric disorders? Lower number of symptoms after menopause]. *Lakartidningen* 1994; **91**:2318–22.

104 Towlerton G, Filshie J, O'Brien M, Duncan A. Acupuncture in the control of vasomotor symptoms caused by tamoxifen. *Palliat Med* 1999; **13**: 445.

105 Hammar M, Frisk J, Grimas O, Hook M, Spetz AC, Wyon Y. Acupuncture treatment of vasomotor symptoms in men with prostatic carcinoma: a pilot study. *J Urol* 1999; **161**: 853–6.

106 Yamashita H, Tsukayama H, Tanno Y, Nishijo K. Adverse events in acupuncture and moxibustion treatment: a six-year survey at a national clinic in Japan. *J Altern Complement Med* 1999; **5**: 229–36.

107 Odsberg A, Schill U, Haker E. Acupuncture treatment: side effects and complications reported by Swedish physiotherapists. *Complement Ther Med* 2001; **9**: 17–20.

108 Cassileth B, Lucarelli C. Herb-Drug Interactions in Oncology. Hamilton, Ontario: BC Decker; 2003.

109 http://nccam.nih.gov. (Accessed on Sept. 29, 2003.)

110 http://www3.cancer.gov/occam. (Accessed on Sept. 29, 2003.)

111 http://www.cancer.gov/cancerinfo/ treatment/cam. (Accessed on Sept. 29, 2003.)

112 http://www.cancer.org/docroot/ETO/ ETO_5.asp?sitearea = ETO. (Accessed on Sept. 29, 2003.)

113 http://www.mdanderson.org/ departments/cimer. (Accessed on Sept. 29, 2003.)

114 http://www.mskcc.org/aboutherbs. (Accessed on Sept. 29, 2003.)

115 http://www.quackwatch.org. (Accessed on Sept. 29, 2003.)

Part 4: Monitoring Progress and Secondary Treatment

15: Radical Prostatectomy After Radical Radiotherapy

Amir Kaisary

Cancer is the second leading cause of death in men. Considered alone, prostate cancer is in the top 10 overall causes of death of men in the United States [1]. The American Cancer Society estimates that in 2004, there will be more than 230 000 new cases of prostate cancer and 29 000 men will die of this disease [2]. Prostate cancer provokes considerable controversial debate in view of the limited data about the natural history of the disease. Increasing public awareness, increasing longevity in men and improved attempts at prostate screening modalities has led to an increase in diagnosis rates of the disease worldwide and has enabled identifying more men with early localised tumour stages. Whether there has been an actual increase in incidence of prostate cancer occurrence or not, is difficult to establish with any certainty as yet. Prospective randomised controlled studies to establish whether early detection (Prostate, Lung, Colon and Ovary Trial) or treatment (Prostate Cancer Intervention versus Observation Trial) of localised prostate cancer decreases the mortality rate from the disease have not yet been completed [3,4]. The treating physicians and their patients face a dilemma with regards to the management of early-diagnosed prostate cancer, whether it is an indolent cancer or a significant one, particularly in men younger than 60 years. The probability of dying from prostate cancer in patients not receiving treatment with curative intent, based on biopsy tumour grades, were studied by Chodak *et al.* (1994), Albertson *et al.* (1995, 1998) and Johansson *et al.* (1997) amongst others. These studies provided strong evidence that clinically localised prostate cancer, although it might be slow growing, can affect a patient's morbidity and mortality [5–8]. Thus there is an understanding that organ-confined prostate cancer diagnosed early (T1–2) should be treated with an intent to cure by aiming to eradicate it. Radiation therapy and surgical radical prostatectomy modalities are offered with possible comparable outcomes of disease control although prospective randomised long-term follow-up trials/studies are lacking. The task of treating physicians is therefore to educate patients by explaining the benefits and risks of possible treatments. This requires adequate consultation time. Patients can be recommended to read educational material. It is always valuable to remember that low-risk tumours in particular, do not require hasty decisions, so physicians and patients can take time to reach a management decision.

External beam radiation therapy and Brachytherapy continue to be commonly used as definitive treatment modalities for localised prostate cancer. Although many patients respond favourably to radiation therapy, treatment failure remains a major problem. The rates of local recurrence and/or persistence of prostate cancer are not clear [9].

Over the last decade, three-dimensional conformal radiation therapy (3D-CRT) and intensity-modulated techniques enabled delivery of considerably higher radiation doses to the prostate, while diminishing the irradiation of surrounding tissues. These developments have dramatically improved cancer control and reduced morbidity [10,11].

Prediction of treatment outcome is central to counselling patients and decision analysis. A nomogram is a graphic representation of a statistical model that incorporates several variables to predict a particular end point. Predictive radiation treatment nomograms make predictions based on the characteristics of individual patient. D'Amico *et al.* (1998) and Kattan *et al.* (2000) developed pre-treatment programs based on clinical stage, biopsy Gleason sum, pre-treatment PSA level, receipt of neo-adjuvant hormonal deprivation therapy and total radiation dose as predictor variables [12,13].

IDENTIFYING LOCAL RECURRENCE OF PROSTATE CANCER

Digital Rectal Examination

Digital rectal examination (DRE) is widely performed for follow-up of patients with localised prostate cancer after definitive therapy. However, its value is limited unless a palpable nodule recurrence is established. Efficacy of DRE surveillance after radiotherapy for prostate cancer was evaluated in a non-randomised study by Johnstone *et al.* (2001). They found no significant correlation between the PSA trend and DRE findings. They concluded that DRE is likely to be helpful only in patients with increasing PSA for whom salvage prostatectomy is an option [14].

Prostate-Specific Antigen

In the modern era, the emergence of the prostate-specific antigen (PSA) led to the concept of early 'Biochemical failure' based on rising PSA. The American Society for Therapeutic Radiology and Oncology Consensus Panel in a consensus statement in 1997, agreed guidelines for using PSA levels in reporting success or failure after irradiation [15]. It is recommended that after the completion of radiation therapy, PSA determinations should be made at 3 or 4 months intervals during the first 2 years and every 6 months thereafter. Three consecutive PSA increases define biochemical failure. However, biochemical failure is not equivalent to clinical failure and is not a justification per se to initiate additional treatment. No definition of PSA failure has been shown to be a surrogate for clinical progression or survival. In addition, while nadir PSA is a strong prognostic factor, there is no absolute valid cut-off level for separating successful and unsuccessful treatments. Thus, it is strongly recommended in clinical practice that the timing and frequency of post-irradiation-treatment PSA measurements is at the discretion of the treating physician. Additional therapy for patients presenting with biochemical PSA progression/failure should then be carefully evaluated. PSA failure was defined as three cumulative increases of serum PSA level, with the failure date designated as the mid-point in time between the first increase and the PSA level before this increase. The American Urological Association (AUA) Best Practice Policy regarding use of PSA in post-treatment management of prostate cancer was subsequently published in 2000 [16] and is summarised in Box 15.1.

Box 15.1 *The AUA Best Practice Policy regarding use of PSA in post-treatment management of prostate cancer [16].*

- Periodic PSA determinations should be offered to detect disease recurrence.
- Serum PSA should decrease and remain undetectable after radical prostatectomy.
- Serum PSA should fall to a low level following radiation and cryotheraphy, and should not rise on successive occasions.
- The pattern of PSA rise after local therapy for prostate cancer can help distinguish between local and distant recurrence.
- The nadir serum PSA and percent decline at 3 and 6 months predict progression-free survival in men with meatstatic prostate cancer treated with androgen deprivation. The degree of PSA decline following second-line treatment of metastatic disease correlates with disease survival.
- Bone scans are indicated for detection of metastases following initial treatment for localised disease. The level of PSA that should prompt a bone scan is uncertain.

Following radical prostatectomy, PSA should fall to an undetectable level within 2–4 weeks provided that all the malignant and benign prostate tissue has been removed [17]. Serum PSA interpretation after External Beam Radiation is more complicated as the prostate, malignant and benign tissue components, stay. PSA elevation occurs during the initial delivery of irradiation and could be attributed to cellular damage, necrosis, inflammation and subsequent PSA release in the circulation [18]. After Brachytherapy, the 'PSA bounce' phenomenon was described: a moderate, inconsequential, temporary rise between 1 and 2 years after seeds implantation. Critz *et al.* (2000) reported a PSA bounce in 273/779 (35%) men with T1–2N0M0 prostate cancer treated with 125 iodine radioactive prostate seed implantation followed by external beam radiation boost. PSA bounce led to anxiety following Brachytherapy treatment by confounding the diagnosis of prostate cancer recurrence [19]. Hence, it is necessary to observe American Society of Therapeutic Radiotherapy and Oncology (ASTRO) recommendations with regards to a PSA recurrence definition, that is, it is not significant until three consecutive increases of PSA occur.

In 2000, Sandler *et al.* reported that a short post-treatment PSA-doubling time (PSA-DT) appeared to identify patients with PSA-defined radiation therapy failure at high risk of subsequent prostate cancer-specific mortality [20]. D'Amico *et al.* (2004) then compiled base line, treatment and follow-up data on 8669 patients with localised prostate cancer treated at multiple institutions in the United States [21]. These included 5918 patients treated with radical prostatectomy and 2751 having received radiation therapy. Treatment was delivered during the period January 1988 and January 2002 for clinical stage T1c–4NxM0. Despite some potential limitations, which were addressed in the analysis, the results indicated that a PSA-DT less than 3 months or the specific PSA-DT value, when it is 3 months or greater, is apparently a surrogate for prostate cancer mortality following surgery or radiation therapy in patients with clinically localised or locally advanced prostate cancer. This is a valuable contribution to the PSA follow-up regimen and its role in recommending the place of further management and its timing in recurrent prostate cancer.

Biopsy Evaluation

With the availability of trans-rectal ultrasound-guided biopsy techniques and serial PSA measurements, early recurrence of prostate cancer after radiation therapy can be achieved. Histological clearance of tumour after radiotherapy is difficult to identify and may take 18 months or longer to occur, owing to ongoing tumour cell death [22]. Histological changes of radiation injury in benign hyperplasia include acinar atrophy and distortion, marked cytological abnormalities of the epithelium, basal cell hyperplasia, stromal fibrosis, decreased ratio of acini to stroma and vascular changes. Marked variation in pleomorphism is seen (Fig. 15.1). Cancer grading usually shows little or no evidence of differentiation post-radiotherapy. Prostatic Intraepithelial

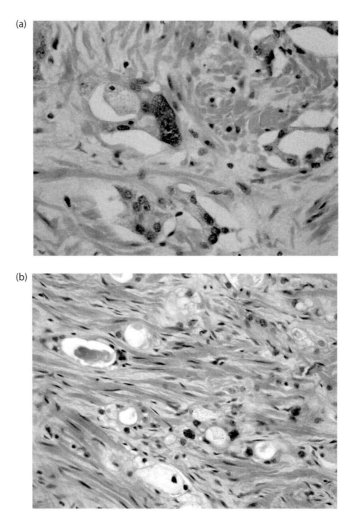

Fig. 15.1 Pathological features in salvage prostatectomy specimens demonstrating variations in pleomorphism. (a) Post-external beam radiotherapy; (b) post-brachytherapy. (Photographs prepared with courtesy from Dr Alan Bates and Dr Martin Young, Consultant Histopathologists, The Royal Free Hospital NHS Trust and University College London and Royal Free Medical School).

Neoplasia (PIN) identified after radiotherapy usually retains the features characteristic of untreated PIN but the prevalence and extent decline. These features include nuclear crowding, nuclear overlapping and stratification, nuclear hyperchromasia and prominent nucleoli. A basal cell layer is usually present but is often fragmented. These features point to the possibility of atypical basal cell hyperplasia as an important differential consideration of high-grade PIN after RT [23,24]. The question remains whether recurrent cancer after irradiation is caused by growth of incompletely eradicated tumour, progression from incompletely eradicated PIN or represents a new tumour *de novo*. In difficult cases, immunostaining of high molecular weight cytokeratin may be helpful in distinguishing basal cell hyperplasia from high-grade PIN.

Gleason grading was designed for untreated prostate cancer and thus should be avoided as it may not be appropriate or applicable to post-radiotherapy biopsies.

Bone Scan

Traditionally, most patients with elevated post-treatment PSA undergo a metastatic screen utilising various modalities. In 1997, Johnstone *et al.* presented the results of a small study assessing the yield of imaging and bone scintigraphy in prostate cancer patients with evidence of biochemical failure. The study included 48 patients: 24 post-radical prostatectomy and 20 post-radiation. Only 5% had a positive bone scan indicating that routine bone scan following early PSA recurrence may not be justified [25]. Cher and Bianco (1998) studied 144 bone scans of 93 patients who had PSA recurrence after radical prostatectomy and found that the lowest PSA value associated with a positive bone scan in the absence of adjuvant hormonal therapy was 46 ng/mL [26].

Computerised Tomography, Position Emission Tomography and Prostacint

Seltzer *et al.* (1999) compared the detection of metastatic disease by helical computerised tomography (CT), positron emission tomography (PET) with F-18 fluorodeoxyglucose and monoclonal antibody scan with 111indium capromab pendetide (ProstaScint scan) in patients with an elevated PSA after treatment for localised prostate cancer [27]. They concluded that CT and PET each showed evidence of metastatic disease in 50% of all patients with a PSA >4 ng/mL, or PSA velocity >0.2 ng/mL/month. However, they were both limited in detecting metastases in patients with low PSA and PSA velocity. Monoclonal antibody scans had a lower detection rate than CT or PET. The utility of ProstaScint for establishing the site of recurrence in men with rising PSA after radiation therapy has been mainly to identify extra-prostatic occult recurrences rather than localised disease [28–30].

Reverse Transcriptase-Polymerase Chain Reaction

Shariat *et al.* (2003) reported that reverse transcriptase-polymerase chain reaction (RT-PCR)/hK2 could detect biologically and clinically significant occult prostate cancer metastases in lymph nodes, which were proven to be normal on routine histology. A strong association was found with prostate cancer progression, failure following salvage radiation therapy, development of clinically evident metastases and prostate cancer-specific mortality after surgery [31].

DNA ploidy

Amling *et al.* (1999) investigated the role of deoxyribonucleic acid in predicting the outcome following salvage radical prostatectomy for radiation-refractory prostate cancer. They reported DNA ploidy to be a strong predictor of cancer-specific and progression-free survival following salvage radical prostatectomy. They recommended that pre-operative consideration of DNA ploidy and serum PSA appear to be the most important predictors of outcome [32].

SELECTION CRITERIA FOR SALVAGE PROSTATECTOMY

Good candidates are young healthy motivated patients who were good candidates for primary prostatectomy and have a life expectancy >10 years. Overall, they should have minimal medical co-morbidities. The results from a bone scan, chest X-ray and CT scan of abdomen and pelvis should provide no evidence of systemic disease or pelvic lymphadenopathy. Minimal to tolerable urinary symptoms are expected in a large number of candidates following irradiation but care should be taken in candidates suffering symptoms of overactive detrusor. Be sure to have a clear and frank discussion explaining the significant potential of peri-operative morbidity and post-operative outcome, particularly incontinence and impotence.

PRE-OPERATIVE PROGNOSTIC FACTORS

Patients who could benefit most from salvage prostatectomy with regards to long-term disease-free survival would include pre-radiation PSA <4 ng/mL [32,33] and pre-radiation clinical stage T1–T2 [34]. Pre-operative favourable parameters include PSA <10 ng/mL [32,34,35], biopsy Gleason score <7 [33,36], clinical stage T1c [33] and diploid DNA [32,37].

PRE-OPERATIVE EVALUATION

Cystoscopy provides the opportunity to identify subtrigonal tumour extension, haemorrhagic cystitis or a concomitant incidental bladder cancer. It also allows bimanual examination under anaesthesia to identify the pliability and softness of the surrounding tissues. The prostate mobility and non-adherance to the overlying rectal mucosa is a promising pre-operative finding. It is not uncommon that patients treated with radiation therapy have a variable degree of lower urinary tract symptoms. Urodynamic study evaluation would be of value to assess bladder capacity and compliance [38]. Patients with poorly compliant bladders or detrusor irritability are poor candidates for salvage prostatectomy alone. As treatment at this stage aims to cure, a modification of the surgical procedure proposed might be considered, namely some patients might be identified to benefit from augmentation cystoplasty and radical prostatectomy or cystoprostatectomy with continent diversion [39–41].

SURGERY

Salvage radical prostatectomy is performed in a similar fashion to a standard radical prostatectomy. The surgical technique should be modified depending on the extent of fibrosis and adhesions encountered. In patients with no previous pelvic surgery, dissection within the retro-pubic space should be performed in a similar fashion to standard surgery. If no previous pelvic lymphadenectomy was carried out, it should be performed. The anatomical planes should be recognised and followed. A combination of ante-grade and retrograde dissection- mobilisation of the prostate should be adapted. After dividing the urethra, sharp dissection is used meticulously and carefully, the plane between the posterior surface of the prostate and anterior wall of the rectum is identified. Blunt dissection could result in rectal tears. A small rectal injury in two layers is repaired with placement interposition of omentum between the anastomotic urethrovesical junction and rectum. If there is any doubt about the rectal tissue viability, or faecal spillage with inadequate pre-operative bowel preparation, the rectal injury is closed and a defunctioning colostomy is fashioned. Preservation of bladder neck is not advocated in view of the possible changes following irradiation damage. Mucousal eversion of the vesical outlet gives the urethrovesical anastomosis the optimal healing outcome. Neuro-vascular bundle preservation might not be feasible in view of the development of dense adhesions. If preservation is attempted, it may not be necessarily successful because of prolonged neuropraxia. Foley catheter drainage is adopted with a recommended minimum of 2 weeks.

OPERATIVE MORBIDITY

Salvage surgery has a significantly higher rate of complications mainly due to radiation fibrosis and loss of anatomical tissue planes. Improvements and refinement in surgical technique have led to decreases in estimated blood loss and blood transfusion requirements [42,43]. The rate of rectal injuries ranges from 0–35% with most injuries occurring in patients with locally advanced disease [35].

POST-OPERATIVE LATE MORBIDITY

Anastomotic urethro-vesical contracture formation ranges between 0% and 28% particularly in men who have had previous trans-urethral resection of the prostate [35]. Some degree of post-operative urinary incontinence is encountered in 30–66% of patients, probably due to radiation effects on the bladder neck/external sphincter mechanism region [32,34–36,43–45]. Nearly all men will become impotent after surgery.

Post-operatively, a favourable pathological parameter is the presence of organ-confined tumour with negative surgical margins. This has been shown in several reports [34,35,37,46,47]. Peri- and post-operative relevant complications in series, where more than 30 patients were reported, are summarised in Table 15.1.

CONCLUSION

Successful treatment outcome from patients undergoing a secondary procedure after relapsing following primary treatment failure is usually measured in terms of morbidity, mortality and impact of subsequent treatment on quality of life [48]. Following salvage radiation or surgery, Tefilli *et al.* (1998) reported that 64–75% of patients were satisfied with their quality of life

Table 15.1 Complications of surgical salvage prostatectomy. Series reporting less than 30 patients are not included.

	Number of patients	Pre-operative outcome		Post-operative outcome	
		EBL	Rectal injury (%)	Incontinence (%)	Anastomotic contracture (%)
Zinke 1992	32	NR	6.3	26.7/Nr[a]	19
Ahlering 1992	34	NR	0	64/Nr[a]	0
Pontes 1993 [36]	43	NR	9	28/17	9
Rogers 1995 [35]	40	910	15	58/Nr[a]	28
Gheiler 1998 [34]	40	1100	7	23/26[a]	13
Amling 1999 [32]	108	NR	6	24/29[a]	21
Eastham 2004 [43]	100	NR	9	38/NR[a]	50

EBL = estimated blood loss; NR = not reported; Urinary incontinence[a] = mild/severe: <2 pads/>2 pads per day.

despite low scores of well being, sexual function and continence. Primary prostatectomy and subsequent salvage radiation, patients seem to report less impact on their quality of life than the converse. It might be very relevant in patients with clinically localised prostate cancer who are at risk of failing primary therapy, to optimise the primary treatment chosen recognising the quality-of-life issues in sequential multimodal therapy options [49].

Salvage prostatectomy should only be considered for patients in good general health with life expectancy longer than 10 years who would have been considered candidates for radical prostatectomy initially. In younger patients with radiation refractory disease and long-life expectancy, salvage prostatectomy may offer the best chance of long-term disease control.

REFERENCES

1 Anderson RN, Smith BL. Death: leading causes for 2001. *Natl Vital Stat Rep* 2003; **52**: 1.

2 American Cancer Society: Cancer Facts & Figures 2004. Atlanta, Georgia: *American Cancer Society* 2004; pp 16–7.

3 Gohagan JK, Prorok PC, Kramer BS, Cornett JE. Prostate cancer screening in prostate, lung, colorectal and ovarian cancer screening trial of National Cancer Institute. *J Urol* 1994; **152**: 1905–9.

4 Wilt TJ, Brawer MK. The prostate cancer intervention versus observation trial (PIVOT). *Oncology* 1997; **11**: 1133–9.

5 Chodak GW, Thisted RA, Gerber GS *et al.* Results of conservative management of clinically localised prostate cancer. *N Engl J Med* 1994; **330**: 242–8.

6 Albertsen PC, Fryback DG, Storer BE, Kolon TF. Long-term survival among men with conservatively treated localised prostate cancer. *JAMA* 1995; **274**: 626–31.

7 Albertson PC, Hanley JA, Gleason DF, Barry MJ. Competing risk analysis of men aged 55 to 74 years at diagnosis managed conservatively for clinically localised prostate cancer. *JAMA* 1998; **280**: 975–80.

8 Johansson JE, Holmberg L, Johansson S *et al.* Fifteen-year survival in prostate cancer. A prospective population-based study in Sweden. *JAMA* 1997; **277**: 467–71.

9 Lee WR, Hanbon AL, Hanks GE. Prostate specific antigen nadir following external beam radiation therapy for clinically localized prostate cancer: the relation between nadir level and disease-free survival. *J Urol* 1996; **156**: 450–3.

10 Perez CA, Michalski JM, Purdy JA *et al.* Three-dimensional conformal radiation therapy (3-D CRT), Brachytherapy and new therapeutic modalities. *Rays* 2000; **25**: 331–43.

11 Bolla M, Collette L, Blank L *et al.* Long term results with immediate androgen suppression and external irradiation in patients with locally advanced prostate cancer (an EORTC study: a phase III randomised trial. *Lancet* 2002; **360**: 103–6.

12 D'Amico AV, Whittington R, Malkowicz SB *et al.* Biochemical outcome after radical prostatectomy, external beam radiation therapy, or interstitial radiation therapy for clinically localised prostate cancer. *JAMA* 1998; **280**: 969–74.

13 Kattan MW, Zelefsky MJ, Kupelian PA *et al.* Pretreatment nomogram for predicting the outcome of three dimensional conformal radiotherapy in prostate cancer. *J Clin Oncol* 2000; **18**: 3352–9.

14 Johnstone PAS, McFarland JT, Riffenburgh RH *et al.* Efficacy of digital rectal examination after radiotherapy for prostate cancer. *J Urol* 2001; **166**: 1684–7.

15 American Society for Therapeutic Radiology and Oncology Consensus

Panel: Consensus statement: guidelines for PSA following radiation therapy. *Int J Radiat Oncol Biol Phys* 1997; **37**: 1035–41.

16 Prostate-specific antigen (PSA) best practice policy. American Urological Association AUA). *Oncology* (Huntingt) 2000; **14**: 267–72, 277–8, 280.

17 Villers A. PSA in a follow up after radical prostatectomy. A review. In: Murphy G, Griffiths K, Denis L, Khoury S, Chatelian C, eds. *Proceedings from the First International Consultation on Prostate Cancer.* Cockett; 1997; AT:112.

18 Zagars CK, Poolack A. The fall and rise of PSA. Kinetics of serum PSA levels after radiation therapy for prostate cance. *Cancer* 1993; **72**: 832–42.

19 Critz FA, William H, Benton JB, Levinson AK, Holladay CT, Halladay D. Prostate specific antigen bounce after radioactive seed implantation followed by external beam radiation for prostate cancer. *J Urol* 2000; **163**: 1085–9.

20 Sandler HM, Dunn RL, McLaughlin PW, Hayman JA, Sullivan MA, Taykaur JM: Overall survival after prostate specific-antigen detected recurrence following conformal radiation therapy. *Int J Radiat Oncol Biol Phys* 2000; **48**: 629–33.

21 D'Amico D'Amico AV, Moul J, Carroll PR, Sun L, Lubeck D, Chen MH. Prostate specific antigen doubling time as a surrogate end point for prostate cancer specific mortality following radical prostatectomy or radiation therapy. *J Urol* 2004; **172**: S42–7.

22 Kuban DA, El-Mahdi AM. Local control after radiation for prostatic carcinoma: significance and assessment. *Semin Radiat Oncol* 1993; **3**: 221–9.

23 Devaraj LT, Bostwick DG. Atypical basal cell hyperplasia of the prostate: immunophenotypic and proposed classification of basal cell proliferations. *Am J Surg Pathol* 1993; **17**: 645–59.

24 Epstein JI, Armas OA. Atypical basal cell hyperplasia of the prostate. *Am J Surg Pathol* 1992; **16**: 1205–14.

25 Johnstone PA, Tarman GJ, Riffenburgh *et al* . Yield of imaging and scintigraphy assessing biochemical failure in prostate cancer patients. *Urol Oncol* 1997; **3**: 108–12.

26 Cher ML, Bianco Jr FJ. Limited role of radionuclide bone scintigraphy in patients with PSA elevations after radical prostatectomy. *J Urol* 1998; **160**: 1387–91.

27 Seltzer MA, Barbaric Z, Belldegrun A *et al.* Comparison of helical computerized tomography, positron emission tomography and monoclonal antibody scans for evaluation of lymph node metastases in patients with prostate specific antigen relapse after treatment for localised prostate cancer. *J Urol* 1999; **162**: 1322–8.

28 Elgamal AA, Troychak MJ, Murphy GP. ProstaScint scan may enhance identification of prostate cancer recurrences after prostatectomy, radiation or hormone therapy: analysis of 136 scans of 100 patients. *Prosate* 1998; **37**: 261–9.

29 Sodee DB, Malguria N, Faulhaber P, Resnick MI. Multicenter ProstaScint imaging findings in 2154 patients with prostate cancer. The ProstaeScint Imaging Centres. *Urology* 2000; **56**: 988–93.

30 Fang DX Stock RG, Stone NN, Krynyckyi BR. Use of radioimmunoscintigraphy with indium-111- labelled CYT-356 (ProstaScint) scan for evaluation of patients for salvage brachytherapy. *Tech Urol.* 2000; **6**: 146–50.

31 Shariat SF, Kattan MW, Erdamar S *et al.* Detection of clinically significant occult prostate cancer metastases in lymph nodes using a splice variant-specific RT-PCR assay for human glandular kallikrein. *J Clin Oncol* 2003; **21**: 1223–31.

32 Amling CL, Seth LE, Martin SK, Slezak JM, Blute ML, Zincke H. Deoxyribonucleic acid ploidy and serum prostate specific antigen predict outcome following salvage radical prostatectomy for radiation refractory prostate cancer. *J Urol* 1999; **161**: 857–62.

33 Cheng L, Sebo TJ, Slezak J *et al.* Predictors of survival for prostate carcinoma patients treated with salvage radical prostatectomy after radiation therapy. *Cancer* 1998; **83**: 2164–71.

34 Gheiler EL, Tefilli MV, Tiguert R *et al.* Predictors for maximal outcome in patients undergoing salvage surgery for

radio-recurrent prostate cancer. *Urology* 1998; **51**: 789–95.

35 Rogers E, Ohori M, Kassabian VS *et al.* Salvage radical prostatectomy: outcome measured by serum prostate specific antigen levels. *J Urol* 1995; **153**: 104–10.

36 Pontes JE, Montie J, Klein E *et al.* Salvage surgery for radiation failure in prostate cancer. *Cancer* 1993; **71**: 976–80.

37 Lerner SE, Blute ML and Zincke H. Critical evaluation of salvage surgery for radio-recurrent/resistant prostate cancer. *J Urol* 1995; **154**: 1103–9.

38 Soloway MS, Pareek K, Sharifi R *et al.* for the Lupron Depot Neoadjuvant Prostate Cancer Study. Neoadjuvant androgen ablation before radical prostatectomy in c2bNxM0: 5-year results. *J Urol* 2002; **167**: 112–6.

39 Gheiler EL, Wood DP Jr, Montie JE, Ponted JE. Orthotopic urinary diversion is a viable option in patients undergoing salvage cystoprostaectomy for recurrent prostate cancer after definitive radiation therapy. *Urology* 1997; **50**: 580–4.

40 Bochner BH, Figueroa AJ, Skinner EC *et al.* Salvage radical cystoprostatectomy and orthotopic urinary diversion following radiation failure. *J Urol* 1998; **160**: 29–3.

41 Pisters LL, English SF, Scott SM, Westney OL, Dinney CPN, McGuire EJ. Salvage prostatectomy with continent catheterizable urinary reconstruction: a novel approach to recurrent prostate cancer after radiation therapy. *J Urol* 2000; **163**: 1771–4.

42 Vidya A, Soloway MS. Salvage radical prostatectomy for radiorecurrent prostate cancer: morbidity revisited. *J Urol* 2000; **164**: 1998–2001.

43 Eastham JA, Scardino PT. Salvage RP: Improving outcome after failed radiation therapy. *Contemporary Urology* 2004; **16**: 34–43.

44 Zinke H. Radical prostatectomy and exenterative procedures for local failure after radiotherapy with curative intent: comparison of outcomes. *J Urol* 1992; **147**: 894–9.

45 Ahlering TE, Lieskovsky G, Skinner DG. Salvage surgery plus androgen deprivation for radioresistant prostatic adenocarcinoma. *J Urol* 1992; **147**: 900–2.

46 Link P, Freiha FS. Radical prostatectomy after definitive radiation therapy for prostate cancer. *Urology* 1991; **37**: 189–92.

47 Garzotto M, Wajsman Z. Androgen deprivation with salvage surgery for radiorecurrent prostate cancer: results at 5-year follow up. *J Urol* 1998; **159**: 950–4.

48 Brazier JE, Harper R, Jones NM *et al.* Validating the SE-36 health survey questionnaire: new outcome measures for primary care. *BMJ* 1992; **305**: 160–4.

49 Tefilli MV, Gheiler EL, Tiguert R *et al.* Quality of life in patients undergoing salvage procedures for locally recurrent prostate cancer. *J Surg Oncol* 1998; **69**: 156–61.

16: Treatment of Renal Impairment Secondary to Locally Advanced Prostate Cancer

Paul Jones and Neil Fenn

INTRODUCTION

Prostate cancer can cause urinary tract obstruction in several ways. Local disease may result in bladder outflow obstruction with subsequent high-pressure chronic retention. Ureteric obstruction can occur either via direct disease extension through the trigone or more proximal extrinsic compression secondary to lymph node metastases. Regardless of its mechanism, urinary tract obstruction and renal failure due to prostate cancer present the patient and clinician with a difficult dilemma regarding treatment.

In this chapter, the incidence, presentation and initial management of both upper and lower urinary tract obstruction resulting from prostate cancer are described. The moral and ethical principles guiding the clinician in their decision making are also explained. In discussing the relative merits, weakness and financial implication of the subsequent treatment options, we hope this chapter will provide the clinician with a management framework to allow the development of appropriate treatment plans for each individual patient in their care.

INCIDENCE

Prostate, cervical and bladder cancer account for 75% of cancers causing urinary tract obstruction. At diagnosis, a considerable proportion of patients with prostate cancer already have voiding difficulties due to locally advanced disease [1,2]. A smaller number of patients will present with symptoms of renal failure as a consequence of their malignancy. Despite treatment, a further 60–70% of patients will develop renal failure within 2 years of initial diagnosis although delays of 20 years have been reported [3].

PRESENTATION

Men with early, localised carcinoma of the prostate are almost always asymptomatic. Lower urinary tract symptoms are common to a variety

193

of urinary tract pathologies and thus not disease specific, however their presence should alert the clinician to the possibility of prostate cancer.

In the majority of patients, the early stages of renal failure are often completely asymptomatic, despite the accumulation of toxic metabolites. Symptoms are common when the blood urea concentration is over 40 mmol/L, but some patients develop uraemic symptoms at lower levels of blood urea. It is not the accumulation of urea itself that causes the symptoms but a combination of multiple metabolic abnormalities, which can often manifest in generalised symptoms of tiredness, lethargy and shortness of breath.

INITIAL MEDICAL TREATMENT

If renal impairment is significant, the standard treatment for renal failure is required. Hyperkalaemia, fluid overload and metabolic acidosis are potentially life threatening and require urgent medical intervention. Insertion of a urethral catheter allows accurate assessment of urine output in the oliguric patient. Hyperkalaemia should be treated with insulin/ dextrose infusions, calcium resonium or salbutamol infusions. Patients failing to respond can be treated with temporary dialysis.

Once a patient is medically stable, the clinician needs to identify those patients who would benefit from relief of obstruction and justify this action. The main objective is to gain as much information about the obstructing process as possible. A thorough physical examination including pelvic and rectal examination are paramount. Appropriate radiology is required in the initial assessment. Accurate diagnosis and staging is reliant on modern imaging techniques of ultrasonography, computerised tomography (CT), magnetic resonance (MR) and isotope bone scanning. When previous tissue diagnosis is not available, then finger or trans-rectal ultrasound-guided prostate biopsies are useful in confirming the diagnosis.

A MULTIDISCIPLINARY TEAM APPROACH

The disease process is not the sole consideration. Comprehensive cancer care requires a team approach at every stage of a patient's illness. In this way, the patient will gain the information they need to help them and their families deal with the issues the illness brings. Locally recurrent prostate cancer is a particular challenge. Patients not only have to deal with a life-limiting illness but also cope with complex symptoms and functional difficulties associated with their disease. This requires a multidisciplinary team including urologists, radiologists, clinical oncologists and palliative care physicians each contributing their expertise.

There are also important ethical issues that can contribute to difficult discussions relating to treatment in these patients. There is a balance between the information a patient wants and what a patient can deal with at a particular time. The urologist involved in the management of bilateral ureteric obstruction in advanced prostate cancer not only has difficult physical clinical issues to deal with, but also the difficulties of dealing directly with physical suffering and supporting the difficult decisions for those who may be approaching the terminal stages of their lives.

Some basic moral principles have been formulated to aid the clinician in making decisions in this area. They emphasise that life is not to be preserved at all cost, and where the means used to sustain life are out of proportion to the life achieved, the mortality of humankind should be accepted and death allowed to take its course [4].

1 Treatment of patients must reflect the inherent dignity of every person, irrespective of age, debility, dependence, race, colour or creed (the value of the person is a separate matter to the question of the usefulness of the treatment: though treatment may stop, tending by medical and nursing staff should never be withdrawn).

2 Actions must reflect the needs of the patient (where he or she is taking into account such issues as the effect on the family, staff, the hospital and the community as well as on resources).

3 Decisions taken must value the person and accept human mortality.

In the United Kingdom, the same basic ethical obligations owed to the patient are clearly defined. In respect of all patients, the General Medical Council informs doctors that they must prescribe only those treatments or drugs that serve the patient's needs and must not subject patients to investigation or treatment that is not in their best interest [5].

Ultimately, the decision rests with the patient and his relatives. For this reason, the clinician should never categorically advise against treatment. It is our belief that the patient and relevant family members should be fully informed of the clinical situation and probable outcome depending on the decision to intervene or not. If the patient has a strong desire to have the obstruction relieved (despite the potential risk and the possibility of surviving only to struggle with symptoms such as pain, nausea, cachexia and external drainage devices) then we believe in respecting their wishes.

TREATMENT OF LOWER URINARY TRACT OBSTRUCTION

Surgery

For patients with obstructive carcinoma of the prostate who are unsuitable for curative treatment, hormone therapy is the treatment of choice

[6–8]. However, 3 months after the commencement of the ablative hormone therapy, one-third of All patients will continue to have persistent obstruction requiring treatment [8,9]. The traditional operative treatment has been a channel trans-urethral resection of the prostate (TURP). Concerns have been raised regarding the oncological safety and high-morbidity rates (up to 20%) quoted for this procedure [10–13]. A number of alternative treatments are available.

Urinary Catheters

For patients with significant co-morbidities, an indwelling catheter may be the only therapeutic option. Long-term catheterisation is sometimes considered a simple and inexpensive option but Booth *et al.* showed that the cost of care for a patient with an indwelling catheter is at least £700 a year [14]. Recurrent catheter blockage, urinary tract infections and haematuria are just some of the side effects that may impair quality of life for these patients.

Prostatic Stents

The success of treating bladder outflow obstruction due to benign prostatic hyperplasia in high-risk patients by the implantation of various permanent metal stent systems has been well reported [15–17]. It is not surprising that attempts to treat obstruction due to carcinoma of the prostate in a similar fashion have been made.

The use of a temporary intraprostatic stents in patients with urinary retention due to adenocarcinoma of the prostate was first described in 1993 by Anson [18]. Ten patients (mean age 72 years) were treated with a combination of flutamide and the insertion of a Porges Urospiral stent. In their series, one patient developed persistent dysuria and urinary frequency necessitating early stent removal and TURP 1 week later. Another patient spontaneously voided his stent 1-month post-insertion. The remaining eight stents were removed 3 months after insertion under sedoanalgesia as day cases. The authors reported that at the 3-month follow-up, all patients had successfully voided following stent removal with adequate flow rates and low post-micturition residuals; they mention only the failure rate and the cost of this combination as disadvantages of the procedure.

Guazzoni *et al.* first advocated the use of a permanent metal stent for obstructive prostatic carcinoma [19]. In their small series of 11 patients, lasting subjective and objective improvement of obstructive symptoms was achieved using the Urolume® Wallstent. Similar early results have been confirmed in larger series, however longer term follow-up using the

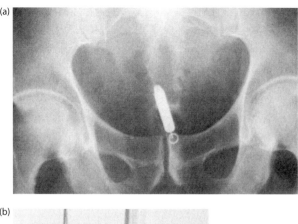

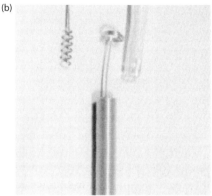

Fig. 16.1 (a) Partial migration of Prostakath®; (b) Gold-plated Prostakath®.

Urolume® stent has revealed problems with epithelial ingrowth, encrustation and stent migration [15,16,20]. The subsequent development of urinary tract infection and lower urinary tract symptoms required stent removal under general anaesthesia [21]. Similarly, the Prosatakath®, a non-epithelialising stent made from rigid gold-plated spiral designed to be easy to insert (Fig. 16.1), suffers from similar problems with over half of patients requiring removal of their stent within the first year due to migration [22].

The Memokath® intraprostatic stent is made of an alloy of nickel and titanium, such that it regains its shape after deformation if it is reheated to a given temperature. The memorised shape of the stent is that of a tight coil opening into a funnel at one end. When unpacked it appears as a straight coil and only assumes the memorised shape when heated to $55°C$ when correctly positioned within the prostate. When cooled using water at $10°C$, it becomes relatively soft and pliable, and can be removed with relative ease under local urethral anaesthesia.

In their series of 200 patients, including patients with carcinoma of the prostate, over 8 years, Perry *et al.* reported over three-quarters of those

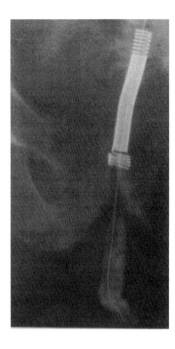

Fig. 16.2 Memokath® *in situ* in the prostate.

patients with a Memokath® stent (Fig. 16.2) described a satisfactory outcome and concluded that it was a safe option particularly for those patients with high co-morbidity [20]. Tissue ingrowth in the prostate cancer group was not a problem. Concern raised regarding the use of radiotherapy following stent insertion has not been substantiated when using conventional multiport radiotherapy treatment protocols.

Despite these favourable results after stent placement, the expense must be considered (~£1200) and also that correct measurement of the length of the prostatic urethra and correct placement of the stent can be a difficult procedure requiring a skilled endoscopic surgeon, who will also have to traverse the individual learning curve. Despite these weaknesses, Perry *et al.* showed that patients undergoing a TURP has less satisfactory than those who received a prostatic stent for their obstruction [20]. Furthermore, the same authors showed that the longer inpatient stay associated with TURP (mean 2.2 days) made the two treatments comparable in price (TURP = £1050 versus. Prostatic Stent = £1200).

TREATMENT OF UPPER URINARY TRACT OBSTRUCTION

Surgical Diversion

Traditionally surgical diversion was used to palliate renal failure due to advance prostatic malignancy. Procedures included open nephrostomy, cutaneous ureterostomy, ileal conduit, intubated ureterotomy, ureterolysis and more recently, laparoscopic bilateral cutaneous ureterostomy [23].

Uraemia is often associated with anaemia, malnourishment and bleeding tendencies rendering the patients a higher operative risk. This was reflected in the high morbidity and mortality in reported series [24–26]. Surgical mortality rates of 3–8% and complication rates as high as 40–50% have been reported [26].

Survival following successful surgical diversion has been addressed by Fallon and associates who reviewed 100 cases of open nephrostomy placement in patients with advanced pelvic malignancy of different histological types [27]. In prostate cancer patients, the average survival from open nephrostomy to death was 12.2 months. This series is now over 20-year old. Improvements in post-operative surgical care and adjuvant treatments are likely to improve the survival time. Contemporary series confirm this with Chiou and associates reporting a median survival time of 21 months after relief of obstruction [28].

These results have made urologists sceptical about palliative surgical diversion although the introduction of laparoscopic techniques has led to some urologists to reconsider the possible advantages of laparoscopic cutaneous ureterostomy (LCU) in patients with advanced cancer [26]. Protagonists of LCU believe that its technical feasibility can be compared directly to percutaneous techniques. The additional general anaesthetic requirements are not significant as none of the patients in the surgical series of Fallon and associates [27] died from intraoperative problems.

Complication rates are not clearly reported for LCU, however, should be lower than the 15% quoted for laparoscopic lymph node dissection, a similar procedure [29]. As with all endourological procedures, complications of LCU are related to the operators' learning curve and also the operating time. In experienced hands, bilateral percutaneous nephrostomies (PCN) can be performed in 30 min and LCU in 1 h [23]. The cost is significantly higher for LCU, especially because of the need for anaesthesia. However, tube dislodgment or obstruction is a common occurrence in PCN, and the cost of repeated tube placement should be taken into account when making comparisons.

Percutaneous Nephrostomy

Until the last decade, nephrostomies were usually inserted by an open surgical technique. Goodwin and colleagues are credited with the first successful attempt, in 1955, to drain a hydronephrotic kidney percutaneously via a nephrostomy tube placed in the renal pelvis [30]. The tube is now placed into the renal pelvis through the renal parenchyma. This has a lower incidence of tearing the renal pelvis and causing urine extravasation.

Advantages include the relative ease of insertion, convenience and low cost compared with open insertion. Furthermore, in patients not fit for an anaesthetic, PCN placement allows stabilisation of the patient and subsequent treatment based on further assessment and quality-of-life issues central to the patient.

Percutaneous nephrostomy significantly reduced the morbidity and mortality from surgical urinary diversion, from 40% to 11% [31]. Culkin and associates quoted the very high perioperative mortality of 11.1% and 29.6% haemorrhage, necessitating transfusion with PCN although the complication rates defined in several larger series testify the safety of the procedure with complication rates being much lower. In these series, mortality was 0.2% owing to haemorrhage in one patient with pre-existing coagulopathy. Significant haemorrhage occurred in 1.3% and sepsis in an additional 1.9% [29,32,33].

As far as the quality of life is concerned, bilateral PCN can be uncomfortable and cumbersome to wear, making it difficult for the patient to sleep in the supine position. Nephrostomy tube-related infection, blockage and dislodgement are commonly reported. Detailed prospective measurements of quality of life are however lacking in the literature. A commonly used surrogate measure is the calculation of the proportion of the patient's remaining lifetime spent as a hospital inpatient. Such values vary widely among the different studies, but serve to illustrate that some patients will spend the majority, or even all, of their remaining days as a hospital inpatient. In the early surgical series previously mentioned, 18–43% of patients died without being discharged from hospital.

The likely duration of survival of patients with obstructive nephropathy due to primary, locally recurrent or metastatic disease has been documented in several retrospective series. Fallon et al. reported a median survival of 7 months for patients with prostate cancer while series that are more recent have consisted largely of patients treated with PCN [27]. The outcome of 37 patients with obstructive nephropathy secondary to prostate cancer was reviewed by Chiou where the overall survival rates at 1 and 2 years were 57% and 29% respectively, with a median survival of 21 months [28]. Dowling et al. reported on 22 patients with hormone-refractory prostate cancer who underwent PCN insertion after the development of obstructive renal failure, of whom 11 subsequently received further therapy [34]. The median survival of all patients was 4 months.

It is important to identify in advance those patients who are unlikely to benefit from PCN so that they can be advised appropriately. Criteria have been identified that are useful in this area. Fallon et al stated that PCN insertion was appropriate in patients with undiagnosed malignant disease, prostate and cervical primary tumours, patients for whom there is an available treatment modality with a reasonable chance of response, patients with localised disease and in patients who request intervention as a means of prolonging life for legal or financial reasons [27]. Feuer *et al.* concluded that the following criteria contra-indicated the placement of PCN: progression of disease while on therapy, potentially life-threatening coincidental medical problems, poor performance status, no available effective salvage therapy, non-compliance with treatment and uncontrolled pain [35].

Harrington *et al.* described PCN placement in 42 patients with obstructive nephropathy secondary to malignancy and concluded that patients likely to benefit from nephrostomy were those for whom there were therapeutic options available for the treatment of their malignancy [36]. Recurrence or progression of obstructive nephropathy contributed significantly to death in 20 of 36 patients, who died with locally progressive disease, despite the presence of PCN. This observation may largely overcome the reservations of other authors in recommending PCN. It is therefore likely that some patients will succumb to a humane uraemic death before the intercession of symptoms relating to disseminated malignant disease.

Harrington *et al.* concluded that the ethics of relieving renal failure in obstructive nephropathy are no longer contentious where, in a group of patients for whom a long period of good quality of life can be achieved. These can be clearly identified using the previously mentioned guidelines as selection criteria and, as such, should not be denied access to the relatively simple procedure of percutaneous nephrostomy.

Paul *et al.* went on to differentiate a further category of selection criteria as a result of their prospective study of 36 patients with bilateral ureteric obstruction in advanced prostate cancer, the majority of whom were treated with PCN decompression [37]. They concluded that in patients for whom hormonal therapy remains an option, upper tract decompression offers a worthwhile improvement in terms of increased survival and reduced inpatient time. However, if ureteric obstruction is diagnosed after hormone manipulation has been used, upper tract decompression has little effect on survival and should only be used in exceptional circumstances.

Double-J stents

The placement of a ureteric stent is probably the oldest procedure available to urologists for the relief of upper tract obstruction. The development of self-retaining double pigtail polyethylene (JJ) stents further enhanced this option. It has been suggested that ureteric stents facilitate urine drainage by causing passive dilatation of the ureter, so that flow occurs alongside rather than through the stent. This may be the case in normal ureters but it is unlikely that in ureters obstructed directly or indirectly (where the ureter is non-pliable), drainage is through the stent. Therefore, it is preferable to insert a fairly large diameter stent whenever possible [38]. Modern materials have a larger internal-to-external diameter ratio and therefore favour drainage through the stent. They are constructed of stronger material with greater memory. Coating with hydrogels has made them easier to insert and less likely to buckle, encrust or become infected.

Ureteric stents can be inserted in a retrograde or antegrade fashion. For retrograde insertion, a general anaesthetic is normally required as passage through the obstruction can be troublesome. Fluoroscopy is advisable to ensure correct positioning of the guidewire and stent. However, placing ureteral stents may not be possible due to bladder mucosal oedema, bladder floor distortion or malignant involvement of the bladder. There are few detailed reports on the patency of double-J catheters [39,40]. Docimo and Dewolf reported poor patency of polyurethane and polyethylene retrograde ureteral stents placed in patients with extrinsic obstruction with a high-failure rate (46–56%) due to recurrent obstruction within 30 days although placing two ipsilateral stents has been shown to produce an improvement in extrinsic compression [39,41]. Furthermore, authors have described additional frequent complications associated with stent placement namely sepsis and dislodgement [39]. Stent irritation can produce urinary frequency, urgency and dysuria, which are also frequently reported.

Percutaneous antegrade stenting is an alternative when retrograde stenting has failed or when converting the external drainage nephrostomy to an internal one.

Antegrade stent insertion performed percutaneously is relatively safe, reliable, cost-effective and relatively easy treatment option that is often possible when retrograde stenting is impossible [38]. Stenting avoids the need for long-term external drainage with its attendant problems and in carefully selected patients offers prevention of progressive renal failure in patients with advanced prostate cancer.

Subcutaneous urinary diversion

Extra-anatomic stents (EAS) have been previously advocated as an alternative treatment [42,43] for those in whom conventional stent insertion has failed or for whom permanent nephrostomy drainage is not acceptable. Minhas et al. in the largest series to date, reported on the use of EAS in patients with impassable ureteric obstruction [43].

In summary, EAS are inserted under a general anaesthetic with ultrasound guidance. The proximal end of a 50 cm 8 F double pigtail-stent

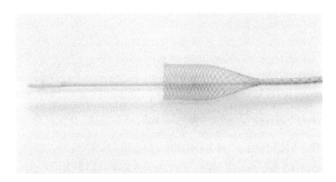

Fig. 16.3 Self-expanding Wallsent® endoprosthesis. The stent reaches its maximum diameter as the plastic cover (rolling membrane) is removed. Simultaneously, a shortening in length takes place.

is placed into the collecting system of the kidney via a percutaneous nephrostomy. A small transverse incision is made over the puncture site and a subcutaneous tunnel created using metal telescopic dilators and sheath to a second incision at the iliac crest. The subcutaneous tunnel is then extended to a third transverse incision in the suprapubic region. The bladder is then filled with saline via a urethral catheter, the bladder punctured under ultrasonographic guidance and the stent passed into the bladder through a 'peel-away' sheath. The incisions were then closed and a radiograph taken to confirm the position of the stent.

Stent change may require routine change every 6 months. The stent is exposed by making a small transverse incision at the site of the previous iliac crest incision. The stent is then cut and a guidewire passed through the proximal portion of the stent, which is then removed. The new stent is passed over the guidewire and the wire withdrawn. The guidewire is then passed into the bladder via the distal end of the old stent, which is then removed. The distal end of the new stent is passed over the wire into the bladder and the guidewire removed cystoscopically from the end of the stent.

The main advantage of this treatment is that it removes the need for external drainage, with its inherent problems of infection, sepsis and displacement. Patients are able to void spontaneously and subsequent adjuvant treatment can be given without complication. Early experience with this method suggests it to be a safe, effective, short-term method of urinary diversion in patients whose long-term outlook is poor, with the aim of improving quality of life.

Ureteric metallic wallstents

The successful insertion of metal wallstents in the vascular and biliary system has led to their use in the urinary system [44,45]. Obstruction due to benign prostatic hyperplasia, urethral stricture and detrusor sphincter dyssnergia have all been treated with stents [46,47]. In the upper urinary tract, metallic stents have been deployed in the ureter, and ureteroileal anastamosis [48].

The main advantage of metal stents in the ureter is the low rate of stent-related complications, due to total incorporation of the stent in the ureteral wall. The mucosa can proliferate through the mesh and cover the surface of the stent, which in turn reduces the danger of infection, encrustation or dislocation. In effect, the morphology produced by the stent approximates the normal morphology of the ureter. Therefore, complications that result from external or internal urinary diversion with a synthetic foreign body can be avoided using metal stents. These devices offer some features that make them more attractive than plastic stents: easy placement in a single step; the possibility of delivery of an endoprosthesis, which is able to reach a greater diameter than the introduction catheter (whose calibre, 7 F is equal to or smaller than the plastic stents); and the self-expanding character that may contribute to maintaining the patency through these lesions of a tough or elastic consistency. The factors limiting the use of these stents in the treatment of ureteral obstructions are the temporary hyperplastic mucosal reaction, the possibility of tumour ingrowth or overgrowth in progressive disease, and the high cost.

In 1990, Gort et al. reported the treatment of a stenotic left ureteroileal anastamosis by antegrade placement of a metallic stent in a 66-year old man [48]. The anastamosis remained patent for 6 months. In 1992, Pauer and Lugmayr first reported the use of metallic Wallstents for the treatment of extrinsic ureteral obstruction in 12 patients (15 ureters) who were followed for 3–31 weeks [49]. During the first month, mucosal hyperplasia occurred causing slight obstruction. However, after 8 weeks the stents became incorporated and the hyperplasia regressed. Complications included haemorrhage in one patient and encrustation in two. The procedure was recommended as a minimally invasive and technically simple intervention.

A number of different metal stents are available, including a Palmaz-Schatz balloon-expandable stent (Johnson and Johnson, Warren, United States), an Accuflex self-expandable stent (Meditech/ Boston-Scientific, Boston, United States) and self-expandable Wallstents (Schneider/ Boston Scientific, Bulach, Switzerland). Wakui et al. reported their experience of using these stents to treat ureteric obstruction and found that the characteristics of the three different types of stents were as follows: The Palmaz-Schatz stent was less flexible than the others and had low radio-opacity; to deploy the stent, balloon dilation with a high pressure was required. The Accuflex stent had the advantage of being flexible and self-expandable but its radio-opacity under fluoroscopic vision was poor. The Wallstent was also flexible and self-expandable; moreover, it was the most radio-opaque of the three under fluoroscopic guidance [50].

The Wallstent is a self-expandable device, made of elastic mesh, woven from stainless cobalt-based alloy filaments mounted on a 7 F catheter. The design and detailed methodology has been previously described [51–53]. Insertion of a Wallstent is initiated with a standard percutaneous nephrostomy followed by fluoroscopy to localise the exact site of the ureteral obstruction. The stenotic segment is crossed by a 0.035-in. hydrophilic guidewire and dilated using a high-pressure balloon (5–6 mm in diameter). Following dilatation, the insertion of the Wallstent is performed along the guidewire.

The stent diameter of 7 mm is marginally greater than the physiological diameter of the ureter. Nevertheless, it is ideal because it can partially compensate for the hyperplastic mucosal reaction. Pauer *et al.* reported that they could prevent the temporary obstruction secondary to mucosal hyperplasia by routine additional implantation of a double-J stent left in place for 4 weeks although several authors have found this unnecessary because most stents used in recent clinical practice possess a marginally greater diameter than the physiological diameter of the ureter, which is thought to, at least, partially compensate for the hyperplastic mucosal reaction and to permit subsequent passage of urological instruments [49].

In 1993, Fluekiger *et al.* reported on the use of Wallstents to bypass malignant ureteral obstruction in 10 patients (13 ureters) [54]. Multiple stents were placed endoscopically to bypass long strictures in four patients. After 1–2 weeks, the lumens of the stent appeared compromised by intimal hyperplasia in four patients and occlusion occurred after 4 weeks in one patient. This temporary obstruction was alleviated with double-J stents. The remaining patients showed no signs of obstruction for 3–14 months of follow-up (average 5.8). Peristalsis was not impaired above or below the metallic stents. Based on their observations, they recommended the use of metallic stents alone or in conjunction with double-J stents to bypass malignant ureteral obstruction and avoid the use of external drainage [53].

Van Sonnenberg *et al.* also recommended the use of metallic stents to bypass ureteral obstruction as a safe and technically easy procedure [53]. They investigated the phenomenon of mucosal hyperplasia with percutaneous intraluminal ultrasound and concluded that intraluminal debris may be the causative factor, with mucosal oedema and hyperplasia being considered mild.

The ease of placing Wallstents via an antegrade approach and the prolonged patency of such stents make this procedure an attractive alternative to surgical diversion of urinary flow in the presence of obstruction due to prostatic malignancies. The lower incidence of complications and feasibility to place such stents in outpatients or with minimal hospitalisation make this a particularly useful technique in patients undergoing chemotherapy or hormonal therapy for advanced carcinoma of the prostate.

CONCLUSIONS

The ethics of relieving renal failure in obstructive nephropathy are no longer contentious. It is apparent that the nature and extent of the obstructing lesion and its potential for further treatment are the major determinants of survival rather than the method used to relieve obstruction. Patients in whom relief of obstruction is likely to produce increased life expectancy with a good quality of life should be offered treatment. Quality of life and global assessment are important in prostate cancer patients, as they are often elderly with a higher incidence of concurrent co-morbidity, which need to be considered.

In considering treatment of urinary obstruction in prostate cancer patient one should be clear about the level of obstruction, the disease and the previous treatments used. Hormone manipulation should be instituted in those patients not already treated [59] Bilateral orchidectomy seems to offer the most reliable and rapid response [59,60]. In these patients, there should be little reservation in the use of upper tract decompression – either in the short term or as a long-term management. On the other hand, when the patient has already had hormone manipulation therapy – that is, the disease has escaped hormone control – the use of decompression offers little improvement in survival or the amount of time spent in hospital. For some patients, the small increase in time at home may be valuable but for most, the kindest course is not to intervene.

The poor results of open urinary diversion cited from earlier articles seem to have clouded clinicians' opinions when contemplating treatment with renal failure arising from prostate cancer. However, multiple minimally invasive techniques now exist to treat this group of patients with substantial improvement in both quality and quantity of expected life. The discussion with the patient will need to take into consideration local availability, expertise and experience to allow an informed decision.

Many advances have been made in the management of bilateral ureteric obstruction in advanced prostate cancer: new techniques, materials and applications in combination with greater understanding of the patients' experience of their illness, and how to manage the complications of the illness. This improved understanding and these advances can be of potential benefit to every patient and should be recognised as integral, when providing care to patients with prostate cancer.

REFERENCES

1 Ortlip SA, Fraley EE. Indications for palliative urinary diversion in patients with cancer. *Urol Clin North America* 1982; **9**: 79–84.

2 Brin EN, Shiff M *et al*. Palliative urinary diversion for pelvic malignancy. *J Urol* 1975; **13**: 619–22.

3 Zadra JA, Jewett MAS *et al*. Nonoperative urinary diversion for malignant ureteric obstruction. *Cancer* 1987; **60**: 1353–7.

4 Jefrey P, Millard PH. An ethical framework for clinical decision making at the end of life. *J R Soc Med* 1997; **90**: 504–6.

5 General Medical Council. Good Medical Practice. London. *GMC*, 2000.

6 Labrie F, Belanger A, Simand J *et al*. Combination therapy for prostate cancer. *Cancer* 1993; **71**: 1059–67.

7 Montie JE. The management of bladder outlet dysfunction due to prostate cancer, untreated and after endocrine treatment. *Prostate* 1992; **54**: 153.

8 Mommsen S, Petersen L. Transurethral catheter removal after bilateral orchidectomy for prostate carcinoma associated with acute urinary retention. *Scand J Urol Nephrol* 1993; **28**: 401–4.

9 Moul JW, Davis R, Vaccaro JA *et al*. Acute urinary retention associated with prostate carcinoma. *J Urol* 1989; 1375–7.

10 Arcangeli G, Micheli A, Verna L *et al*. Prognostic impact of transurethral resection on patients irradiated for localised prostate cancer. *Radiother Oncol*. 1995; **35**: 123–8.

11 Sandler HM, Hanks GE. Analysis of the possibility that transurethral resection promotes metastases in prostate cancer. *Cancer* 1988; **62**: 6222.

12 Doll HA, Black NA, Mc Pherson K *et al*. Mortality, morbidity and complications following transurethral resection of the prostate for benign prostatic hypertrophy. *J Urol* 1992; **147**: 1566–73.

13 Mebust WK, Holtgrewe HL *et al*. Transurethral prostatectomy: immediate and postoperative complications. A co-operative study of 13 participating institutions evaluating 3,885 patients. *J Urol* 1989; **141**: 243–7.

14 Booth CM, Chaudry AA, Lyth DR. Alternative prostatic treatments. Stent or catheter for the frail? *J Managed Care* 1997; **1**: 24–6.

15 Kaplan SA, Merrill DC *et al*. The titanium intraprostatic stent: the United States experience. *J Urol* 1993; **150**: 1624–9.

16 Kirby RS, Heard SR *et al*. Use of the ASI titanium stent in the management of bladder outflow obstruction. *J Urol* 1992; **148**: 1195–7.

17 Milroy E, Chapple CR. The urolume stent in the management of benign prostatic hyperplasia. *J Urol* 1993; **150**: 1630–5.

18 Anson KM, Barnes DG *et al*. Temporary prostatic stenting and androgen suppression: a new minimally invasive approach to malignant prostatic retention. *J R Soc Med* 1993; **86**: 634–6.

19 Perry MJA, Roodhouse AB *et al*. Thermo-expandable intraprostatic stents in bladder outlet obstruction: an 8 year study. *BJU* 2002; **90**: 216–23.

20 Guazzoni G, Montorsi F *et al*. Prostatic Urolume Wallstent for Urinary retention due to advanced prostate cancer. A 1 year follow-up. *J Urol* 1994; **152**: 1530–2.

21 Anjum MI, Palmer JH. A technique for removal of the Urolume endourethral wallstent prosthesis. *BJU* 1995; **76**: 655–6.

22 Nordling J, Ovensen H, Poulsen Al. The intraprostatic spiral: clinical results in 150 consecutive patients. *J Urol* 1992; **147**: 645–7.

23 Puppo P, Perachino M *et al*. Laparoscopic Bilateral Cutaneous Ureterostomy for Palliation of Ureteral Obstruction Caused by Advanced Pelvic Cancer. *J Endourol* 1994; **8**: 425–8.

24 Brin EN, Shiff M *et al*. Palliative urinary diversion form pelvic malignancy. *J Urol* 1975; **13**: 619–22.

25 Meyer J, Yatsuhashi M *et al*. Palliative urinary diversion in patients with advanced pelvic malignancy. *Cancer* 1980; **45**: 2698–701.

26 Sharer W, Grayhack J *et al*. Palliative urinary diversion for malignant ureteral obstruction. *J Urol* 1978; **120**: 162–6.

27 Fallon B, Olney L *et al.* Nephrostomy in cancer patients: to do or not to do? *Br J Urol* 1980; **52**: 237.

28 Chiou RK, Chang W *et al.* Ureteral obstruction associated with prostate cancer: the outcome after percutaneous nephrostomy. *J Urol* 1990; **143**: 957.

29 Kavoussi LR, Sosa E *et al.* Complications of laparoscopic pelvic lymph node dissection. *J Urol* 1993; **149**: 322.

30 Goodwin WE, Casey WC *et al.* Percutaneous trocar (needle) nephrostomy in hydronephrosis. *JAMA* 1955; **157**: 891–4.

31 Culkin DJ, Wheeler *et al.* Percutaneous nephrostomy for palliation of metastatic ureteral obstruction. *Urology* 1987; **30**: 229.

32 Holden S, McPhee M *et al.* The rationale of urinary diversion in cancer patients. *J Urol* 1990; **143**: 957.

33 Brin EN, Schiff M *et al.* Palliative urinary diversion for pelvic malignancy. *J Urol* 1975;**113**: 619.

34 Dowling RA, Carrasco CH *et al.* Percutaneous urinary diversion in patients with hormone refractory prostate cancer. *Urology* 1991; **37**: 89–91.

35 Feuer GA, Fruchter R *et al.* Selection for percutaneous nephrosotomy in gynaecological cancer patients. *Gynaecol Oncol* 1991; **42**: 60–3.

36 Harrington KJ, Pandha HS *et al.* Palliation of obstructive nephropathy due to malignancy. *Br J Urol* 1995; **76**: 101–7.

37 Paul AB, Love C *et al.* The management of bilateral ureteric obstruction and renal failure in advanced prostate cancer. *Br J Urol* 1994; **74**: 642–5.

38 Harding JR. Percutaneous antegrade ureteric stent insertion in malignant disease. *J Roy Soc Med* 1993; **86**: 511–3.

39 Docimo SG, Dewolf WC. High failure rate of indwelling ureteral stents in patients with extrinsic obstruction: experience at 2 institutions. *J Urol* 1989; **142**: 277.

40 Rackson ME, Mitty HA *et al.* Biocompatible copolymer ureteral stent: maintenance of patency beyond 6 months. *Am J Radiol* 1989; **153**: 783–4.

41 Liu JS, Hrebinko RL. The use of 2 ipsilateral stents for relief of ureteral obstruction from extrinsic compression. *J Urol* 1998; **159**: 179–81.

42 Ahmadzadeh M. Clinical experience with subcutaneous urinary diversion: new approach using a double pigtail stent. *Br J Urol* 1991; **67**: 596–9.

43 Minhas S, Irving H.Extra-anatomic stents in ureteric obstruction: experience and complications. *Br J Urol* 1999; **84**: 762–4.

44 Sigwart U, Puel J *et al.* Intravascular stents to prevent occlusion and restenosis after transluminal angioplasty. *New Engl. J Med* 1987; **316**: 701.

45 Adam A, Chetty N *et al.* Self expandable steel endoprosthesis for treatment of malignant bile duct obstruction. *Amer J Radiol* 1991; **156**: 321.

46 Guazzoni G, Pansadoro V *et al.* A modified prostatic Urolume Wallstent For healthy patients with symptomatic benign prostatic hyperplasia: a European multicenter study. *Urology* 1994; **44**: 364–70.

47 Milroy E, Allen A. Long-term results of Urolume urethral stent for recurrent urethral strictures *J Urol* 1996; **155**: 904–8.

48 Gort H, Mali W. Metallic self-expandable stenting of a ureteroileal stricture. *AJR* 1990; **155**: 422.

49 Pauer W, Lugmayr H. Metallic Wallstents: a new therapy for extrinsic ureteral obstruction. *J Urol* 1992; **148**: 281.

50 Wakui M, Takeuchi J. Metallic stents for malignant and benign ureteric obstruction. *Br J Urol* 2000; **85**: 227–32.

51 Ringel A, Richter S. Late complications of Ureteral stents. *Endourology* 2000; **38**: 41–44.

52 Barbalias G, Siablis D. Metal stents: A new treatment of malignant ureteral obstruction. *J Urol* 1997; **158**: 54–8.

53 Van Sonnenberg E, D'Agostino H. Malignant ureteral obstruction: treatment with metal stents – technique, results and observations with percutaneous intraluminal US. *Radiology* 1994; **191**: 764.

54 Fluekiger F, Lammer J *et al.* Malignant ureteral obstruction: treatment with metal stents: preliminary results of treatment with metallic self-expandable stents. *Radiology* 1993; **186**: 169.

17: Open Radical Prostatectomy: How Can Intra-operative, Peri-operative and Post-operative Complications Be Prevented?

Robert P. Myers, R. Houston Thompson, Stephen M. Schatz and Michael L. Blute

INTRODUCTION

Widespread testing of serum prostate-specific antigen (PSA) has led to an increased diagnosis of clinically localised prostate cancer. Most of the patients confirmed on subsequent biopsy to have localised prostate cancer will be asymptomatic with respect to their disease. Once the diagnosis is established, the prospect of any definitive treatment beyond conservative 'watchful waiting' raises possible diminution in health-related quality of life. For patients who elect surgery, peri-operative complications, including loss of life, must be considered and proper care taken to avoid them. Furthermore, surgical technique must be precise or patients may be saddled with any one of the feared long-term complications or serious functional deficits including urinary incontinence, erectile dysfunction and faecal soiling.

This chapter focuses on practical measures to reduce or prevent complications in open radical retropubic prostatectomy (RRP) and thus maximise return of health-related quality of life. Unique morbidity, specifically associated with other forms of radical prostatectomy, namely, radical perineal and laparoscopic, including robotic laparoscopic, are not addressed. However, many of the guidelines herein applicable to RRP can be readily applied to other approaches.

CURRENT COMPLICATION RATES

Since 1987, when PSA testing became widely used for prostate cancer screening, the number of RRPs performed has increased dramatically. Many of the complications associated with RRP, including the long-term health-related quality-of-life side effects, can be diminished with proper attention to surgical technique and peri-operative care. Blood loss varies from 530 to 1500 mL, depending on the reporting institution [1–5]. The remaining reported complications include rectal injury 0.05–2.9%, urethral injury 0–1.6%, deep venous thrombosis 0.6–7.8%, pulmonary complications (including embolus and acute respiratory distress syndrome) 0.7–2.7%, cardiovascular events (including myocardial infarction, arrhythmia or cerebrovascular accident) 0–1.8%, lymphocele 0.1–22.3% (maximum diagnosed with ultrasonography), urine leak 0.1–21.7%, wound complication (including infection) 0–2.6%, gastrointestinal effects (including protracted ileus, gastrointestinal bleed, ulcer disease and small bowel obstruction) 0.2–1.7%, nerve compression (brachial plexus and ulnar, radial, femoral, or peroneal nerves) injury 0.1–1.1% and peri-operative mortality 0–0.5%. These data show that the rate of complications of a specific nature is exceedingly low, but nevertheless present. For 11 522 patients older than 65 years who underwent RRP between 1992 and 1996, the peri-operative mortality was 0.5% and the approximate overall rate of 'post-operative complications' was 30%. Odd and exceedingly rare complications have been reported, including non-arteritic anterior ischemic optic neuropathy with visual loss [6], a complication possibly related to operating in an anaesthetic environment of deliberately controlled hypotension. In addition, hypotension is a particular risk to patients with aortic stenosis [7,8].

We recently reviewed our own institutional RRP complication rate, comparing intra-operative, early (≤30 days) and late (>30 days) complications [9]. This contemporary cohort included 1 860 consecutive patients who underwent RRP from January 1, 1999, through December 31, 2001. The total number of surgeons were 16, including the category 'chief resident'. Only seven of these surgeons performed more than 50 RRPs during the study period. There were no intra-operative or hospital deaths. Two patients (aged 70 and 77 years) died of a myocardial infarction in the early complication period. The hospital transfusion rate was 12%, and the rate of intra-operative rectal injury was less than 1%. Wound infection or separation was the most common early complication, occurring in 1.7% of patients. All other early complications, including myocardial infarction, deep venous thrombosis, pulmonary embolism, sepsis, urinary tract infection and urinary retention occurred in <1% of patients. Bladder neck contracture was the most common late complication, developing in 2.7% of patients. Other late complications, such as deep venous thrombosis, pulmonary embolism, pelvic abscess and lymphocele, occurred in <1% of patients.

In the same study, we assessed post-operative urinary continence but not erectile function. From the third-party, but not validated questionnaire used for the study, it was possible to extract single-surgeon (Robert P. Myers, MD) outcome with respect to urinary continence for 383 consecutive patients who underwent open RRP; this analysis showed a relationship between age and outcome. The message from the study is that older patients are more likely to require protective pads during the first 12 months after RRP (Table 17.1). Patients older than 70 years at operation often have visible striated urethral

Table 17.1 Urinary continence status ($n = 383$) at 1 year after RRP

Status	Age group										Total no. of Patients
	<55		≥55–<60		≥60–<65		≥65–<70		≥70		
	No.	%	No.	%	No.	%	No.	%	No.	%	
No pads required	82	96.47	89	97.80	75	89.29	85	93.41	27	84.38	358
Security pad	1	1.18	1	1.10	5	5.95	3	3.30	5	15.63	15
1–2 pads per day	1	1.18	1	1.10	3	3.57	3	3.30	0	0	8
≥3 pads per day	0	0	0	0	0	0	0	0	0	0	0
Artificial sphincter	0	0	0	0	0	0	0	0	0	0	0
Incontinence, not otherwise specified	1	1.18	0	0	1	1.19	0	0	0	0	2
Total	85		91		84		91		32		383

sphincter atrophy. This phenomenon in combination with greater detrusor instability in older patients in general is the likely cause for the observable increased need for pad protection in this age group.

In another retrospective questionnaire study approved by the Mayo Foundation Institutional Review Board, 187 of 211 consecutive patients (89%) undergoing bilateral nerve-bundle-preserving RRP by a single surgeon (R.P.M.) from August 1998 through September 1999 were assessed. The questionnaire mailed in September 2000 by the Mayo Clinic Survey Research Center simply asked whether patients were able to have successful intercourse and also whether they were using any assistance. The mean age of the patients was 57 years (range, 45–76 years), and the level of preoperative sexual function was not elicited. Of the 187 patients, 157 (84%) claimed satisfactory intercourse after RRP with or without erectile function assistance: 61% of the 157 replied they had no need for help, but 17% of these admitted to supplementary sildenafil for improved performance. Thus, only 44% were satisfied with nothing, 29% found sildenafil necessary, 7% needed intra-cavernosal pharmacotherapy and 3% were combining methods or using a vacuum device. This study provided a breakdown of aids with respect to achieving satisfactory intercourse, but it lacked the power of prospective assessment with a validated questionnaire and therefore, on this basis, was not submitted for potential inclusion in peer-reviewed literature.

Prospective studies have special merit [10–12], but no study to date is perfect for several reasons. An ideal study might include (1) a prospective assessment of erectile status, libido and partner availability; (2) a suitable number of consecutive patients; (3) a serial functional assessment to monitor changes over time; (4) use of validated questionnaires; (5) an objective measure of erectile function post-operatively; (6) an outcome of satisfactory intercourse, not just rigidity sufficient for penetration; (7) partner validation of reported results and (8) independent third-party control of data collection. The study by Catalona *et al.* [10] is notable for the sheer number of patients ($n = 1800$), but a validated questionnaire was not used. Walsh *et al.* [11] used a validated instrument and third-party control, but the study ceased after the accumulation of only 64 patients. Despite the best intentions, it is very difficult to achieve patient co-operation in research studies of such a sensitive nature. The study by Rabbani *et al.* [12] of 314 patients highlighted the status of pre-operative erectile function. By using Kaplan–Meier analysis, they determined outcomes based on those with pre-operative full erections, those with recently diminished erections and those with partial erections. This comparison is important because cross-sectional analysis shows progressive deterioration of sexual function with age: 26% with erectile dysfunction in men 50–59 years old and an increase to 40% in men 60–69 years old [13].

In considering patients potent only if they achieved unassisted intercourse, Chauveau *et al.* [14] reported 38% potent at 12 months, 56% at 18 months and 70% at 24 months in a study of 200 consecutive patients, who were potent pre-operatively. These results included 87% undergoing bilateral neurovascular bundle preservation and 13% unilateral. Furthermore, pre-operatively, 82% of patients claimed normal erectile function and 18% moderate erectile dysfunction. Use of a validated instrument was not mentioned, but the study gives a sense of what can be expected without the use of assistance, and the improvement after 1 year is remarkable. Noldus *et al.* [15], using the International Index of Erectile Function (IIEF5) in 406 patients with 'good pre-operative erections', showed that at 12 months after bilateral neurovascular bundle preservation, IIEF5 scores for degree of erectile dysfunction (ED) were 5–7 (severe ED) in 34.7%, 8–21 (moderate to mild ED) in 34.1%, and 22–25 (no ED) in 31.2% for ability to achieve unassisted intercourse. One concludes from these two studies that 1-year results are premature and that assistance of some form, for example, a phosphodiesterase-5 inhibitor (sildenafil, tadalafil, vardenafil), could theoretically improve the situation for many patients.

PATIENT SELECTION

The best way to minimise complications is to select patients who, by the nature of their general health, physical examination and laboratory data, are not only suitable but also ideal candidates for the procedure. It is well recognised that in the absence of serious competing morbidity, patients should be expected to have more than a 10-year life expectancy, barring some unforeseen incident. There is a prevalent notion that patients 70 years or older should not be offered RRP, but that cut-off is chronologic, not biologic. In general, it has been emphasised that men who are 70 years or older tend to die of diseases other than prostate cancer, a fact that has led many urologists to deny radical prostatectomy to men of this age [16]. However, Aus *et al.* [17] showed that patients in their 70s who were treated expectantly (watchful waiting) could expect to die of their disease at an alarming rate. Furthermore, a recent study concluded that age should not be a barrier to 'potentially curative therapy . . . for older men with few comorbidities and moderately or poorly differentiated localised prostate cancer' [18]. Patients up to an age of 80 years with poorly differentiated disease benefited in terms of both life expectancy and quality-adjusted life expectancy.

Before any operation is contemplated, the goal is to carefully assess for significant competing morbidity, including coronary artery disease, hypertension, diabetes, morbid obesity and sedentary lifestyle. Patients should pass the 'eyeball test', meaning that the 70-year-old who looks and acts like a 60-year-old is very likely a better candidate than a wisened 70-year-old who looks and acts like an 80-year-old. On digital rectal examination, the prostate should be mobile and the cancer palpably intra-capsular and sufficiently removed from the apex. Sulci lateral to the prostate should be free of significant extraprostatic extension. Palpable apical cancers are best not treated with radical prostatectomy because affected patients are almost certain to have significant positive apical margins and likely will need radiotherapy, anyway. Furthermore, wide resection of the apex poses a substantial risk of subsequent and unacceptable urinary incontinence. Prostates with large palpable cancers judged to be close to the capsular surface, the bladder base, or apex, fixation denoting extra-capsular extension (T3 disease) with discrete loss of portions of peripheral sulci on digital rectal examination, high pre-biopsy PSA values or multiple bilateral positive cores on biopsy may all augur positive surgical margins. Moreover, large-volume cancers are widely recognised to have a much higher incidence of seminal vesical invasion and lymph node metastasis, both of which, similar to a high Gleason score, are independent predictors of treatment failure.

PATIENT PREPARATION

Timing of the operation relative to the date of the biopsy is important. Very simply, patients should tolerate operation and recover their pre-operative vigour more quickly if they seek to achieve the best physical condition possible pre-operatively. Post-biopsy inflammatory adhesion of the prostate to adjacent tissues obliterates otherwise easily developed tissue planes. There-fore, it is prudent to delay operation for 6 to 8 weeks after biopsy to re-establish the critical tissue planes between the neurovascular bundles and prostate capsule, as well as the plane between the rectal surface and the pro-statoseminal vesicular (Denonvilliers') fascia. The ability to achieve negative surgical margins and recovery of both urinary control and erectile function is directly related to the ease with which the prostate and seminal vesicles can be extracted without damage to the distal striated and smooth muscle urethral sphincters and the neurovascular bundles.

The waiting period also allows the patient to engage in cardiovascular conditioning with an aerobic exercise program and weight loss, if neces-sary. An exception might include performing the operation in a fit patient within a week of biopsy before the development of significant peri-prostatic inflammation.

All patients should undergo a thorough medical evaluation to determine their tolerability of general anaesthesia. For sedentary patients with suspec-ted borderline coronary artery disease, a functional cardiac study should be considered to evaluate for sub-clinical ischemia. Occasionally, but not surprisingly, patients in this age group wanting prostate removal may find themselves undergoing coronary artery stent placement.

If the patient has a Gleason score of 7 or more, bicalutamide 50 mg per day with its known minimal adverse effects on erectile function might be considered before RRP. Although there is no current randomised, prospect-ive study to justify its efficacy, bicalutamide has the potential to both arrest cancer growth during the 6- to 8-week waiting period and to pacify the anxi-eties of the patient and spouse or partner. Patients should be forewarned that breast tenderness might develop.

EXERCISE AND DIET

During the 6- to 8-week period after biopsy, patients should be encouraged to pursue a programme of cardiovascular conditioning and diet to be as thin as possible between the navel and pubis on the day of operation. Patients should be told that being thin significantly improves access to the prostate and makes the operation technically easier. No surgeon enjoys working at the bottom of a well. Furthermore, smokers should be encouraged to quit; nicotine skin patches or nicotine-containing chewing gum may facilitate the process.

A daily aerobic exercise programme is proposed to the patient to reduce the incidence of intra-operative cardiovascular and anaesthetic complica-tions, to speed post-operative recovery, and thereby to allow return to work as soon as possible. For those who lead sedentary lives, such a programme

---

Box 17.1 *Suggestions for exercise before RRP*

1. Fast walking up to 3 miles per day with good hiking shoes (include walking up and down hills, if possible)
2. Use of a treadmill at a rate of 3 to 3.5 mph up to 30 min twice a day. Younger patients may want to increase their rate to 4 to 4.5 mph during a portion of their 30 min programme
3. For patients who know how to swim and are confident of their swimming ability, breaststroke laps in a local swimming pool at least 30 min per day. Swimming is particularly advantageous for patients with arthritis in knees or hips who need weight-bearing restriction
4. Stair climbing, stepping machine, stationary cross-country ski machine and stationary bicycle may be appropriate activities for some individuals

---

should be introduced with caution and not adopted too suddenly. The patient's goal then is to increase cardiovascular endurance gradually and thereby avoid fatal stress on the heart. If there is any question about exercise limitation, patients should consult their general physician and in some cases obtain the advice of a cardiologist. Personal trainers can help the physically unfit. Some patients will require β-adrenergic blockers.

Suggested forms of exercise to 'burn' calories and to improve fitness for patients who are able are included in Box 17.1.

For the morbidly obese patient who is at greater risk for peri-operative complications, dietary calorie restriction (Box 17.2) (including reduction of carbohydrates, especially refined sugar and fat) may benefit both the intra-operative and peri-operative course.

IMMEDIATE PRE-OPERATIVE MEASURES

An orderly transition from outside the hospital to the operating room involves some simple guidelines. The patient should be advised to stay well hydrated. The patient should eat a soft diet on the day before operation and should be told, 'If you have to chew it, don't eat it'. This step will ease the resumption of normal bowel movements post-operatively. If the surgeon is inexperienced, a mechanical bowel preparation, including antibiotics, should be used so that the rectum, if entered, can be closed primarily and, in most cases, save the patient from a temporary colostomy. If the surgeon has exceptional experience, a phophosoda enema programme (until clean) may be sufficient, if rectal entry is not a significant risk. Necessary oral

---

Box 17.2 *Dietary suggestions when weight reduction is paramount to prepare for surgery*

Breakfast: bowl of oatmeal with sliced banana and skimmed milk.

Lunch and dinner: vegetables emphasised: green beans, peas, carrots, tomatoes, leaf spinach, broccoli, cauliflower, lettuce, cabbage. (Avoid starchy vegetables such as squash.) Boiled lentils (mung beans or mung dahl) are an excellent protein source. Eat modest portions of a relatively low glycemic rice, such as basmati, as the main carbohydrate, not pasta or bread

   Meat choices: chicken, white meat and skinless; fish, broiled; pork tenderloin, broiled

   Avoid milk products except for skim milk

   Drink plenty of water and do not become dehydrated

Dessert: single piece of fresh fruit, for example, an apple, a pear or a peach

Add daily multivitamin if not taking one

Avoid: potatoes, buttered bread, fried food, fast food, pastries, pizza, ice cream, honey, chocolate, mayonnaise, oil, red meat including pork (except for pork tenderloin), nuts, chips, sugar-containing soda pop and alcohol

---

medications for comorbidities, for example, a β-adrenergic blocker, should be taken on the morning of operation with a sip of water. Most hospitals have special protocols for patients with diabetes. All patients should be instructed to come to the hospital in clean clothes after being fully showered or bathed with soap and shampoo. Fingernails and toenails should be cleaned and trimmed.

ANAESTHESIA PREPARATION

The method of anaesthesia used for RRP largely depends on the preference of the surgeon, anaesthesiologist and patient, with no strong evidence supporting one method over another. Reports that epidural anaesthesia is associated with less blood loss have not been substantiated [19]. General endotracheal anaesthesia is most commonly used for RRP at the authors' institution, but some urologists use a spinal anaesthetic and general anaesthesia in a programme of pre-emptive analgesia (see below).

   Mortality from anaesthesia alone is rare. The rate of death due solely to anaesthesia is about 1 in 200 000 patients [20]. Adverse respiratory events, including inadequate ventilation, oesophageal intubation and aspiration, account for the majority of anaesthetic deaths [21]. In non-cardiac surgery, between 0.1% and 0.7% of patients have a myocardial infarction [22,23]. Patients with a history of myocardial infarction are at significantly greater risk for reinfarction, occurring in 4–6% after 6 months of myocardial stabilisation [22,23]. It is not advisable to perform RRP within 6 months of myocardial infarction. Peri-operative β-adrenergic blockade reduces cardiac morbidity and mortality in patients at risk for coronary artery disease [24]. Cardiac risk factors include age above 65 years, hypertension, history of smoking, hypercholesterolemia and diabetes mellitus. Adverse drug reactions, including malignant hyperthermia and anaphylaxis, are other potential serious anaesthetic concerns.

Peri-operative blood transfusions are needed in about 1 in 10 patients undergoing RRP. With the advent of nucleic acid testing, the risk of infectious transmission of known viruses is rare. Mathematical models now estimate transmission rates per unit of blood to be 1 in 220 000 for hepatitis B virus, 1 in 1 600 000 for hepatitis C virus and 1 in 1 800 000 for human immunodeficiency virus [25]. With improved anatomical dissection and control of the dorsal vascular complex [26], severe blood loss is rare, and most patients do not require invasive monitoring such as a central venous catheter or arterial line. Invasive anaesthetic monitoring may have adverse effects and should not be used without a good indication. In general, most patients who are appropriate candidates for RRP should not require invasive monitoring.

IN-HOSPITAL MEASURES

All patients should conform to a careful administrative admissions protocol that includes a confirmed recent satisfactory history and physical examination.

1 All patients should enter the operating room well hydrated to minimise hypotension during induction. This may require that intra-venous fluids be given well before the patient actually enters the operating room.

2 Consider, on call to the operating room, a systemic broad-spectrum antibiotic, for example, an intra-venously administered cephalosporin, if no known allergy, and an antacid regimen to prevent post-operative gastric or duodenal ulcer disease.

3 For relatively quick dismissal from hospital, generally in 24–48 h, with minimal post-operative pain or narcotic requirement and subsequent rapid dietary progression, consider an anesthesia program that includes pre-emptive analgesia. (One such programme used at our institution currently includes a spinal anaesthetic with bupivacaine 0.75% 2 mL, clonidine 50 μg and hydromorphone 40 μg.) After endotracheal intubation, patients

then require only light levels of sevoflurane or isoflurane, nitrous oxide and oxygen as a general anaesthetic. Cisatracurium is used as a systemic skeletal muscle relaxant. Ketorolac 15 to 30 mg is given intra-muscularly on induction and at the end of the procedure and then intra-venously every 6 h for 48 h. Ketorolac is alternated with 1 g of acetaminophen orally every 6 h so that the patient receives an analgesic every 3 h until dismissal. Nausea and pruritus are countered by prophylactic dexamethasone 8 mg intra-venously at the beginning of the procedure and then with ondansetron 4 mg intra-venously when the prostate is removed. The short-acting opioid fentanyl, 25 μg intra-venously, is used as needed for breakthrough pain. The spinal anaesthetic at the appropriate vertebral level provides sympathetic blockade, spares the parasympathetic autonomic nervous system and allows patients to eat and drink with very rapid dietary progression to solid food. Patient-controlled narcotic analgesia is discouraged because it provokes ileus and delays dismissal. For patients who cannot tolerate ketorolac, tramadol 50–75 mg every 6 h may be a suitable alternative. Acetaminophen 0.5–1.0 g orally as needed every 6 hours is recommended as outpatient postoperative analgesia, but patients sometimes require something stronger, such as propoxyphene napsylate with acetaminophen 1–2 pills orally every 6 h as needed.

Throughout the operation and in the immediate post-operative period, an active programme should be instituted to prevent lower extremity and pelvic venous thromboembolism. This should include a support hose up to mid-thigh, leg elevation ('heels higher than heart'), active leg and ankle movement in bed and early ambulation. Although useful sometimes, passive compression devices may discourage leg movement. If used, they must be adjusted properly to minimise the risk of inducing compartment syndrome.

Patients who require warfarin anticoagulation daily are a special perioperative challenge to the surgeon. Those at risk for thromboembolic complications with cessation of anticoagulation usually can be divided into low- and high-risk groups (Box 17.3). In general, patients are asked to discontinue use of clopidogrel (Plavix) 14 days before RRP, aspirin and ticlopidine (Ticlid) 7–10 days before RRP, and non-steroidal anti-inflammatory agents 3–4 days before RRP. Dipyridamole (Persantine) and pentoxifylline (Trental) use does not need to be discontinued. An international normalised ratio of 1.4 or less is adequate for near-normal hemostasis. Anticoagulation can be initiated as soon as 8 h after RRP provided that the haemoglobin level is stable and haematuria is absent. Generally, patients in the low-risk group can discontinue use of warfarin 5 days before RRP and initiate its use without a loading dose the evening after RRP. Warfarin usually takes 2–3 days to be therapeutic and can be a procoagulant initially.

Box 17.3 *Risk of thrombotic complications after cessation of warfarin therapy*

Low risk
  Isolated aortic valve prosthesis
  Deep venous thrombosis more than 3 months ago
  Asymptomatic atrial fibrillation
  Left ventricular aneurysm
  Congestive heart failure with left ventricular dilatation
  Inferior vena cava filter
  Peripheral synthetic vascular graft
High risk
  Mitral valve prosthesis
  Deep venous thrombosis less than 3 months ago
  Atrial fibrillation with other cardiovascular co-morbidities (cerebro-vascular accident, transient ischaemic attack, thrombus)
  Inherited thrombotic deficiency (such as antiphospholipid, factor V Leiden)
  Any two or more of the low-risk group

Peri-operative low molecular weight heparin can be used on an outpatient basis, the last pre-operative dose being given at least 24 h before RRP. We emphasise that peri-operative anticoagulation often must be individualised and communication with the patient's primary care physician, cardiologist or thrombophilia specialist is required [26–28].

ON THE OPERATING ROOM TABLE

Fastidious supine positioning will prevent nerve-related injury. Flexing the table enhances pelvic exposure; however, over-flexion may produce severe post-operative lumbosacral nerve root irritation. Patients then should be queried pre-operatively about the status of their low back. Arms should not be placed straight out at 90° but should rest well supported at an angle of approximately 30° from straight out in order to prevent brachial plexus stretch and injury. Elbows and forearms should be luxuriously padded to protect the ulnar and median nerves. Straps used to immobilise the lower legs should avoid the peroneal nerves and thus prevent footdrop.

INTRA-OPERATIVE MEASURES

Technical ability and the technique used are absolutely crucial to achieving the well-recognised outcomes of (1) negative surgical margins, (2) pad-free

(a)

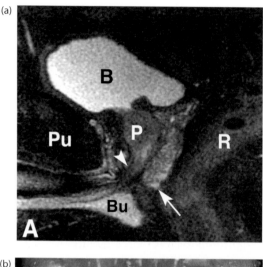

(b)

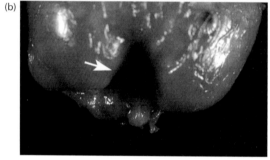

Fig. 17.1 (a), Posterior lip-anterior apical notch prostate apex as seen in 3-Tesla coil mid-sagittal T2-weighted MRI. Lip extends distally behind sphincteric (membranous) urethra, thereby complicating optimal urethral transection. B, bladder; Pu, pubis; P, prostate; Bu, bulb; R, rectum; arrowhead, urethra; arrow, posterior apical lip of prostate. (b), Radical prostatectomy specimen with anterior apical notch and posterior lip (arrow) that complicated the satisfactory release of and preservation of an adequate urethral stump.

urinary control and (3) resumption of erectile function at presurgical capacity. RRP is a very challenging operation. Complicating factors include (1) exogenous obesity, (2) deep android pelvis with narrow pubic arch, (3) anterior aberrant or accessory pudendal arteries that should be saved, (4) atypical, profuse, large dorsal vein and peri-prostatic venous plexus, (5) prostate gland size less than 15 g or more than 80 g, (6) sphincteric (membranous) urethral length less than 1.5 cm and (7) anterior apical notch-posterior lip prostate apex [29] (Fig. 17.1). This apical configuration variant may be responsible for most cases of post-operative stress incontinence because the urethra has been transected at a point too distal and significant sphincteric tissue situated on the posterior lip is inadvertently sacrificed.

If radical prostatectomy is to be done by the open retropubic approach, the incision should be substantial enough to allow the surgeon to palpate the apex of the prostate with both index fingers. Apical configuration (such as doughnut versus croissant [29]) then can be appreciated before and during apical dissection. Once the incision is made, any abdominal wall retractor should be placed with thought to prevent compression injury of femoral and lateral femoral cutaneous nerves.

During pelvic lymphadenectomy, thought must be given to avoid vascular, ureteral and obturator nerve injury. Compulsive occlusion of lymphatics will help avert subsequent lymphocele formation.

Control of what is popularly known as the dorsal vein complex of the penis is more accurately termed control of the 'pudendal vascular complex anterior to the prostatourethral junction'. Veins in this location exist in a sinusoidal network with arteries of variable calibre and some tiny nerves. Frequently observable asymmetry with respect to the underlying prostate is captured in Müller's 'plexus pubicus impar', 'impar' meaning unequal [30]. Meticulous haemostasis will minimise the need for transfusion and allow clear visualisation of the critical apical dissection and mobilisation of the nerve bundles as intact as possible. How vascular control is conducted may affect return of erectile function. Aberrant pudendal arteries in the 2- to 4-mm calibre range should be preserved. But, in some cases, there may be several even smaller arteries that are sacrificed; their attrition in the act of haemostasis may play a role in post-operative erectile dysfunction. Erectile dysfunction sometimes blamed on 'venous leak' may be the result of compromised arterial inflow.

Individual variation at the apex with respect to vessels, nerves and prostate parenchymal configuration in relation to the striated urethral sphincter demands adequate exposure and visualisation of prostate size and contour. This is aided by bunching the pre-prostatic pudendal vascular plexus and intervening detrusor apron into a mid-line bundle anterior to the anterior commissure (isthmus) of the prostate [31,32]. One or two long 'sponge sticks', held either by the surgeon or assistant depending on the situation, are very useful to retract and to rotate the prostate in the axial, coronal or sagittal plane, depending on what is needed to visualise precisely the point of dissection. In the course of dissection, the croissant versus dough nut apex or other variations should be appreciated and steps taken to optimise urethral transection. The goal should be to deliver a cylinder of urethral stump that protrudes cephalad from the point of entry of the neurovascular bundles. We recommend the optimal transection point to be through the urethral wall 5 mm proximal to the beginning of the striated urethral sphincter. This means that subsequent individual anastomotic sutures will be embedded in the proximal 5 mm of urethral wall and only 2–3 mm of striated urethral sphincter. For visualisation of the optimal transection point, it may be necessary to retract the prostate in the mid-line away from the urethra once the prostatourethral junction is clearly determined. This is easier when an element of benign prostatic hyperplasia is present.

Preservation of the neurovascular bundles at the apex is critical in the nerve-sparing operation. The bundles should be identified at the prostatourethral junction and carefully released so that the urethra can be circumscribed and isolated with a vascular tape before urethral transection. During mobilisation of the prostate from the rectal surface and away from the posterolateral neurovascular bundles, the prostate is palpated between thumb and forefinger for any suspicious induration close to the capsule and the neurovascular bundle, a manoeuvre that thereby allows appropriate wider resection. With a guiding index finger interposed between the rectal surface and prostatoseminal vesicular (Denonvilliers') fascia, the neurovascular bundle is thus allowed to roll-off the posterolateral prostate with minimal stretching or injury to the bundle itself. The roll-off is facilitated with blunt push-off using a small right-angle forceps or Kitner dissector. In this manoeuvre, care must be taken not to enter inadvertently the plane between benign prostatic hyperplasia and the peripheral zone of the prostate.

Final intra-operative commentary relates to successful vesicourethral anastomosis after resection of the prostate from the vesical neck. We recommend mucosal eversion and plication of the bladder neck to a calibre no less than 24 to 26 Ch. The subsequent anastomosis must be watertight and the catheter irrigated at the end of the procedure to confirm no leakage before wound closure. Any extravasation of urine into the pelvis increases the risk of subsequent vesical neck contracture. For anastomosis, use monofilament suture (for example, 00 or 000 poliglecaprone [Monocryl]) is used and a slip-slip-square-square knot tie-down is done of each anastomotic suture with the index fingernail against the urethra about 1 cm beyond the knot. Tension to snug each individual throw is applied with the up hand, not with the down or lead hand. Tie-down should be tension free, and perineal pressure may help. Tying over the Foley balloon on traction is to be avoided, because the tie-down may be more difficult and less certain. The more substantial anterior sutures should be tied first because tension will then be relieved from the more tenuous posterior sutures. To relieve tension during the tie-down, an assistant can hold a Babcock clamp that grasps the catheter through the wall of the bladder distal to the balloon and 5 cm proximal to the bladder neck. The assistant then approximates the bladder neck to the urethral stump, which is made more visible by simultaneous perineal pressure from another assistant's sponge stick applying cephalad pressure to the perineal skin overlying the pubic arch.

The more sutures used for anastomosis, the more likely the development of a ring of fibrosis. Four sutures placed at the 2-, 5-, 7- and 10-o'clock positions should be sufficient for a watertight anastomosis and to protect full-length urethral stump viability. The sutures should avoid the neurovascular bundles and the adjacent levator muscle that is involved in the quick stop of urination and the support of the vesicourethral anastomosis [33]. Anastomotic sutures placed first at the bladder neck outside-in and then into the urethral stump inside-out using a smooth indwelling 18-F urethral Van Buren sound avoids the trauma of a larger grooved sound. Rotation of a grooved sound may damage natural mucosal infoldings (mucosal seal aspect of the distal continence mechanism). Furthermore, sounds larger than 18 to 20 Ch may unduly stretch urethral wall's elastic tissue and delay time to pad-free status. The indwelling urethral Foley catheter diameter should then be 20 Ch or less.

A temporary closed-system placement of pelvic drains not only will help to prevent lymphocele formation after pelvic lymphadenectomy but also will drain urine in the event of unsatisfactory anastomosis.

POST-OPERATIVE MEASURES

In addition to the in-hospital measures mentioned above, there is the question of the proper timing for drain and catheter removal. It is recommended that drains stay in place until there is less than 20 mL per drain per 48 h. The current popular movement is to remove the Foley catheter as soon as possible. However, early catheter removal is associated with catheter re-insertion in some patients and the need for cystography, both of which can be avoided by adhering to normal principles of wound healing. Approximately 50% of collagen will be laid down by 9 days and 100% by 14 to 17 days, and beginning collagen remodelling and strengthening in most cases will occur by day 21. Most patients should do well if their catheters are removed in 18 to 21 days post-operatively without need for any secondary procedures. Patients should be taught to apply 0.5% to 1% hydrocortisone plus broad-spectrum antibiotic creams daily to the urethral meatus to prevent stenosis.

When the catheter is removed, some patients will have immediate control but others will take longer. Patients should be encouraged to perform sets of pelvic floor exercises (puborectalis–bulbospongiosus contractions), preferably before bed and not throughout the entire day so as to fatigue the muscle in a counterproductive way. If present, detrusor hyperreflexia sometimes can be ameliorated by prescribing oxybutynin 2.5 mg paired with imipramine 10 mg orally three times per day.

REFERENCES

1 Shekarriz B, Upadhyay J, Wood DP. Intraoperative, perioperative, and long-term complications of radical prostatectomy. *Urol Clin North Am* 2001; **28**: 639–53.

2 Lerner SE, Blute ML, Lieber MM, Zincke H. Morbidity of contemporary radical retropubic prostatectomy for localized prostate cancer. *Oncology (Huntingt)* 1995; **9**: 379–82.

3 Dillioglugil O, Leibman BD, Leibman NS, Kattan MW, Rosas AL, Scardino PT. Risk factors for complications and morbidity after radical retropubic prostatectomy. *J Urol* 1997; **157**: 1760–7.

4 Lepor H, Nieder AM, Ferrandino MN. Intraoperative and postoperative complications of radical retropubic prostatectomy in a consecutive series of 1,000 cases. *J Urol* 2001; **166**: 1729–33.

5 Begg CB, Riedel ER, Bach PB *et al.* Variations in morbidity after radical prostatectomy. *N Engl J Med* 2002; **346**: 1138–44.

6 Williams GC, Lee AG, Adler HL *et al.* Bilateral anterior ischemic optic neuropathy and branch retinal artery occlusion after radical prostatectomy. *J Urol* 1999; **162**: 1384–5.

7 Stoelting RK, Dierdorf SF (eds.). *Anesthesia and co-existing disease*, 3rd edn. Churchill Livingstone, New York, 1993.

8 Benumof JL, Saidman LJ (eds.). *Anesthesia and perioperative complications*, 2nd edn. Mosby, St. Louis, Mo, 1999.

9 Schenk GS, Zincke H, Slezak JM, Bergstralh EJ, Blute ML. Updated morbidity of radical retropubic prostatectomy for localized prostate cancer [abstract]. *J Urol* 2004; **171**: 212–3.

10 Catalona WJ, Carvalhal GF, Mager DE, Smith DS. Potency, continence and complication rates in 1870 consecutive radical retropubic prostatectomies. *J Urol* 1999; **162**: 433–8.

11 Walsh PC, Marschke P, Ricker D, Burnett AL. Patient-reported urinary continence and sexual function after anatomic radical prostatectomy. *Urology* 2000; **55**: 58–61.

12 Rabbani F, Stapleton AM, Kattan MW, Wheeler TM, Scardino PT. Factors predicting recovery of erections after radical prostatectomy. *J Urol* 2000; **164**: 1929–34.

13 Bacon CG, Mittleman MA, Kawachi I, Giovannucci E, Glasser DB, Rimm EB. Sexual function in men older than 50 years of age: results from the Health Professionals Follow-up Study. *Ann Intern Med* 2003; **139**: 161–8.

14 Chauveau P, Barre C, Herve P. Predictive factors of potency recovery after nerve-sparing (NS) radical retropubic prostatectomy (RRP) [abstract]. *J Urol* 2003; **169**; 441.

15 Noldus J, Palisaar J, Michl UG, Graefen M, Haese A, Huland H. Potency after radical retropubic prostatectomy (RRP): evaluation using the IIEF5 questionnaire (index of erectile function) [abstract]. *J Urol* 2003; **169**: 438.

16 Corriere JN Jr, Cornog JL, Murphy JJ. Prognosis in patients with carcinoma of the prostate. *Cancer* 1970; **25**: 911–8.

17 Aus G, Hugosson J, Norlen L. Long-term survival and mortality in prostate cancer treated with noncurative intent. *J Urol* 1995; **154**: 460–5.

18 Alibhai SM, Naglie G, Nam R, Trachtenberg J, Krahn MD. Do older men benefit from curative therapy of localized prostate cancer? *J Clin Oncol* 2003; **21**: 3318–27.

19 Shir Y, Raja SN, Frank SM, Brendler CB. Intraoperative blood loss during radical retropubic prostatectomy: epidural versus general anesthesia. *Urology* 1995; **45**: 993–9.

20 Eichhorn JH. Prevention of intraoperative anesthesia accidents and related severe injury through safety monitoring. *Anesthesiology* 1989; **70**: 572–7.

21 Tiret L, Desmonts JM, Hatton F, Vourc'h G. Complications associated with anaesthesia: a prospective survey in France. *Can Anaesth Soc J* 1986; **33**: 336–44.

22 Mangano DT. Perioperative cardiac morbidity. *Anesthesiology* 1990; **72**: 153–84.

23 Roberts SL, Tinker JH. Perioperative myocardial infarction. In: Gravenstein N, Kirby RR, eds. *Complications in anesthesiology*, 2nd edn. Lippincott-Raven, Philadelphia, 1996, 335–49.

24 Mangano DT, Layug EL, Wallace A, Tateo I, for the Multicenter Study of Perioperative Ischemia Research Group. Effect of atenolol on mortality and cardiovascular morbidity after noncardiac surgery. *N Engl J Med.* 1996; **335**: 1713–20. Erratum in: *N Engl J Med* 1997; **336**: 1039.

25 Busch MP, Kleinman SH, Nemo GJ. Current and emerging infectious risks of blood transfusions. *JAMA* 2003; **289**: 959–62.

26 Heit JA. Perioperative management of the chronically anticoagulated patient. *J Thromb Thrombolysis* 2001; **12**: 81–7.

27 Brown JA, Heit JA, Novicki DE. Urologic Surgery and the Anticoagulated Patient, *AUA Update Series – Lesson 19* 1998; **17**: 146–51.

28 Rosenblum N, Lepor H. Radical retropubic prostatectomy: preoperative management. *Urol Clin North Am* 2001; **28**: 499–507.

29 Myers RP. Practical surgical anatomy for radical prostatectomy. *Urol Clin North Am* 2001; **28**: 473–90.

30 Müller J. *Über die organischen Nerven der erectilen männlichen Geschlectsorgane des Menschen und der Säugethiere.* (Concerning the autonomic nerves of the male erectile genital organs of man and mammals.) Berlin: F. Dummler, 1836.

31 Myers RP. The surgical management of prostate cancer: radical retropubic and radical perineal prostatectomy. In Lepor H, ed. *Prostatic diseases*, W. B. Saunders Company, Philadelphia, 2000, 410–43.

32 Myers RP. Detrusor apron, associated vascular plexus, and avascular plane: relevance to radical retropubic prostatectomy: anatomic and surgical commentary. *Urology* 2002; **59**: 472–9.

33 Myers RP, Cahill DR, Kay PA, *et al.* Puboperineales: muscular boundaries of the male urogenital hiatus in 3D from magnetic resonance imaging. *J Urol* 2000; **164**: 1412–5.

18: Documenting Prostate Cancer: Epidemiology and Treatment

Leslie Moffat

For thousands of years, governments have required to know basic statistics about their people. Censuses were well known in Roman times, we have it on good authority that one of the first early and important censuses was carried out during the reign of Caesar Augustus, and the reason was stated that the world was to be taxed! It is likely that taxation and military service provided the main stimulus for this type of recording.

The system of registration of deaths in England and Wales started as a result of the Births and Deaths Registration Act of 1836 [1]. Failure to registrar a death became the subject of possible penalty some 38 years later. This then allowed mortality data to be compiled from the cause of death stated by the informant to the Registrar. There is provision for a change in the cause of death after the performance of a post-mortem. The informant must give details of the deceased' place and date of birth, occupation and usual address. These figures thus allow epidemiological information (*epi* – upon or among, *demos* – the people, *logos* – study) and this allows interested parties to describe disease, in terms of its natural history and possible risk factors, trend prediction and look at the effects of any form of intervention. In terms of deriving incidence data, it is important that the total number of people at potential risk of the disease is known before an incidence risk and a prevalence rate can be calculated.

CANCER REGISTRATION

With Cancer Registration originally, the authorities merely wished to know the causes of death where there were possible implications, in terms of accidents or potential murders. In England, the Ministry of Health set up a system in 1923 to follow up patients treated with radium [1]. A Radium Commission was set up in 1947, and finally it was agreed that

On behalf of Scottish Urological Cancer Audit (SUCA).

epidemiological studies and the causes of cancer should be added to cancer registration.

A scheme for cancer registration was started around 1958, but it was not until 1962 that this extended to regions in England and Wales, when a national scheme was started. The data was collected through regional cancer registries, which then forwarded the material to OPCS in England and Wales and to the Information Services Division of the Common Services Agency in Scotland. The Cancer Registration Scheme started in Northern Ireland in 1959 [1]. From 1971 onwards, cancer patients were registered on the NHS Central Register. This simple system allows the calculation of survival for all patients with cancer.

From time to time, efforts have been made to check the completeness of data and although the percentage of total cases continues to rise, registration is usually achieved by a linkage of multiple source records, using probability matching, followed by manual verification of diagnosis and other variables by Cancer Registration Officers in the field [2].

In Scotland, dates of death supplied by the Registrar General for Scotland are added to the cancer file on a continuous basis by registration staff both for Scotland and for those who died elsewhere. Upto four causes of death are added to the Cancer Registration File and once again probability matching issues. The NHS Central Registrar is available to reduce the number of lost-traces of registration through, for example, emigration and linkage failure [3]. Further systems have been developed using hospital activity analysis (HAA) and this has been shown to increase registration rates. Statistics are necessary to show where an attribution of death is by death certificate only (DCO) or takes into account other factors, such as post-mortem.

INTERNATIONAL CANCER REGISTRATION

Examining the coverage of world population, there has been a drive to stand-ardise registration methods and definitions of registration and coding. The International Classification of Diseases (ICD) has been the most extensive classification system of all diseases, including cancers and appears to have stood the test of time.

In any study, it is necessary to state which ICD codes were used with which set of data since definitions have been added to and occasionally changed. It is therefore necessary when comparing data from different coun-tries, to ensure that the classification used in incidence tables is the same. Although it is not a problem for prostate cancer, it is important that all histological groups are compared on an equal basis.

It is also necessary to establish whether a cancer has been detected by chance at post-mortem, or whether it has presented as a clinical problem.

Sometimes this can lead to re-coding of data, where new data becomes available. Cancer Registration is therefore a dynamic process and incidence rates may appear to change when new data becomes available.

Registries tend to include tumours diagnosed during screening programmes and this effect was seen when mammographic screening for cancer was introduced. This effect was also noted in the United Kingdom and other countries when trans-urethral prostatectomy (TURP) became more popular and some small asymptomatic cancers were detected at histological examination [4,5].

Completeness of registration of cases is a major problem and also steps must be taken to avoid duplicate registration of the same case. There are ways of assessing the completeness of data and various indices can be used such as the proportion of cases histologically verified, the mortality to incidence ratio, the stability of incidence rates over time and incidences in different populations. In addition, age-specific incidence can be generated [5].

Quality Control

Quality control can be carried out to check the validity of the proportion of cases and a data set, which truly have the feature that is recorded and this can be examined in terms of internal consistency, histological verification, attested by death certificate only disease and patients with unknown ages.

A census has taken place every 10 years in the United Kingdom since 1801, with the exception of 1941. The 1991 census was the first to include a question on ethnic groups. The non-white population comprises of around 6% of the population of the United Kingdom [6].

Postcodes in the United Kingdom

Postcode is based on an eight-character designation. The first two letters indicate the postcode of the area, which are 120 in the country. The next two numbers are the postcode of the district. The next number is the postcode sector within a district and the final two letters indicate the geographical area, with around 15 houses. Postcodes can therefore be used for very close analysis of geographical location.

Deprivation Measures

Because it is now possible to localise areas of residence, it is possible to identify areas that are considered to be deprived. There are a number of such deprivation indices and the names of Townsend and Garman are relatively well known [7,8].

Death Certification and Cause of Death in the United Kingdom

The death certificate is divided into two parts. The first part asks for the direct cause of death, along with any other conditions leading to the direct cause of death – Parts 1a, 1b and 1c. Part two requests significant contributing conditions, but that are not directly a consequence of death.

Crude-Death Rate

Crude-death rate measures the number of deaths that take place in a period, per 1000 of the population. The mid-year population is used, and this single figure is derived by comparison with mortality within an area over a period. If the age and sex structure of the population change, the results may vary and this is the main disadvantage. This method does not allow group comparison between different areas with respect to age distribution.

Standardised rates

Standardisation allows comparison of two or more populations using a single standardised death rate, where allowance has been made for the age structure of the population [6]. The standardised mortality ratio (SMR) is the ratio of the observed death to the expected deaths and is expressed as a percentage. The standard population has an SMR of 100% and the observed and the expected deaths are the same. This allows a detailed comparison of geographical areas, taking into account the different age structure.

Hospital-Based Systems

Data can be collected on a number of deaths in the hospital, but this is clearly the imperfect system of comparison, in that the caseload and the severity of disease in one hospital may be very much greater than in another. In particular, patients may be referred who are more seriously ill or have been referred for major procedures that are not available in smaller hospitals.

Hospital Episode Statistics

This data was developed particularly in response to purchaser provider and can record the number of finished consultant episodes (FCE's) with respect to disease group.

Korner Data

This is the main system in the United Kingdom for recording health service activity, named after the Chairman of the Steering Group, it collects information on a wide range of patient activities in hospitals in England. It allows comparison of activity between different hospitals.

International Classification of Diseases

The World Health Organisation arranged an International Classification of Diseases (ICD) and related to health problems. This has gone through many revisions and the current revision of the ICD is known as ICD-10. Diseases of the genito-urinary system N00 – N99 provides a rate of codes of diseases.

Classification of Surgical Procedures

Surgical procedures can occasionally be difficult to classify and the most accepted classification is that of the fourth revision of the classification of surgical operations and procedures, now known as OPCS-4. The Read code system seems to have lost popularity.

AUDIT AND DATA COLLECTION

NHS data that are collected centrally are often insufficiently detailed to allow medical audit. The British Association of Urological Surgeons (BAUS) in the United Kingdom set up a system of voluntary surgical recording of patient information to facilitate audit. The Clinical Resource and Audit Department (CRAG) of the Scottish Office commissioned a similar audit for Scotland, the Scottish Urological Cancer Audit (SUCA).

BAUS Cancer Registry

The BAUS section of Oncology was formed in November 1997, at a meeting held in Leeds. At that time, it was decided that one of the main activities of the section would be to start a national registry of newly diagnosed urological tumours and this was piloted for a 6-month period in 1998 (1.4.98 – 30.9.98). The results were presented at the first AGM in November, when data from 203 consultants was presented.

Each subsequent year, the dataset has increased/modified slightly and all definitions correspond to those within the national guidelines, where appropriate. Analyses have now been published for the full years 1999, 2000 and 2001 and all documents are available to download from the BAUS website (www.baus.org.uk). The original objectives are printed in the data dictionary that is produced for each year's dataset and are as follows:

- To establish a database of all newly presenting urological cancers.
- To establish continuous data collection with regular analyses and reports.
- To develop detailed datasets for specific cancers.

- To develop electronic methods of data collection and reporting applicable to all members of the section.
- To foster responsibility for data collection by senior clinicians.
- To enable workload analyses for section members and their centers.
- To ensure confidentiality and integrity of the data under the guidance of the executive committee.

During this course of 2002, the database has been given the name : BAUS Cancer Registry (BCR) – the new term reflecting the broad-base of contributors, many of whom are not members of the section of oncology of BAUS. The BCR involves all urological cancers, but prostate cancer represents a sizeable proportion of the work of the BAUS members.

The SUCA Analysis

At the request of the Scottish Office, SUCA was established. It was agreed by all the Scottish members who deal with urological cancer that this audit be supported, giving the Scottish Office details of performance issues, such as delays, difficulties in obtaining imaging, etc.

As an integral part of this, the data required by the BAUS Cancer Registry is being forwarded automatically, thus the patients only need to be registered with one of the audit groups.

The SUCA Audit

The aim of the SUCA describes the delivery of investigations and treatments to patients with urological cancer within Scotland and to audit these in terms of outcome. It was envisaged that they should form a basis for the implementation of any future guidelines produced for the management of urological cancer.

In particular, the audit will identify variations of clinical practice in investigation and treatment of urological cancer in Scotland, identify good and inappropriate practice based on clinical outcomes and identify possible reasons for this and also identify areas that require further investigation. A steering group was set up and the audit was carried out on the practice of delivery of care of the prostate, kidney, testes, bladder, renal pelvis, ureters and penile cancers. The oncology service delivery is also audited by oncologists. There were two steering group members tasked with overseeing prostate audit. Numerous steering group meetings took place to draft questions and to agree data definitions. Six treatment data sets were prepared of all the main cancers, and in particular for prostate cancer. The prostate cancer data included the BAUS data set, so that Scottish office of SUCA would send data to BAUS, to avoid duplication of effort by clinicians. The prostate set required 9 drafts.

A pilot study was taken in three hospitals (Aberdeen Royal Infirmary, Western General Hospital Edinburgh and Ayr Hospital). This took place over a 4-week period.

The study was then opened widely. Consultant consent was then obtained by data managers travelling throughout their regions and visiting hospitals. The most common difficulty encountered was that many consultants did not have the time or the resources to help completing the forms. However, almost all consultants consented for the data to be collected. The initial study required consultants to register their patients. However, due to the difficulties in registering all the patients, back-up systems were introduced. Information was obtained from biochemistry departments of high PSAs (prostate-specific antigen), which had not previously been recorded and a print out was obtained of all PSA results greater than 100. This of course would miss a number of patients with prostate cancer, but in the first instance, it was felt important to capture all the patients with advanced cancer, who were not necessarily being treated by a consultant urologist/surgeon.

All the Records Departments/Information Departments were contacted throughout Scotland and they were requested to provide printouts of all patients coded upon discharge with prostate cancer. Records managers were also contacted throughout Scotland to request access to medical records, so that data managers could examine the case notes. Information and Standard Division (ISD) were contacted to provide us with data from their Cancer Registration Department. Application was made to the Privacy Advisory Committee, who approved the application and permitted data to be sent.

Data definitions

To ensure that all clinicians and data managers were collecting the same data, data definitions were agreed. The data definitions required considerable refinement. The data managers were all provided with a set of the data definitions and each data set has a definitions appendix for clinician reference.

Preparation of database

Many consultants expressed their wish to input the data straight on to the database, instead of completing forms. The budget did not contain money for database design, but one of the data managers designed an initial basic database. This database was expanded and had the necessary validations and queries built in. The database was then distributed to consultants.

Confidentiality

Due to the Data Protection Act of 1998, the Caldicott Report, the GMC Guidance Booklet on confidentiality and possibly other factors, there was an interruption in data capture. There were some issues as to whether e-mails were considered a secure way of transferring data. The present position is that e-mails are not considered secure enough, without data encryption, under the terms of the Data Protection Act 1998. The project was of course registered with the Data Protection Group.

SUCA QUESTIONS IN PROSTATE CANCER

Q1
Source of referral? GP/Urologist/Other
Date of referral?

Q2
Priority of Referral?
With suspicion of cancer
Routine
Discovered during follow-up

Q3
Were there any symptoms at time of referral?
Yes/No/Not Known
If yes, duration of symptoms? weeks.
If more than 4 weeks, delay in referral due to; GP/Patient/Not Known

Q4
Date seen by first hospital clinician?
Date of first consultation with surgeon?

Q5
Diagnosis
Date of definitive diagnosis?

What information is diagnosis based on?
Histology
Cytology
Radiology
Clinical

Tumour marker
Other – specify

If histology, what is the basis of histological diagnosis?
TURP
Prostatectomy
Needle biopsy (not TRUS)
TRUS – Urologist/Radiology
Other – specify

Q6
Histology
Weight of prostate resection gram/not recorded
Tumour type: Adenocarcinoma
Others – specify

PIN:
None
Low Grade
High Grade
Not stated

Gleason Score:
major component + minor component = Total Gleason

Grade (UICC 1997):
GX (grade cannot be assessed)
G1 (well differentiated)
G2 (moderately differentiated)
G3–4 (poorly differentiated/undifferentiated)

Q7
Clinical Staging (UICC 1997)

Clinical:
T
N
M

Pathological:
pT
pN
pM

Radiology for clinical staging:
Plain Radiography

MRI
CT
Bone scan
TRUS
None

PSA at time of diagnosis?

Q8
Initial treatment intention
Curative
Palliative
Surveillance only
Not recorded

Q9
Treatment type(s)
Surgery:
TURP
Radical prostatectomy
   Retropubic
   Perineal
   Node dissection
   Other

Orchidectomy:
Subcapsular
Total
Other
Other treatment:
Radiotherapy
   Radical to prostate
   Palliative to prostate
   Palliative to bone
IV chemotherapy

Oncology Clinician referred to
Hospital

Hormone:
LH RH (Gonadorelin) analogue
Anti-androgen
Other

Q10
Treatment delay
Date of starting definitive treatment:
NB: This is date of the first surgical procedure or therapy treatment

Was there a delay of more than 2 weeks between diagnosis and definitive treatment?
Yes
No

If yes, then delay due to:
Imaging delay
In-Patient waiting time – specify
Patient factor
Others – specify

Q11
Is patient currently involved in clinical trial?
Yes
No
Not aware of any relevant current trial
If yes, state trial:

If no, give reason:
Patient not eligible for current trial
Patient eligible but has been refused
Lack of local support
Surgeon's decision

Q12
Date form completed.

DATA DEFINITIONS PROSTATE

Basis of Histological Diagnosis

Definition

The initial method used to confirm the histological diagnosis of prostate cancer.

Notes for users

Record the initial diagnostic procedure performed confirming prostate cancer by histology. If multiple diagnostic methods have been reported, the initial diagnostic procedure confirming histological diagnosis is recorded.

TURP stands for transurethral resection of prostate, which is carried out using an instrument introduced via the urethra, and does not involve cutting of the skin. Prostatectomy implies some form of open removal of prostatic tissue. Needle biopsy implies the introduction of a needle into the prostate to sample prostate tissue. TRUS stands for trans-rectal ultrasound and is a way of imaging the prostate, which can be done by either the urologist or in the radiology department. Selected areas of the prostate can be biopsied using a needle gun. Other basis of histological diagnosis includes a tru-cut biopsy or a cystectomy with prostatic biopsy.

Coding details

If there is no histological diagnosis, record as 'inapplicable'.

If a patient never sees a urologist or surgeon for the management or treatment of their urological cancer, record as 'inapplicable'.

If a patient is diagnosed by post-mortem, record the histological basis of diagnosis as other and record in the specify box 'diagnosed by post-mortem'.

Code	Description
1	TURP
2	Prostatectomy
3	Needle biopsy (not TRUS)
4	Urologist – TRUS
5	Radiology – TRUS
6	Other
1010	Inapplicable
9999	Not recorded

Notes by users

WEIGHT OF PROSTATE RESECTION

Definition

This is the weight of the pathological chips in grams.

Notes for users

Pathological tumour weight is in grams and is recorded by the pathologist. If the pathologist does not record this, use the weight as measured in the theatre.

Coding details

If there is no histological diagnosis, record 1010.

If a patient never sees a urologist or surgeon for the management or treatment of their urological cancer, record 1010.

If the measurement is not stated, record 9999.

Notes by users

PIN

Prostate

Definition

Prostatic Intraepithelial Neoplasia. A pre-malignant change arising in the prostatic epithelium, the most likely precursor of prostatic adenocarcinoma.

Notes for users

This will be a diagnosis on the pathology report.

Coding details

If there is no histological diagnosis, record as 'inapplicable'.

If a patient never sees a urologist or surgeon for the management or treatment of their urological cancer, record as 'inapplicable'.

Code	Description
1	None
2	Low grade
3	High grade
4	Not stated by pathologist
1010	Inapplicable
9999	Not recorded

Notes by users

GLEASON SCORE

Definition

Gleason is a scoring method based on low-power visualisation of prostatic tissue by the pathologist.

Notes for users

The pathologist will quote the most predominant pattern of tumour seen and the second most predominant pattern, with the two scores being added to produce the total Gleason.

Coding details

If the pathologist records the total gleason score only, record 9999 for the major and minor components. If two different scores are quoted (e.g. $4 + 2$ and $3 + 3$), record the combined overall gleason score, which the pathologist should state in the report. If this is not stated, consult the pathologist concerned.

If there is no histological diagnosis, record 1010.

If a patient never sees a urologist or surgeon for the management or treatment of their urological cancer, record 1010.

If the Gleason scores are not available record 9999.

Notes by users

RADIOLOGY FOR CLINICAL STAGING

Prostate

Definition

This defines which method of Radiology was used to stage the tumour.

Notes for users

None.

Coding details

If a patient is diagnosed by post-mortem, record as 'inapplicable'.

Code	Description
1	Yes
2	No
1010	Inapplicable

Notes by users

PSA AT TIME OF DIAGNOSIS

Prostate

Definition

Prostate-specific antigen. A biochemical test measuring a specific antigen normally secreted by the prostate.

Notes for users

Record the PSA result at the date of diagnosis or at the time diagnostic procedures were undertaken. If there are multiple PSA results available at the time of diagnosis, record the result closest to the date of diagnosis and then the highest result. If a PSA test is not performed as part of diagnostic procedures, record the latest PSA performed between referral and diagnosis.

Coding details

If a PSA test was not performed, record as 101010.
  If a PSA result is not available, record as 99999.
  If a patient is diagnosed by post-mortem, record as 101010.

Notes by users

SURGERY

Prostate

Definition

This is the surgery performed on the patient for treatment of their prostate cancer.

Notes for users

Combinations of treatment types can be selected. TURP stands for trans-urethral resection of prostate, which is carried out using an instrument introduced via the urethra with no cutting of skin. Radical prostatectomy is the removal of the entire prostate and its capsule plus seminal vesicles. This can be removed retropubically at an open operation or through the perineum. Lymph nodes may be removed at the retropubic prostatectomy (node dissection). Orchiectomy is used to deprive the tumour of male sexual hormone, removing all testicular tissue. Subcapsular orchiectomy is the removal of testicular tissue but with retention of the testicular capsule to retain a small area of non-functioning tissue within the scrotum.

....

Coding details

If a patient has a TURP, which is just for diagnostic purposes, this should not be considered as surgery.

If no surgery was performed on the patient, record as 'inapplicable'.

If a patient is diagnosed by post-mortem, record as 'inapplicable'.

Code	Description
1	Yes
2	No
1010	Inapplicable

Notes by users

OTHER TREATMENT

Prostate

Definition

This is the therapy given for treatment of their prostate cancer.

Notes for users

Combinations of treatment types can be selected. Radiotherapy is the treatment of disease by radiation. Radical treatment goes to the root and therefore aims for an absolute cure. Palliative treatment is a dosage that may not cure but may control local progression. Chemotherapy is the type of course of cytotoxic drugs, which destroys cells. Hormone therapy is the treatment of cancer by alteration of the hormonal balance. Some cancers, will only grow in the presence of certain hormones. LHRH (Gonadorelin) analogue injections are given 1 or 3-monthly to lower the output of testosterone; buserelin (Suprefact), goserelin (Zoladex), leuprorelin (Prostap), triptorelin (De-capeptyl). Anti-androgen tablets are given to interfere with the action of male sexual hormones; cyproterone (Cyprostat), flutamide (Drogenil), bicalutamide (Casodex).

Coding details

If the type of Oncology treatment is not indicated on the form, record as 'unrecorded'.

If no other treatment was given to the patient, record as 'inapplicable'.

If the patient is referred for other treatment but dies before being seen, the treatment the patient is referred for should still be recorded. If referred for radiotherapy or chemotherapy, the oncology form will then state 'no treatment prescribed' with the reason being death of patient. If referred for any other treatment, record in the 'comments' box that the patient did not receive treatment as planned due to death of patient.

If a patient is diagnosed by post-mortem, record as 'inapplicable'.

Code	Description
1	Yes
2	No
3	Oncologist's decision
9999	Unrecorded
1010	Inapplicable

Notes by users

DATE OF STARTING DEFINITIVE TREATMENT

Prostate

Definition

This is the date of the definitive surgical procedure or therapy treatment.

Notes for users

This is the major treatment element involved in removing the tumour. A biopsy would not be considered definitive treatment.

Coding details

The format should be DDMMCCYY.

If a patient has a TURP that is just for diagnostic purposes, this should not be considered as surgery and therefore should not be used as date of starting definitive treatment.

If the patient did not receive treatment or the patient refused treatment, record 10/10/1910.

For exact dates unknown, record 09/09/1909.

If a patient is diagnosed by post-mortem, record as 10/10/1910.

Notes by users

DELAY BETWEEN DIAGNOSIS AND DEFINITIVE TREATMENT

Prostate

Definition

This is the timescale between date of diagnosis, described elsewhere, and date of starting definitive treatment, described elsewhere.

Notes for users

If the delay between date of diagnosis and starting definitive treatment is more than 2 weeks, the reason should be coded accordingly:
- delayed Imaging – delay by the imaging department, or
- waiting times (in-patient) – delay in surgery due to shortage of beds, staff or lack of operating time, etc, or
- patient factor delay – treatment cancelled by patient for personal reasons, or
- other, specify – any other reason not covered by the previous points.

Coding details

Delay in treatment; if the patient did not receive treatment or the patient refused treatment, record as 'inapplicable'.

If either the date of diagnosis or the date of starting definitive treatment is unknown, record as 'dates unknown'.

If a patient is diagnosed by post-mortem, record as 'inapplicable'.

Code	Description
1	Yes
2	No
3	Dates unknown
1010	Inapplicable
9999	Not recorded

Reasons for delay

If the patient did not receive treatment or the patient refused treatment, record as 'inapplicable'.

If the dates are unknown, record as 'inapplicable'.

If a patient is diagnosed by post-mortem, record as 'inapplicable'.

Code	Description
1	Delayed imaging
2	Waiting times (in-patient)
3	Patient factor
4	Other
1010	Inapplicable
9999	Not recorded

Notes by users

ENVOI

The increased interest by government and public in prostate cancer has allowed the construction of increasingly robust measurements of epidemiology related to treatment process and outcomes, and will inform and shape better management regimes for our patients.

ACKNOWLEDGEMENTS

The combined input of all participating urologists, radiotherapists and other participating clinicians is kindly and gratefully acknowledged. The data definitions were drafted by Nikki Burgess, Chris Goodman and Bob Meddings and members of the SUCA Steering Committee. The help of Mrs Sarah Fowler, the BAUS Cancer Registry Manager, is gratefully acknowledged. The help of Ms Michaela Rodger of the SUCA is also acknowledged.

REFERENCES

1 Alderson MR, Holland WW, Detels R, Knox G. Oxford Text Book of Public Health. Oxford, OUP: 1985.

2 Kendrick S, Clarke J. Scottish Record Linkage System. *Health Bulletin.* (Edinburgh) 1993; **51**: 72–9.

3 Harris V, Sandridge AL, Black RJ, Brewster DH, Gould A. Cancer Registration Statistics Scotland 1986–95. ISD Scotland Publications, Edinburgh, 1998.

4 Potosky AL, Miller BA, Albertsen PC, Kramer BS. The role of increasing

detection in the rising incidence of prostate cancer. *JAMA* 1995; **273**: 548–52.

5 Parkin DM, Chen VW, Ferlay J, Galceran J, Storm HH, Wheelan SL. Comparability and quality control in cancer registration. (IARC Technical Reports 19) 1994 Lyon IARC.

6 Donaldson LJ, Donaldson RJ. *Essential Public Health*. 2nd Edition. Petroc Press, London, 2000.

7 Townsend P, Phillimore P, Beattie A. *Health and Deprivation: Inequality and the North*. Rotledge, London, 1988.

8 Garman B. Identification of underprivileged areas. *Brit Med J* 1983; **286**: 1705–9.

19: Trends in Prostate Cancer Incidence and Mortality

Steven Oliver, Rhidian Hurle and Owen Hughes

INTRODUCTION

Prostate cancer is an important health problem and is emerging as the most common life-threatening cancer in men in the majority of Western Countries [1]. Estimates of global cancer incidence show that prostate cancer has become the second most common cancer in men with in excess of 679 000 new cases worldwide and over 221 000 deaths (Globocan 2002). Despite its major impact on public health, the aetiology of prostate cancer is poorly understood, with the only recognised risk factors being age, family history and ethnicity [2]. The lifetime risk of being diagnosed with prostate cancer is 1 in 14 (7%). Incident rates are very low below the age of 50 but rise steeply with age with rates in men above 85 being 70 times higher than that in men aged 50–54 years [2]. This has major significance in light of the predicted demographic population changes with a shift to an increasingly aged population. In 2002, the number of persons worldwide aged 60 years or older was estimated to be 629 million and is projected to grow to almost 2 billion by 2050. By this time the population over the age of 60 will be larger than the population of children (0–14 years) for the first time in human history.

At present there is a 30-fold variation in prostate cancer incidence rates reported between populations from the highest rates in the United States, particularly among African Americans, and the lowest seen in Asian countries (Fig. 19.1 Prostate Cancer Age-Standardised Incidence rate per 100 000 Globocan 2002, IARC).

The majority of the world's older persons currently reside in Asia (54%), while Europe has the next largest share (24%). One of every 10 persons is now aged 60 years or older; by 2050, the United Nations predicts that one fifth, and by 2150 on third, of people will be aged 60 years or older. The percentage is currently much higher in the more developed than in the less developed regions, but the pace of ageing in developing countries is more rapid. Their transition from a young to an old age structure will be more compressed in time.

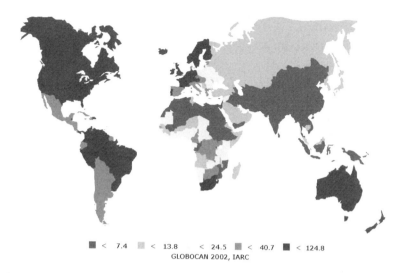

■ < 7.4   ▒ < 13.8   < 24.5 ▓ < 40.7 ■ < 124.8
GLOBOCAN 2002, IARC

Fig. 19.1 GLOBOCAN 2002 http://www-dep.iarc.fr/. International Agency for Research on Cancer, Lyon, France presents estimates for the year 2002. However, although the populations of the different countries are those estimated for the middle of 2002, the disease rates are not those for the year 2002, but from the most recent data available, generally 2–5 years earlier).

In the United Kingdom, recent cancer registry statistics indicate that there were over 30 000 new cases and more than 10 000 deaths in 2003 (Cancer Research UK, 2005). With an ageing population and the continuing decline in other common cancers such as those of stomach and lung, prostate cancer is now the most common cancer among men in the United Kingdom.

Studies of familial risk of prostate cancer show a trend of higher risk with increasing number of affected relatives and an earlier age of diagnosis in those relatives. Men with three or more relatives with prostate cancer have a 35–45% risk of developing prostate cancer. Men whose fathers or brothers had prostate cancer are, on average, diagnosed 6 to 7 years earlier than men with no family history of this disease. Research suggests that one or more autosomal dominant genes may lead to early onset of prostate cancer. However, this is thought to account for no more than 10% of prostate cancers.

The paucity of identified risk factors limits the opportunity for primary prevention and attempts to reduce the burden of prostate cancer morbidity and mortality have increasingly focused on secondary prevention through early detection and treatment. Early detection is now largely achieved through the use of the prostate-specific antigen (PSA) blood test, augmented with digital rectal examination and trans-rectal ultrasound. The aim of this form of cancer screening is the avoidance of prostate cancer as a cause of death. While the PSA test makes population screening possible, the question of whether early detection will lead to a sufficient reduction in deaths from prostate cancer, to outweigh adverse consequences of over-detection and morbidity of treatment, remains open. The only meaningful method to answer this question is through well-conducted randomised controlled trials (RCTs), and two such studies are underway in North America [3] and Europe [4]. A further RCT of treatment 'ProtecT' in the United Kingdom in screen detected cases is currently recruiting and will also provide evidence on the relative benefit of early treatment.

RECENT TRENDS IN PROSTATE CANCER INCIDENCE

The worldwide incidence of prostate cancer has dramatically increased in recent years in both high- and low-incidence countries. In both the United Kingdom and United States, a steady rise was present during the 1980s with the widespread use of transurethral resection of prostate (TURP). A sharp increase in incidence was observed in both countries during the early 1990s at a time when PSA testing became routinely available (see Fig. 19.2). The effect of PSA testing on incidence rate was pronounced in the United States where widespread PSA testing was employed in 1987 for detecting early cancers in asymptomatic men. The subsequent fall in incidence after 1996 was probably due to removal of prevalent cases diagnosed. Mortality rates are less sensitive to diagnostic practices and so provide a more accurate reflection of the true underlying variation in rates of prostate cancer between countries.

RECENT TRENDS IN PROSTATE CANCER MORTALITY

Until the late 1980s prostate cancer mortality as well as incidence were both rising in most countries [5]. However, from the mid 1990s onwards it became clear that death rates were falling in some parts of the world [6,7]. The greatest interest has focused on mortality trends in the United States, where a dramatic peak in prostate cancer incidence followed the introduction of the PSA test in 1985 [7,9]. Since 1991, a fall in mortality has been seen in the United States, and there has been debate over the extent to which this may be a consequence of PSA screening [9]. In England and Wales, where national health policy has discouraged PSA screening [6], a similar decline in mortality have also been observed [10]. Reports of falling prostate cancer death rates have also come from Scotland [11] and Canada [12].

WHY DO TRENDS IN INCIDENCE AND MORTALITY MATTER?

Given that the results of RCTs are going to be the only reliable source of evidence on the effectiveness of screening what can we learn from examining trends in mortality? The variation in PSA testing intensity both over time

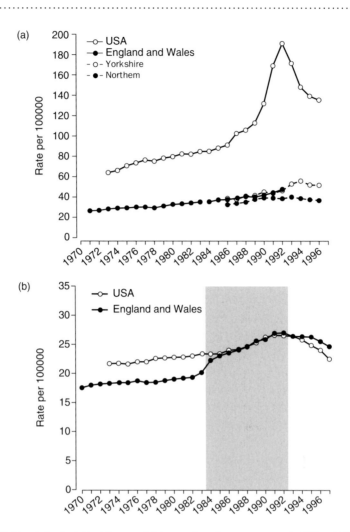

Fig. 19.2 Trends in the (a) incidence and (b) mortality of prostate cancer in UK and USA. The shaded area in (b) indicates a time period when the classification of cause of death was changed in England and Wales.

and between populations provides a number of 'natural experiments' and an opportunity for observational epidemiological study. While these studies may give an insight into what might occur at a population level in the event of screening, they are open to bias, and it is always important to recall that non-randomised populations may differ in other ways than in screening uptake. However, in the final event the true impact of screening can only be measured through changes in mortality at a population level. An understanding of how mortality patterns are changing over time is therefore vital in setting the results of experimental studies in context. Mortality trends also have an impact on the design of RCT of screening, death rates in the control population are an important determinant of the power of any screening study.

A SYSTEMATIC REVIEW OF MORTALITY TRENDS IN INDUSTRIALISED COUNTRIES

In 2000, a systematic review of trends in mortality from prostate cancer within industrialised countries was conducted [13]. Mortality and population data were extracted from the World Health Organisation Mortality Database for the period 1979–97. Countries were included in analyses if:

1   they had at least 200 deaths from prostate cancer per year;
2   mortality data were available for at least 9 years in the period 1979–97;
3   they had systems of death certification in which cause of death was assigned by a medical practitioner in ≥95% of cases, and coverage was considered good.

Deaths coded to prostate cancer using the 9th revision of the International Classification of Disease were used in analyses (ICD9 185). Age-standardised death rates were calculated for the range 50–79 years in 5 year age bands, using the European standard population. Deaths in the population aged over 79 years were excluded as death certification is known to be less accurate in older individuals [14]. Mortality and population data from the former German Democratic Republic and the Federal Republic of Germany for the years 1979–89 were combined to give a single rate for Germany.

Trends in age-specific and age-standardised mortality were calculated using join point regression [15]. This is a form of regression analysis in which trend data can be described by a number of contiguous linear segments and 'join points' at which trends change. The regression model also estimates the annual percentage change (APC) in rates, the number and location of join points and confidence intervals (CI) for these parameters.

There was a more than five-fold difference between the lowest (Japan 1994, 15.1 per 100 000) and highest (Sweden 1996, 81.5 per 100 000) age-standardised rates at the end of the time series. The lowest death rates were seen in Japan and the Southern European countries (Greece, Spain, Portugal and Italy) and the highest in Scandinavia and North America. Most countries experienced a constant increase in prostate cancer mortality over the years studied. In seven countries: Canada, USA, Austria, France, Germany, Italy and the United Kingdom, mortality trends showed a down-turn in recent years. In Belgium and Hungary trends were static.

Estimates of the year when changes in the trend in prostate cancer mortality occurred, and of the annual percentage change in prostate cancer mortality between these years, are shown in Table 19.1. Mortality rates increased at between 1–2% per year in most countries during the study period. Japan, with the lowest initial mortality rate, had one of the highest rates of increase at 2.6% per year. In those countries where a down-turn in

Table 19.1 Summary of the APC and join points for trends in age-standardised prostate cancer mortality (50–79 years) in 24 countries. (When more than one join point was identified in the trend for a country, the APC between join points is given)

Country (range of years)	APC (95% ci)	Join point (95% ci)	APC (95% ci)	Join point (95% ci)	APC (95% ci)
Two join points					
USA (1979–87)	0.5 (0.1 to 1.0)	1988 (1981–1990)	3.6 (−1.0 to 8.4)	1991 (1989–1993)	−3.6 (−4.3 to −2.8)
UK (1979–97)	0.1 (−5.5 to 6.0)	1981 (1981–1992)	3.2 (2.7 to 3.7)	1991 (1989–1995)	−2.1 (−2.9 to −1.3)
One join point					
Canada (1979–97)	1.7 (1.2 to 2.3)	1991 (1988–1992)	−3.0 (−4.3 to −1.6)		
Austria (1980–97)	1.0 (0.2 to 1.9)	1991 (1989–1994)	−2.5 (−4.5 to −0.3)		
France (1979–95)	1.1 (0.6 to 1.6)	1989 (1987–1990)	−2.9 (−3.7 to −2.0)		
Germany (1980–97)	0.5 (0.3 to 0.8)	1995 (1993–1995)	−6.0 (−11.5 to −0.1)		
Italy (1979–95)	1.0 (0.1 to 1.7)	1988 (1986–1991)	−2.1 (−3.3 to −1.0)		
No join point					
Belgium (1979–97)	−0.1 (−0.5 to 0.4)				
Finland (1987–95)	1.1 (−0.4 to 2.6)				
Greece (1979–97)	1.0 (0.5 to 1.4)				
Ireland (1979–96)	1.8 (1.0 to 2.7)				
Netherlands (1979–95)	0.9 (0.5 to 1.2)				
Norway (1986–95)	0.4 (−0.3 to 1.1)				
Portugal (1980–97)	1.4 (1.0 to 1.8)				
Spain (1980–95)	0.3 (0.01 to 0.5)				
Sweden (1987–96)	1.3 (0.5 to 2.2)				
Bulgaria (1979–95)	0.9 (0.5 to 1.2)				
Hungary (1979–95)	−0.02 (−0.4 to 0.4)				
Poland (1980–96)	1.8 (1.4 to 2.1)				
Romania (1979–97)	1.0 (0.5 to 1.4)				
Israel (1979–96)	1.8 (0.8 to 2.8)				
Japan (1979–94)	2.6 (2.3 to 3.0)				
Australia (1979–95)	1.7 (1.3 to 2.1)				
New Zealand (1979–96)	1.1 (0.4 to 1.8)				

trend was identified, join points for this clustered in the time period 1988–91, the earliest reversal in trend was seen in Italy (1988, 95% CI, 1986 to 1991). Following the reversal in trend, the annual percentage change ranged from falls of 2.1% per year in the United Kingdom (95% CI, 1.3 to 2.9) and Italy (95% CI, 1.0 to 3.3) to 6% (95% CI, 0.1 to 11.5) in Germany.

In Canada, United States, France, Italy and the United Kingdom a reversal in mortality trends was seen in each 5 years age-group from 60–79 years. The timing of these changes in age-specific trends ranged from 1986 to 1992, consistent with a calendar period effect. Trends in age-specific rates were less consistent in Germany and Austria where changes were observed mainly in the 74–79 years age-bands.

MORTALITY TRENDS WITHIN COUNTRIES

Two recent papers have used the opportunities provided by 'natural experiments' in which the intensity of PSA testing has varied within countries to examine the possible impact of screening on mortality. In Austria, PSA testing was made freely available to men aged 45–75 in the Tyrol region in 1993 [16]. In the following 5 years approximately two-thirds of the population of the region (c. 65 000 men in the age range 45–75 years) had at least one PSA test. Mortality rates within the region were seen to fall significantly faster than in the rest of Austria. The authors of the study concluded that PSA testing and subsequent management of screen-detected cancer was probably the cause for the decline in mortality. However, they also concluded that the very short lead time between introduction of PSA testing and changes in mortality suggested that improved death rates might result from downstaging and successful treatment, rather than through detection and treatment of early cancers.

In contrast, a recent paper from North America observed no difference in mortality trends between regions with very different intensities of PSA testing and aggressive treatment. On the basis of data on men over the age of 65 years, Lu-Yao and colleagues compared mortality rates amongst men living in Seattle and Connecticut [17]. In Seattle, rates of PSA testing in the period 1988–90 were over five times higher than in the region of Connecticut, in addition rates of biopsy and potentially curative treatment were also higher. However, review of mortality rates over the period 1987–97 showed no evidence of a difference in death rates between these regions.

MORTALITY TRENDS AND SCREENING

Recent trends in prostate cancer mortality reveal marked differences amongst industrialised nations. In most countries, the long-term trend of rising death rates has persisted over the last 20 years, in others there is evidence of a decline over the last decade. These observed declines in mortality could result from any combination of either artefact, reduction in prostate cancer incidence, a rise in competing causes of death or changes in the risk of death from prostate cancer.

Artefact

Because of its relatively slow progression, and peak incidence in an elderly population, attribution of cause of death in men with prostate cancer poses particular difficulties. Changes in the interpretation of WHO rules on assigning underlying cause of death have resulted in spurious changes in prostate cancer mortality trends in England and Wales [6]. Two recent studies from the United States suggest that 10–20% of prostate cancer deaths may be mis-attributed [18,19]. In a study comparing patterns of non-prostate cancer deaths in cohorts of men with and without prostate cancer, Newshaffer and colleagues reported that attribution of cause of death in men with prostate cancer could have been influenced by knowledge of previous treatment. Prior beliefs about the effectiveness of radical treatment may have lead to a reluctance to attribute death to prostate cancer in men who had undergone 'aggressive' interventions [19].

Changes in Incidence

Trends in mortality could fall if the underlying incidence of aggressive prostate tumours was decreasing, possibly in response to changes in environmental risk factors such as diet. Such changes are hard to detect as overall estimates of incidence are heavily influenced by methods of case detection, particularly with the advent of PSA testing. However, age-specific death rates in most countries experiencing apparent falls in mortality appear consistent with a period effect, with rates declining at similar times in different age-bands. Changes in chronic disease incidence are more commonly reflected in mortality trends as cohort effects, unless the latent time between exposure and outcome is short and all age groups experience a simultaneous change in exposure. Apart from the short-term changes in incidence driven by PSA testing there is as yet little evidence that prostate cancer incidence is in decline in those countries where mortality trends have reversed [5].

Competing Causes

It is also unlikely that reductions in prostate cancer mortality are due to a real increase in the incidence of competing causes of death. Life expectancy in the age range (50–79) is increasing in those countries experiencing a reversal in trend (WHO, 1998) and this hypothesis is not consistent with knowledge about trends in the other major life-threatening conditions.

Increased Survival – Impact of Health Care

The earlier detection of prostate cancer following introduction of PSA testing distorts analyses of survival (lead-time bias) and makes comparisons of recent data on survival between countries and over time very difficult. Given the apparent period effects in age-specific prostate cancer death rates, the most likely cause of the observed down-turns in mortality is the impact of some form of therapeutic intervention. Two recent changes in the management of prostate cancer could account for this. First, in countries such as the United States the rapid rise in incidence was accompanied by an increase in the utilisation of radical surgery and radiotherapy. However, it appears unlikely that the results of radical treatments alone could have caused the observed changes in death rates. Using a simulation model of prostate cancer mortality, including varying estimates of treatment efficacy and screening lead time, Etzioni and colleagues estimated the possible impact of radical treatments on death rates in the United States [20]. Only when the effectiveness of radical treatments was set at its highest level (relative risk reduction of 0.5) and lead time at its lowest (3 years) could use of such treatments account for the observed mortality change in the United States. In the United Kingdom the extent of radical treatment has been far lower, but a similar down-turn in mortality has been observed [6].

Second, developments in the management of advanced prostate cancer also occurred in the 1980s with the introduction of medical anti-androgen therapies. While the effectiveness of drug-induced androgen deprivation is similar to the traditional approach of surgical castration [21], increased uptake of more acceptable medical therapies could extend population survival by deferring death from prostate cancer sufficiently for competing causes to intervene. Initiation of hormone treatment earlier in the course of advanced disease might also have an influence on death rates [22]. However, it is also worth observing that any unrecognised adverse effects of therapy, if they induced competing causes of death such as thromboembolic disease or other malignancies, would be translated into reductions in prostate cancer-specific death rates. International and secular variation in health-care interventions for prostate cancer are not well described, and it is unclear whether the patterns in observed mortality trends are matched by differences in treatment.

IMPACT OF PSA SCREENING

The relationship between the observed national mortality trends and the known uptake of PSA testing raises some paradoxes. Mortality rates are falling in the United States, where PSA screening is common [9], but not in Australia where uptake has also been high [23,24]. In contrast in the United Kingdom, where screening uptake is low [6], mortality rates are declining. Published reports of prostate cancer screening in other countries are limited. PSA testing was thought to have had an impact on prostate cancer incidence by 1988 in at least one area in France [25], while in the Italian region of Tuscany, PSA was first being used in the early 1990s [26]. Feasibility studies for prostate cancer screening are also ongoing in Austria [27], and Italy [28], and centres in Belgium, Finland, Italy, the Netherlands and Sweden are participating in the European Randomised Study of Screening for Prostate Cancer [29]. The lack of a consistent association between PSA uptake and mortality trends highlight the limitations of observational data in assessing the effectiveness of cancer screening, which awaits the results of ongoing randomised trials.

CONCLUSION

Data on trends in death rates suggest that important changes have happened recently in several countries, which may be a result of health-care activity. However evidence from mortality trends is not sufficient to answer the question of the effectiveness of population screening, which can still only come from randomised controlled trials. The burden of prostate cancer morbidity and mortality continues to rise in most parts of the world, and research into isolating the contributing causes of observed declines in mortality should have high priority.

REFERENCES

1 Cancer in five Continents vol. VII. Lyon: IARCPress, 1997.

2 Selley S, Donovan J, Faulkner A, Coast J, Gillat D. Diagnosis, Management and Screening of early localised prostate cancer. *HTA*, 1997.

3 Gohagan JK, Prorok PC, Kramer BS, Cornett JE. Prostate cancer screening in the prostate, lung, colorectal and ovarian cancer screening trial of the National Cancer Institute. *J Urol* 1994; **152**: 1905–9.

4 Auvinen A, Rietbergen JB, Denis LJ, Schroder FH, Prorok PC. Prospective evaluation plan for randomised trials of prostate cancer screening. The International Prostate Cancer Screening Trial Evaluation Group. *J Med Screen* 1996; **3**: 97–104.

5 Hsing AW, Tsao L, Devesa SS. International trends and patterns of prostate cancer incidence and mortality. *Int J Cancer* 2000; **85**: 60–7.

6 Oliver SE, Gunnell D, Donovan JL. Comparison of trends in prostate-cancer mortality in England and Wales and the USA. *Lancet* 2000; **355**: 1788–9.

7 Mettlin CJ, Murphy GP. Why is the prostate cancer death rate declining in the United States? *Cancer* 1998; **82**: 249–51.

8 Farkas A, Schneider D, Perrotti M, Cummings KB, Ward WS. National trends in the epidemiology of prostate cancer, 1973 to 1994: evidence for the effectiveness of prostate-specific antigen screening. *Urology* 1998; **52**: 444–8.

9 Hankey BF, Feuer EJ, Clegg LX *et al.* Cancer surveillance series: interpreting trends in prostate cancer–part I: Evidence of the effects of screening in recent prostate cancer incidence, mortality, and survival rates. *J Natl Cancer Inst* 1999; **91**: 1017–24.

10 Majeed A, Babb P, Jones J, Quinn M. Trends in prostate cancer incidence, mortality and survival in England and Wales 1971–98. *BJU Int* 2000; **85**: 1058–62.

11 Brewster DH, Fraser LA, Harris V, Black RJ. Rising incidence of prostate cancer in Scotland: increased risk or increased detection? *BJU Int* 2000; **85**: 463–72.

12 Meyer F, Moore L, Bairati I, Fradet Y. Downward trend in prostate cancer mortality in Quebec and Canada. *J Urol* 1999; **161**: 1189–91.

13 Oliver SE, May MT, Gunnell D. International trends in prostate-cancer mortality in the "PSA ERA". *Int J Cancer* 2001; **92**:893–8.

14 Grulich AE, Swerdlow AJ, dos SS, I, Beral V. Is the apparent rise in cancer mortality in the elderly real? Analysis of changes in certification and coding of cause of death in England and Wales, 1970–1990. *Int J Cancer* 1995; **63**: 164–8.

15 Kim HJ, Fay MP, Feuer EJ, Midthune DN. Permutation tests for join point regression with applications to cancer rates. *Stat Med* 2000; **19**: 335–51.

16 Bartsch G, Horninger W, Klocker H *et al.* Prostate cancer mortality after introduction of prostate-specific antigen mass screening in the Federal State of Tyrol, Austria. *Urology* 2001; **58**: 417–24.

17 Lu-Yao GL, Albertsen PC, Stanford JL, Stukel TA, Walker-Corkery ES, Barry MJ. Natural experiment examining impact of aggressive screening and treatment on prostate cancer mortality in two fixed cohorts from Seattle area and Connecticut. *BMJ* 2002; **325**: 740–3.

18 Albertsen PC, Walters S, Hanley JA. A comparison of cause of death determination in men previously diagnosed with prostate cancer who died in 1985 or 1995. *J Urol* 2000; **163**: 519–23.

19 Newschaffer CJ, Otani K, McDonald MK, Penberthy LT. Causes of death in elderly prostate cancer patients and in a comparison non prostate cancer cohort. *J Natl Cancer Inst* 2000; **92**: 613–21.

20 Etzioni R, Legler JM, Feuer EJ, Merrill RM, Cronin KA, Hankey BF. Cancer surveillance series: interpreting trends in prostate cancer – part III: Quantifying the link between population prostate-specific antigen testing and recent declines in prostate cancer mortality. *J Natl Cancer Inst* 1999; **91**: 1033–9.

21 Chamberlain J, Melia J, Moss S, Brown J. Report prepared for the Health Technology Assessment panel of the NHS Executive on the diagnosis, management, treatment and costs of prostate cancer in England and Wales. *Br J Urol* 1997; **79**: 1–32.

22 Anonymous. Immediate versus deferred treatment for advanced prostatic cancer: initial results of the Medical Research Council Trial. The Medical Research Council Prostate Cancer Working Party Investigators Group. *Br J Urol* 1997; **79**: 235–46.

23 Slevin TJ, Donnelly N, Clarkson JP, English DR, Ward JE. Prostate cancer testing: behaviour, motivation and attitudes among Western Australian men. *Med J Aust* 1999; **171**: 185–8.

24 Smith DP, Armstrong BK. Prostate-specific antigen testing in Australia and association with prostate cancer incidence in New South Wales. *Med J Aust* 1998; **169**: 17–20.

25 Menegoz F, Colonna M, Exbrayat C, Mousseau M, Orfeuvre H, Schaerer R. A recent increase in the incidence of prostatic carcinoma in a French population: role of ultrasonography and prostatic specific antigen. *Eur J Cancer* 1995; **31A**: 55–8.

26 Barchielli A, Crocetti E, Zappa M. Has the PSA wave already crashed upon us? Changes in the epidemiology of prostate cancer from 1985 to 1994 in central Italy. *Ann Oncol* 1999; **10**: 361–2.

27 Reissigl A, Horninger W, Fink K, Klocker, Bartsch G. Prostate carcinoma screening in the county of Tyrol,

Austria: experience and results. *Cancer* 1997; **80**: 1818–29.

28 Ciatto S, Bonardi R, Mazzotta A, Zappa M. Evidence and feasibility of prostate cancer screening. *Cancer J* 1995; **8**: 33–5.

29 Schroder FH, Denis LJ, Kirkels W, de Koning HJ, Standaert B. European randomized study of screening for prostate cancer. Progress report of Antwerp and Rotterdam pilot studies. *Cancer* 1995; **76**: 129–34.

20: Chemotherapy in Prostate Cancer

Jason Lester and Emma Hudson

INTRODUCTION

Prostate cancer has overtaken lung cancer as the most common male malignancy in the United Kingdom, with 24 708 new cases registered in 1999 [1]. The increasing use of serum prostatic-specific antigen (PSA) for early detection has resulted in a stage shift at diagnosis towards more organ-confined disease. Despite this, nearly one in five patients have stage 4 disease at diagnosis [2]. In addition, over half of the patients will develop metastases at some point during the course of their disease [3]. Hormonal therapy remains the mainstay of treatment for patients with locally advanced or metastatic prostate cancer. However, the median duration of response to androgen deprivation is only 18 months [3]. Second-line hormonal therapy may have a transient effect, but inevitably the disease escapes hormonal control and progresses. Historically, the median survival of patients with metastatic hormone-refractory prostate cancer (HRPC) was around 8 months [4], and hence effective systemic therapy is needed to improve the outcome of these patients.

Methods

Studies were identified on Medline using the keywords 'prostate', 'chemotherapy' and the individual generic names of cytotoxic chemotherapy agents. Abstract lists from major conferences were also searched. All contemporary published phase III trials identified were included in the review, as were selected phase II trials deemed relevant.

Early Work (1970 to 89)

Early clinical studies using single agent cytotoxic chemotherapy in metastatic HRPC were hindered by a lack of reliable objective measures of disease activity. The skeleton is often the only site of metastases, and the measurement of bone changes in response to treatment is difficult to quantify radiologically [5,6].

One approach to this problem was to enrol patients with bidimensionally measurable disease (e.g. lymph node, pulmonary or visceral metastases) into trials. In fact, the presence of extra-osseous metastases is infrequent in advanced prostate cancer making this approach impractical. It is also possible that these patients have a worse prognosis compared to those with bone-only metastases, and are therefore unrepresentative of the patient group as a whole [7]. In addition serum acid phosphatase, the most widely used biochemical marker to monitor disease, has only limited sensitivity and specificity for prostate cancer. The lack of accurate reproducible objective measures of response to treatment lead to a host of indirect measures being used, including quality-of-life (QOL) scales, weight change, analgesic use and performance status [8–10]. Diverse combinations of these direct and often invalidated indirect measures were incorporated into many response criteria. As a consequence, authors reported a large variability in response rates for the same drug making any meaningful interpretation of results difficult. In many of the early trials, patients with clinically or radiologically stable disease (SD) were often included in the overall response (OR) category for statistical analysis. It is well known that a proportion of patients with metastatic HRPC have relatively quiescent disease. This combined with a lack of precision in assessing treatment response led to the mistaken belief that cancer had stabilised as a result of treatment in many patients. Hence, these early studies reported very encouraging response rates of up to 31%. In 1985, many of the early studies were re-evaluated using criteria that were more stringent, and an overall objective response rate (excluding SD) of only 4.5% was reported [11]. In addition, it was clear that the treatment was poorly tolerated, responses were not sustained and there was no survival advantage. The disappointing results achieved with single agents led to combination chemotherapy being evaluated. A number of randomised trials compared regimens of two or more drugs with single-agent chemotherapy, but unfortunately none of the combinations used had any major impact on response rates or survival [12,13]. Consequently, the interest in treating HRPC with chemotherapy declined.

Later Work (1990 to Present)

In the 1990s, the role of chemotherapy in metastatic HRPC was revisited. New, less toxic chemotherapy agents became available and, importantly, assessing objective response to treatment became easier with the widespread introduction of serum PSA. PSA is a glycoprotein found almost exclusively in prostate cells and seminal fluid [14]. Although there is variation in PSA production between individual tumours evidence demonstrates that serum PSA levels correlate with tumour burden [15]. Serum PSA levels have now become an integral component of assessing response to therapy in advanced prostate cancer. This use of PSA as a surrogate end point has been justified by the demonstration of an association between a reduction in PSA of ≥50% with therapy and longer survival [16]. The use of PSA to assess response is controversial, however. *In vitro* studies using the anti-angiogenic agent suramin have demonstrated a reduction in PSA secretion by prostate cancer cells without evidence of tumour cell destruction [17]. It is possible that in some cases a falling serum PSA represents a reduction in PSA secretion by viable cancer cells, and not a reduction in tumour burden. Thus, the validity of serum PSA as a measure of response may depend on the particular treatment agent being used. In addition, several phase III trials have shown a significant reduction in serum PSA with chemotherapy, without an associated significant increase in survival (Table 20.1) [18–20].

Despite these limitations, a decrease in pre-treatment serum PSA of ≥50% serves as a primary end point in many contemporary trials. Indeed, trials have reported up to a ≥50% PSA reduction in up to 76% of patients with advanced HRPC treated with newer cytotoxic chemotherapy agents [21]. It would seem, these results compare very favourably with studies using older drugs. However, such comparisons must be made with caution. Pre-PSA studies depended on radiographically measurable disease to assess response, which as stated previously is fraught with difficulties. When PSA reduction was counted as a response to treatment, response rates increased. This increase seen with newer chemotherapy agents may in part therefore be due to the alteration in definition of response.

This chapter aims to provide an overview of chemotherapy in advanced HRPC. Treatment for non-acinar tumours such as squamous cell and small-cell cancers will not be discussed.

MITOXANTRONE

Mitoxantrone, an anthracenedione structurally similar to doxorubicin, was synthesised in the 1970s. The exact mechanism of action is unknown but includes intercalation with DNA to cause inter/intrastrand cross-linking. It also causes DNA strand breaks by binding with the phosphate backbone of DNA. It is associated with cardiac toxicity, although at a substantially lower rate than doxorubicin [22]. Small phase II studies in metastatic HRPC demonstrated mitoxantrone had a low toxicity profile, and there was

Table 20.1 Recent randomised phase III trials in HRPC.

Author	Regimen	n	Palliative response	PSA reduction ≥50%	Survival (months)
Tannock [25]	Mitoxantrone-P versus P	161	Pain relief: 29% versus 12%, $p = 0.01$	33% versus 22% (NS)	NS
Kantoff [19]	Mitoxantrone-H versus H	242	NS	38% versus 22%, $p = 0.008$	12.3 versus 12.6 (NS)
Berry [18]	Mitoxantrone-P versus P	120	Not assessed	48% versus 24%, $p = 0.007$	23 versus 19 (NS)
Hudes [20,37]	Vinblastine–EMP versus vinblastine	201	NS	25% versus 3%, $p < 0.0001$	12.5 versus 9.4 (NS)
Abratt [42]	Vinorelbine-H versus H	414	31% versus 19%, $p = 0.01$	30% versus 19%, $p = 0.01$	14.7 versus 15.2 (NS)
SWOG [52] $p = 0.02$	Docetaxel-EMP versus mitoxantrone-P	674	NS	50% versus 27%, $p = 0.001$	17.5 versus 15.6
TAX 327 [53] $p = 0.009$	Docetaxel-P versus mitoxantrone-P	1006	Pain relief: 35% versus 22%, $p = 0.001$	45% versus 32%, $p < 0.001$	18.9 versus 16.5

P = prednisolone; H = hydrocortisone; EMP = estramustinephosphate; NS = not significant.

a suggestion of some palliative benefit in metastatic HRPC [23,24]. Following these encouraging results, two important randomised studies were started in the early 1990s comparing mitoxantrone plus a corticosteroid with a corticosteroid alone in men with metastatic HRPC.

A phase III Canadian study randomised 161 symptomatic HRPC patients to oral prednisolone 10 mg daily plus mitoxantrone 12 mg/m^2 intravenous (IV) every 21 days or oral prednisolone 10 mg daily [25]. The primary end point was a palliative response defined by a decrease in pain using a validated pain monitoring instrument [26]. There was a statistically significant decrease in pain (29% versus 12%, $p = 0.01$) and a longer duration of response (43 versus 18 weeks, $p < 0.0001$) in the mitoxantrone plus prednisolone arm compared to the prednisolone only arm. Patients randomised to the combined arm also reported prolonged improvement in physical and social functioning, global QOL, anorexia, drowsiness, constipation and other symptoms. Reduction in serum PSA level of $\geq 50\%$ was seen in 33% in the chemotherapy arm and 22% in the prednisolone only arm ($p = 0.11$). The toxicity associated with mitoxantrone was minimal, and there were no treatment-related deaths. Two patients did develop symptomatic congestive cardiac failure with a cumulative dose of mitoxantrone > 100 mg/m^2. There was no significant difference in survival between the two arms. This may in part have been due to the small size of the study and the cross-over design; 50 patients randomised to receive prednisolone alone subsequently received mitoxantrone due to non-response or progressive symptoms.

A larger phase III cancer and leukaemia group B (CALGB) study randomised 242 patients with metastatic HRPC to receive either oral hydrocortisone 40 mg daily plus mitoxantrone 14 mg/m^2 IV every 3 weeks or oral hydrocortisone 40 mg daily [19]. The primary end point of this study was overall survival. Rather optimistically, the study was designed to detect a 50% increase in survival in the combined arm despite no previous studies demonstrating a survival advantage with chemotherapy. No significant difference in median survival was demonstrated between the two treatment arms. Median survival in the mitoxantrone arm was 12.3 months compared to 12.6 months for the hydrocortisone alone arm ($p = 0.77$). The mitoxantrone arm was associated with a significant improvement in time to disease progression (3.7 months versus 2.3 months, $p = 0.02$), and significantly more patients achieved a $\geq 50\%$ reduction in serum PSA levels (38% versus 22%, $p = 0.008$). Although this study did not demonstrate a significant improvement in overall QOL there was a trend towards improved pain scores in the chemotherapy arm, supporting the Canadian study. Treatment toxicity was minimal, although using a higher dose of mitoxantrone (14 mg/m^2 versus 12 mg/m^2) the CALGB study reported higher rates of grade 3 and 4 neutropenia compared to the Canadian study (63% versus 45%). The lack of improvement in QOL in the CALGB trial may in part be due to the differences in trial population between the two studies. The presence of symptoms was not an entry prerequisite in CALGB, unlike the Canadian study. Indeed, more than a third of patients at baseline had no pain or pain that did not warrant analgesia. This is emphasised by the fact that 18 patients (22%) in each arm of the Canadian study were ECOG (Eastern Cooperative Oncology Group) performance status (PS) 3. In contrast, 85% in the CALGB study were PS 0 or 1, and no PS 3 patients were included.

A more recent phase III American trial randomised 120 men with asymptomatic progressive HRPC to oral prednisolone 10 mg daily or oral prednisolone 10 mg daily plus mitoxantrone 12 mg/m^2 IV every 3 weeks [18]. Median time to progression was significantly longer in the chemotherapy arm (8.1 months versus 4.1 months, $p = 0.018$), and more patients achieved a $\geq 50\%$ reduction in serum PSA levels (48% versus 24%, $p = 0.007$). There was no QOL assessment included. As in the previous two randomised trials there was no significant difference in survival between the two arms (23 months versus 19 months).

Evidence suggested therefore that mitoxantrone plus a corticosteroid prolongs time to disease progression and lowers serum PSA levels, but provides no survival benefit compared to steroid therapy alone. Despite no survival benefit mitoxantrone palliates a significant minority of patients, is well tolerated and hence became the standard of care for patients with symptomatic HRPC.

ESTRAMUSTINE

Estramustine is an oral agent, which is a synthetic fusion of oestradiol with a nitrogen mustard [27]. It was designed specifically for the treatment of prostate cancer; the oestradiol moiety facilitating drug uptake via steroid receptors on the surface of prostate cancer cells allowing the intracellular release of the nitrogen mustard. The mechanism of action of estramustine has been extensively studied, and it appears to have a wide spectrum of effects including microtubular inhibition and an oestrogenic effect [28,29]. Initial studies using relatively high doses of single agent estramustine demonstrated only modest response rates of between 5% and 19% in metastatic HRPC [30,31]. In addition, side effects to the treatment were considerable including nausea, vomiting and high incidence of thromboembolic events [32]. Subsequently, *in vitro* studies demonstrated synergy between estramustine and other microtubular toxins including the *Vinca* alkaloids, etoposide and the taxanes [33,34]. These *in vitro* synergies lead to the clinical evaluation of lower doses of estramustine in combination with various chemotherapeutic agents (described below).

VINCA ALKALOIDS

Vinblastine

Vinblastine, an extract of the periwinkle plant, was the first of the microtubular toxins to be evaluated in combination with estramustine. Phase II studies demonstrated a reduction in PSA of $\geq$50% in 54–61.1% of patients [35,36]. Following these results a randomised phase III trial assessing oral estramustine plus vinblastine IV versus vinblastine IV alone in 201 patients with metastatic HRPC was carried out by the Hoosier Oncology Group [20]. A significantly greater proportion of patients in the combined arm had a $\geq$50% reduction in PSA levels (25.2% versus 3.2%, $p < 0.0001$). Compliance for pain and QOL assessments was poor making any robust analysis of the data impossible. Median time to progression was significantly longer in the combined arm (3.7 months versus 2.2 months, $p = 0.0004$). The difference in median survival did not reach statistical significance (12.5 months versus 9.4 months, $p = 0.051$) [37].

Vinorelbine

Vinorelbine is a semisynthetic *Vinca* alkaloid derived from vinblastine, and is less neurotoxic than its predecessor. Phase II studies using various weekly vinorelbine IV plus estramustine regimens have demonstrated PSA response rates of $\geq$50% in 24–61% of patients [38,39]. Small phase II studies demonstrated weekly vinorelbine IV also has single agent activity in HRPC with $\geq$50% PSA response rates of 17–36%. The treatment appeared well tolerated with some symptomatic benefit to patients [40,41].

Following these phase II studies, Abratt *et al.* reported a multicentre phase III study of vinorelbine 30 mg/m^2 IV days one and eight in a 21-day cycle plus oral hydrocortisone 40 mg/day $\pm$ aminoglutethimide 1000 mg daily versus oral hydrocortisone 40 mg/day $\pm$ aminoglutethimide 1000 mg daily in 414 metastatic HRPC patients [42]. Clinical benefit was assessed from changes in a pain index and the Karnofsky performance score. PSA response was significantly higher in the vinorelbine arm (30.1% versus 19.2%, $p = 0.01$) as was clinical benefit response (30.6% versus 19.2%, $p = 0.01$). Like all other previous phase III trials there was no significant difference in median survival between the two arms (14.7 months versus 15.2 months). Toxicity in the vinorelbine arm included grade 3 or 4 neutropenia in 25.6% of cases, and neutropenic infection in 3% of cases.

ETOPOSIDE

The Michigan Prostate Institute carried out a phase II study using oral etoposide in combination with oral estramustine in 62 patients with HRPC [43]. Among these, 22 had received prior chemotherapy regimens; 39% of patients had a $\geq 50\%$ decrease in pre-treatment PSA levels and median overall survival was 13 months. There was no difference in survival or response in patients treated with previous chemotherapy compared to those who were chemotherapy naïve. These results were supported by a parallel phase II study of similar size using a comparable regimen at the University of Athens School Of Medicine, Greece [44].

TAXANES

Paclitaxel

Paclitaxel is derived from the needles of the European yew tree. Hudes *et al.* reported on 34 metastatic HRPC patients who received paclitaxel 120 mg/m^2 by 96-h IV infusion starting on day one of a 21-day cycle together with oral estramustine 600 mg/m^2/day continuously [45]. Overall, 17 of 32 patients (53.1%) with an elevated pre-treatment PSA level had a $\geq 50\%$ PSA response with an overall median survival of 69 weeks. Grade 3 or 4 leucopenia occurred in seven patients (21%). Three patients (9%) developed subclavian thromboses associated with a central venous access device, and one of these also had an ischaemic stroke. There were no treatment-related deaths. The relatively high levels of toxicity using the 3-weekly schedule led to the development of weekly regimens and shorter courses of estramustine in an attempt to make the treatment more tolerable.

The same author subsequently reported an ECOG trial in 63 metastatic HRPC patients receiving weekly paclitaxel 90 mg/m^2 IV on day two plus oral estramustine 280 mg BD days one to three every 6 out of 8 weeks [46]. Of 62 patients with an elevated PSA 36 had a $\geq 50\%$ PSA response with treatment (58%). At the time of presentation median survival had not been observed. This regimen was moderately less toxic than the 3-weekly paclitaxel, with four patients (6%) developing grade 3 or 4 neutropenia and four patients (6%) thromboembolic disease. There was one treatment-related death.

Berry *et al.* have reported a randomised phase II trial of 163 HRPC patients treated with weekly paclitaxel IV and oral estramustine versus weekly paclitaxel IV alone [47]. The PSA response rate in the combined arm was significantly greater than in the single agent paclitaxel arm (47% versus 27%, $p < 0.01$). Median survival in the combined arm was 16.1 months compared to 13.1 months in the paclitaxel alone arm. The high rate of thromboembolic events in the combined arm (7.5%) led the authors to suggest that prophylactic anticoagulation should be considered when using estramustine. There are no published phase III trials evaluating the paclitaxel–estramustine combination.

Docetaxel

Docetaxel is a semi-synthetic drug also derived from the needles of the European yew tree. Both paclitaxel and docetaxel bind the same microtubule site. A CALGB phase II study in 46 men with HRPC investigated the combination of docetaxel 70 mg/m^2 day two IV, oral estramustine 3.3 mg/kg three times per day, days one to five, and oral hydrocortisone 40 mg daily in a 21-day cycle [48]. Overall 68% of patients with an elevated pre-treatment PSA had a $\geq$50% reduction in PSA. The median survival was 20 months. The predominant toxicity was haematological with 56% of patients developing grade 3 or 4 neutropenia. Thromboembolic events were reported in four patients (9%). There were no treatment-related deaths. Petrylak *et al.* used a combination of docetaxel 70 mg/m^2 IV on day two and oral estramustine 280 mg TDS days one to five of a 21-day cycle. In this study of 35 chemotherapy naïve patients 74% of patients had a PSA response, and the 1-year survival was 77% [49]. Despite using a regimen similar to the CALGB study toxicity was greater; 22(63%) patients developed grade 3 or 4 neutropenia with two(6%) deaths from neutropenic sepsis. Two patients suffered strokes and there were two deep venous thromboses. The high rate of vascular events resulted in aspirin and low-dose warfarin being added to the protocol after the trial had started. In addition several other small phase II studies using single agent docetaxel showed a 50% or greater decline in PSA levels in up to 50% of patients [50,51]. These data along with other supporting studies led to two large phase III trials being established; Southwest Oncology Group (SWOG) trial 9916 compared docetaxel and estramustine with mitoxantrone and prednisolone in men with androgen-independent prostate cancer [52] and TAX 327 a 3-arm trial that compared 3-weekly or weekly docetaxel with mitoxantrone and prednisolone[53]. TAX 327 aimed to answer two questions; was docetaxel more effective than the current standard of care in HRPC (mitoxantrone and prednisolone) and, if so, should it be administered 3-weekly or weekly? In SWOG 9916, 674 men were randomly allocated to docetaxel 60 mg/m^2 IV day two and estramustine 280 mg TDS days one to five or mitoxantrone 12 mg/m^2 IV plus prednisolone 5 mg BD orally daily, both in a 21-day cycle. The docetaxel was preceded by 60 mg of dexamethasone in divided doses starting the night before chemotherapy. Treatment continued until disease progression, unacceptable toxicity or a maximum of 12 cycles had been administered. Median survival was significantly longer in the docetaxel arm (17.5 months versus 15.6 months, $p = 0.002$). A PSA decrease of $\geq 50\%$ occurred more frequently in the docetaxel arm (50% versus 27%, $p < 0.001$). There was no significant difference in pain relief between the two arms. Docetaxel and estramustine resulted in significantly more grade 3 and 4 toxicity with higher rates of neutropenic fever (5% versus 2%), cardiovascular events (15% versus 7%), metabolic disturbances (6% versus 1%) and neurological events (7% versus 2%). There were eight treatment-related deaths in the docetaxel arm compared to four in the mitoxantrone arm. Quality-of-life data were not collected.

In TAX 327, 1006 men with metastatic HRPC were randomly allocated to docetaxel 75 mg/m^2 IV on day one of a 21-day cycle, docetaxel 30 mg/m^2 IV days 1, 8, 15, 22 and 29 of a 6-week cycle or mitoxantrone 12 mg/m^2 IV on day one of a 21-day cycle. All patients received prednisolone 5 mg BD orally from day one. Dexamethasone premedication was given to the patients receiving docetaxel. Compared to the mitoxantrone group median survival was significantly longer in the 3-weekly docetaxel group (18.9 months versus 16.5 months, $p = 0.009$) but not in the weekly docetaxel group (17.4 months versus 16.5 months, $p = 0.36$). A PSA decrease of $\geq 50\%$ occurred in 45% of patients who were given 3-weekly docetaxel and 48% given weekly docetaxel. Both of these results were significantly higher than the 32% response seen in the mitoxantrone group ($p < 0.001$ for both comparisons). A reduction in pain was seen more frequently in the 3-weekly docetaxel group than in the mitoxantrone group (35% versus 22%, $p = 0.01$). The reduction in pain seen with weekly docetaxel was not significantly better than in the mitoxantrone group (31% versus 22%, $p = 0.08$). Quality of life was improved significantly in both docetaxel groups (22% for 3-weekly, 23% weekly) compared to the mitoxantrone group (13%, $p = 0.009$ and 0.005 respectively). Grade 3 or 4 toxicity was higher with both docetaxel regimens than with mitoxantrone, particularly alopecia, diarrhoea, sensory neuropathy, stomatitis and peripheral oedema. As expected, weekly docetaxel had a significantly lower incidence of neutropenia compared to 3-weekly docetaxel or mitoxantrone but there was no significant difference in the incidence of neutropenic pyrexia. There were three treatment-related deaths in the mitoxantrone group and one in each of the docetaxel groups.

The weekly docetaxel group in TAX 327 did not demonstrate a survival advantage over mitoxantrone nor was there less treatment-related toxicity than in the 3-weekly docetaxel group. Weekly docetaxel is less convenient than 3-weekly schedules, and therefore probably has little role to play in the management of patients with HRPC.

It is of note that only the docetaxel groups in both trials received dexamethasone premedication. The safe administration of docetaxel requires this premedication but corticosteroids can have a PSA-lowering effect in prostate cancer [18,19,25]. Was the benefit seen with docetaxel simply the result of higher doses of corticosteroid compared to the mitoxantrone groups? Only one small series has been published looking at the effect of cyclical high-dose dexamethasone in HRPC [54]. None of the 12 patients treated had a significant PSA response but certainly a steroid effect cannot be dismissed as possibly contributing to the additional benefit seen with docetaxel over mitoxantrone.

Should 3-weekly docetaxel be combined with estramustine? It is interesting to compare the docetaxel–estramustine group in SWOG 9916 with the 3-weekly docetaxel group in TAX 327. The patients in both trial groups were very similar with respect to the number of patients (330 versus 332), median age (70 versus 68) and proportion with bone metastases (84% versus 90%). In addition, most patients in both groups were of good performance status (90% PS 0–1 in SWOG 9916 and 87% Karnofsky ≥70 in TAX 327). Median baseline PSA was higher in the SWOG 9916 group (84 versus 114 ng/ml).

The treatment outcomes in the two groups were also similar with respect to PSA response rate (50% versus 45%) and median survival (17.5 months versus 18.7 months). It is clear that in both trials there was a greater incidence of adverse effects in the docetaxel groups compared to the mitoxantrone groups. It is not possible to say, however, whether docetaxel–estramustine or single agent docetaxel is better tolerated; toxicity data are difficult to compare as different adverse events were reported in the two trials. Unlike in the TAX 327, the SWOG 9916 did collect data on vascular complications in some detail because of the known association with estramustine. Grade 3 or worse vascular events occurred in 14% of patients in the SWOG 9916 docetaxel–estramustine group. In addition, there were more treatment-related deaths in the SWOG 9916 group compared to the TAX 327 group (eight patients versus one patient). It is probable, therefore that the addition of estramustine to 3-weekly docetaxel does not significantly increase PSA response or survival, and may be associated with increased toxicity.

OTHER COMBINATION REGIMENS

The palliative efficacy of mitoxantrone has lead to its combination with newer chemotherapy agents. Heidenreich [55] reported on a phase II trial of 72 patients with metastatic HRPC and asymptomatic PSA progression given docetaxel 60 mg/m^2 IV plus mitoxantrone 8 mg/m^2 IV 3-weekly. A PSA response of ≥50% was achieved in 62% of patients. Haematological toxicity was mild. There were, however, three treatment-related deaths. A variety of three-drug regimens incorporating newer agents has also been developed including estramustine, etoposide and vinorelbine [56], and paclitaxel, estramustine and carboplatin [57]. Although demonstrating significant activity in phase II studies with respect to PSA response, the value of triplets versus doublets has yet to be established with respect to improvement in QOL or survival, and hence they should not be considered standard treatment for HRPC.

CONCLUSION

For many years the aim of treatment given to patients with HRPC was to alleviate symptoms and improve QOL only; no treatment had been shown to improve survival. In 1996, evidence from a small randomised trial in patients with symptomatic HRPC suggested that mitoxantrone plus a corticosteroid lowered serum PSA levels and palliated a significant minority of patients but provided no survival benefit compared to steroid therapy alone [25]. Data from subsequent similar trials also failed to show a survival benefit but confirmed the tolerability of mitoxantrone, which became the standard of care for patients with symptomatic HRPC fit enough for chemotherapy.

In October 2004, the results of SWOG 9916 and TAX 327 were published simultaneously [52,53]. They are the only randomised trials to show a survival advantage with any therapy in HRPC. TAX 327 showed that compared to mitoxantrone 3-weekly single agent docetaxel increased median survival by 2.5 months, improved pain control and QOL. The benefits were however at the expense of increased treatment-related toxicity. SWOG 9916 showed that compared to mitoxantrone, 3-weekly docetaxel plus estramustine increased median survival by nearly 2 months but again, like TAX 327, at the expense of increased treatment-related toxicity. There were more treatment-related deaths in the SWOG trial and overall results were similar suggesting the addition of estramustine to docetaxel provides no additional benefit and may increase toxicity.

Despite these encouraging results the treatment of HRPC remains a challenge. The survival benefits seen with docetaxel are modest, and come at the price of increased toxicity. Many patients with HRPC are older and have significant cormorbid illnesses, which may preclude docetaxel. In fitter patients, docetaxel should be considered as a therapeutic option as it is the only treatment to show a significant survival advantage in patients with HRPC. For the less robust, mitoxantrone and prednisolone remains an appropriate treatment option.

REFERENCES

1 Cancer Research UK Scientific Yearbook 2002/3, Cancer Research UK, London, 2–3.

2 Evans HS, Moller H. Recent trends in prostate cancer incidence and mortality in Southeast England. *Eur Urol* 2003; **43**: 337–41.

3 Gittes RF. Carcinoma of the prostate. *N Engl J Med* 1991; **324**: 236–45.

4 Raghavan D. Non-hormone chemotherapy for prostate cancer: principles of treatment and application to the testing of new drugs. *Semin Oncol* 1998; **15**: 371–89.

5 Sabbatini P, Larson SM, Kremer A *et al.* Prognostic significance of extent of disease in bone in patients with androgen-independent prostate cancer. *J Clin Oncol* 1999; **17**: 948–57.

6 Smith PH, Bono PA, Calais da Silva F *et al.* Some limitations of the radioisotope bone scan in patients with metastatic prostate cancer. A subanalysis of EORTC trial 30853. *Cancer* 1990; **66**: 1009–16.

7 Hussain M, Wolf M, Marshall E *et al.* Effects of continued androgen-deprived therapy and other prognostic factors on response and survival in phase II chemotherapy trials for hormone-refractory prostate cancer: a Southwest Oncology Group report. *J Clin Oncol* 1994; **12**: 1868–75.

8 Yagoda A. Non-hormonal cytotoxic agents in the treatment of prostatic adenocarcinoma. *Cancer* 1973; **32**: 1131–40.

9 Yagoda A. Cytotoxic agents in prostate cancer: an enigma. *Semin Urol* 1983; **1**: 311–20.

10 Eisenberger MA, Abrams JS. Chemotherapy for prostatic carcinoma. *Semin Urol* 1988; **6**: 303–10.

11 Eisenberger MA, Simon R, O'Dwyer PJ *et al.* A re-evaluation of nonhormonal cytotoxic chemotherapy in the treatment of prostatic carcinoma. *J Clin Oncol* 1985; **3**: 827–41.

12 Chlebowski RT, Hestorff R, Sardoff L *et al.* Cyclophosphamide versus the combination of Adriamycin, 5-fluorouracil and cyclophosphamide in the treatment of metastatic prostate cancer – a randomized trial. *Cancer* 1978; **42**: 546–52.

13 Herr HW. Cyclophosphamide, methotrexate and 5-fluorouracil combination chemotherapy versus chlorethyl-cyclohexy-nitrosourea in the treatment of metastatic prostate cancer. *J Urol* 1982; **127**: 462–5.

14 Wung MC, Valenzuela LA, Murphy GP *et al.* Purificaton of a human prostate specific antigen. *Invest Urol* 1979; **17**: 159–63.

15 Chybowski FM, Keller JJ, Bergstralh EJ *et al.* Predicting radionuclide bone scan findings in patients with newly diagnosed, untreated prostate cancer: prostate specific antigen is superior to all other clinical parameters. *J Urol* 1991; **145**: 313–8.

16 Scher HI, Kelly WM, Zhang ZF *et al.* Post-therapy serum prostate-specific antigen level and survival in patients with androgen-independent prostate cancer. *J Natl Cancer Inst* 1999; **91**: 244–51.

17 Thalmann GN, Sikes RA, Chang SM *et al.* Suramin-induced decrease in prostate-specific antigen expression with no effect on tumour growth in the LNCaP model of human prostate cancer. *J Natl Cancer Inst* 1996; **88**: 794–801.

18 Berry W, Dakhil S, Modiano M *et al.* Phase III study of mitoxantrone plus low dose prednisone versus low dose prednisone alone in patients with asymptomatic hormone refractory prostate cancer. *J Urol* 2002; **168**: 2439–43.

19 Kantoff PW, Halabi S, Conaway M *et al.* Hydrocortisone with or without mitoxantrone in men with hormone-refractory prostate cancer: results of the Cancer and Leukaemia Group B 9182 study 1. *J Clin Oncol* 1999; **17**: 2506–13.

20 Hudes G, Einhorn L, Ross E *et al.* Vinblastine versus vinblastine plus oral estramustine phosphate for patients with hormone-refractory prostate cancer: a Hoosier Oncology Group and Fox Chase Network phase III trial. *J Clin Oncol* 1999; **17**: 3160–6.

21 Copur MS, Ledakis P, Lynch J et al. Weekly docetaxel and estramustine in patients with hormone-refractory prostate cancer. *Semin Oncol* 2001; **28**: 16–21.

22 Calabresi P, Chabner BA. Antineoplastic agents. In: Gilman AG, Rall TW, Nies AS et al., eds. *Goodman and Gilman's The Pharmacological Basis of Therapeutics,* McGraw-Hill Inc, San Francisco, 1993: 1241–4.

23 Moore MJ, Osoba D, Murphy K et al. Use of palliative endpoints to evaluate the effects of mitoxantrone and low dose prednisolone in patients with hormonally resistant prostate cancer. *J Clin Oncol* 1994; **12**: 689–94.

24 Kantoff PW, Block C, Letvak L et al. 14-Day continuous infusion of mitoxantrone in hormone-refractory metastatic adenocarcinoma of the prostate. *Am J Clin Oncol* 1993; **16**: 489–91.

25 Tannock IF, Osoba D, Stockler MR et al. Chemotherapy with mitoxantrone plus prednisone or prednisone alone for symptomatic hormone-resistant prostate cancer: a Canadian randomized trial with palliative end points. *J Clin Oncol* 1996; **14**: 1756–64.

26 Tannock IF, Gospodarowicz M, Meakin W et al. Treatment of metastatic prostate cancer with low-dose prednisone: Evaluation of pain and quality of life as pragmatic indices of response. *J Clin Oncol* 1989; **7**: 590–7.

27 Tew KD, Stearns ME. Estramustine: a nitrogen mustard/steroid with antimicrotubule properties. *Pharmacol Ther* 1989; **43**: 299–319.

28 Mareel MM, Storme GA, Dragonetti CH et al. Antiinvasive activity of estramustine on malignant MO4 mouse cells and on DU-145 human prostate carcinoma cells *in vitro. Cancer Res* 1988; **48**: 1842–9.

29 Hudes G. Estramustine-based chemotherapy. *Semin Urol Oncol* 1997; **15**: 13–19.

30 Culine S, Droz JP. Chemotherapy in androgen-independent prostate cancer 1990–1999: a decade of progress? *Ann Oncol* 2000; **11**: 1523–30.

31 Benson R, Hartley-Asp B. Mechanisms of action and clinical uses of estramustine. *Cancer Invest* 1990; **8**: 375–80.

32 de Kernion JN, Murphy GP, Priore R et al. Comparison of flutamide and Emcyt in hormone-refractory metastatic prostate cancer. *Urology* 1988; **31**: 312–7.

33 Speicher LA, Barone L, Tew KD et al. Combined antimicrotubule activity of estramustine and Taxol in human prostatic carcinoma cell lines. *Cancer Res* 1992; **52**: 4433–40.

34 Kreis W, Budman DR, Calabro A. Unique synergism or antagonism of combinations of chemotherapeutic and hormonal agents in human prostate cancer cell lines. *Br J Urol* 1997; **79**: 196–202.

35 Hudes GR, Greenberg R, Krigel RL et al. Phase II study of estramustine and vinblastine, two microtubule inhibitors, in hormone refractory-prostate cancer. *J Clin Oncol* 1992; **10**: 1754–61.

36 Seidman AD, Scher HI, Petrylak D et al. Estramustine and vinblastine: use of prostate specific antigen as a clinical trial end point for hormone refractory prostate cancer. *J Urol* 1992; **147**: 931–4.

37 Hudes G, Ross E, Roth B et al. Improved survival for patients with hormone-refractory prostate cancer receiving estramustine-based antimicrotubule therapy: final report of a Hoosier Oncology Group and Fox Chase Network phase III trial comparing vinblastine and vinblastine plus oral estramustine phosphate. *Proc Am Soc Clin Oncol* 2002; 704a.

38 Sweeney CJ, Monaco FJ, Jung SH et al. A phase II Hoosier Oncology Group study of vinorelbine and estramustine phosphate in hormone-refractory prostate cancer. *Ann Oncol* 2002; **13**: 435–40.

39 Smith MR, Kaufman D, Oh W et al. Vinorelbine and estramustine in androgen-independent metastatic prostate cancer: a phase II study. *Cancer* 2000; **89**: 1824–8.

40 Tralongo P, Bollina R, Aiello R. Vinorelbine and prednisolone in older cancer patients with hormone-refractory metastatic prostate cancer. A Phase II study. *Tumori* 2003; **89**: 26–30.

41 Oudard S, Caty A, Humblet Y et al. Phase II study of vinorelbine in patients with androgen-independent prostate cancer. *Ann Oncol* 2001; **12**: 847–52.

42 Abratt RP, Brune D, Dimopoulos MA *et al*. Randomized phase III study of intravenous vinorelbine plus hormonetherapy versus hormonetherapy alone in hormone-refractory prostate cancer. *Ann Oncol* 2003; **22**: 382.

43 Pienta KJ, Redman BG, Bandekar R *et al*. A phase II trial of oral estramustine and oral etoposide in hormone refractory prostate cancer. *Urology* 1997; **50**: 401–6.

44 Dimopoulos MA, Panopoulos C, Bamia C *et al*. Oral estramustine and oral etoposide for hormone-refractory prostate cancer. *Urology* 1997; **50**: 754–8.

45 Hudes GR, Nathan F, Khater C *et al*. Phase II trial of 96-hour paclitaxel plus oral estramustine phosphate in metastatic hormone-refractory prostate cancer. *J Clin Oncol* 1997; **15**: 3156–63.

46 Hudes GR, Manola J, Conroy J *et al*. Phase II study of weekly paclitaxel by 1-hour infusion plus reduced-dose oral estramustine in metastatic hormone-refractory prostate carcinoma: a trial of the Eastern Cooperative Oncology Group. *Proc Am Soc Clin Oncol* 2001; 697a.

47 Berry WR, Hathorn JW, Dakhil SR *et al*. Phase II randomized trial of weekly paclitaxel with or without estramustine phosphate in progressive, metastatic, hormone-refractory, prostate cancer. *Clin Prostate Cancer* 2004; **3**: 104–11.

48 Savarese DM, Halabi S, Hars V *et al*. Phase II study of docetaxel, estramustine, and low-dose hydrocortisone in men with hormone-refractory prostate cancer: a final report of CALGB 9780. *J Clin Oncol* 2001; **9**: 2509–16.

49 Petrylak DP, Shelton GB, England-Owen C *et al*. Response and preliminary survival results of a phase II study of docetaxel and estramustine in patients with androgen-independent prostate cancer. *Proc Am Soc Clin Oncol* 2000; **19**: 334a.

50 Beer TM, Pierce WC, Lowe BA *et al*. Phase II study of weekly docetaxel in symptomatic androgen-independent prostate cancer. *Ann Oncol* 2001; **12**, 1273–9.

51 Berry W, Dakhil S, Gregurich MA *et al*. Phase II trial of weekly single agent docetaxel in hormone-refractory, symptomatic, metastatic carcinoma of the prostate. *Semin Oncol* 2001; **28**: 8–15.

52 Petrylak DP, Tangen CM, Hussain, MHA, *et al*. Docetaxel and Estramustine Compared with Mitoxantrone and Prednisolone for Advanced Refractory Prostate Cancer. *N Engl J Med* 2004; **351**: 1513–1519.

53 Tannock, IF, de Wit R, Berry WR *et al*. Docetaxel plus prednisolone or mitoxantrone plus prednisolone for advanced prostate cancer. *N Engl J Med* 2004; **351**: 1502–12.

54 Weitzman AL, Shelton G, Zuech N *et al*. Dexamethasone does not significantly contribute to the response rate of docetaxel and estramustine in androgen-independent prostrate cancer. *J Urol* 2000; **163**: 834–7.

55 Heidenreich A, Carl S, Gleissner O *et al*. Docetaxel and mitoxantrone in the management of hormone-refractory prostate cancer. *Proc Am Soc Clin Oncol* 2003; 1655a.

56 Colleoni M, Graiff C, Vicario G. Phase II study of estramustine, oral etoposide, and vinorelbine in hormone-refractory prostate cancer. *J Clin Oncol* 1997; **20**: 383–6.

57 Urakami S, Igawa M, Kikuno N *et al*. Combination chemotherapy with paclitaxel, estramustine and carboplatin for hormone-refractory prostate cancer. *J Urol* 2002; **168**: 2451–3.

Index